# THE
# HORMONE
# CONNECTION

The Comprehensive Hormone Health Handbook for Women

# THE HORMONE CONNECTION

How to Achieve a Better Hormone Balance: a Major
Resource for Every Woman

GALE MALESKEY & MARY KITTEL AND THE EDITORS OF

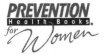

RODALE

This edition first published in the UK in 2003 by
Rodale Ltd
7–10 Chandos Place
London W1G 9AD
*www.rodale.co.uk*

Printed and bound in the UK by CPI Bath using acid-free paper from sustainable sources
3 5 7 9 8 6 4 2

A CIP record for this book is available from the British Library
ISBN 1–4050—0674–9

**This paperback edition distributed to the book trade by Pan Macmillan Ltd**

The relaxation exercise on page 279 was excerpted from pages xviii to xxiii of *The Relaxation Response* by Herbert Benson, M.D., with Miriam Z. Klipper. © William Morrow and Company. Reprinted by permission of HarperCollins Publishers, Inc./William Morrow.

## Acknowledgments

The publisher thanks the many health care professionals, researchers and clinicians who contributed their expertise to the development and creation of this book. While the views presented do not necessarily reflect a consensus among all the experts cited, we appreciate and respect input from all who were consulted.

In particular, we would like to thank the following for the special assistance they gave to our writers and researchers for information related to their specialties.

**Connie Catellani, M.D.**
Director, the Miro Center for Integrative Medicine
Evanston, Illinois, USA

**Larrian Gillespie, M.D.**
Author of *The Menopause Diet*, *The Goddess Diet* and *The Gladiator Diet*
Beverly Hills, California, USA

**Geoffrey P. Redmond, M.D.**
Director, Hormone Center of New York
President, Center for Health Research
New York City, USA

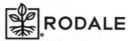

**RODALE**
WE **INSPIRE** AND **ENABLE** PEOPLE TO IMPROVE
THEIR LIVES AND THE WORLD AROUND THEM

## About *Prevention* Health Books

The editors of *Prevention* Health Books are dedicated to providing you with authoritative, trustworthy and innovative advice for a healthy, active lifestyle. In all of our books, our goal is to keep you thoroughly informed about the latest breakthroughs in natural healing, medical research, alternative health, herbs, nutrition, fitness and weight loss. We cut through the confusion of today's conflicting health reports to deliver clear, concise and definitive health information that you can trust. And we explain in practical terms what each new breakthrough means to you, so you can take immediate, practical steps to improve your health and well-being.

Every recommendation in *Prevention* Health Books is based upon reliable sources, including interviews with qualified health authorities. In addition, we retain top-level health practitioners who serve on the Rodale Books Board of Advisors. *Prevention* Health Books are thoroughly fact-checked for accuracy, and we make every effort to verify recommendations, dosages and cautions.

The advice in this book will help keep you well-informed about your personal choices in health care – to help you lead a happier, healthier, and longer life.

# Board of Advisors

# Contents

## PART 1

## Your "Invisible" Health System

Provides a "crash course" on hormones. Learn what hormones are, what they do, how they interact, how they affect women at different stages of their lives, and why they go out of whack.

Explains how you can take advantage of what's new in hormone research and apply breakthrough discoveries to your own health. Emphasizes the need to keep all your hormones in balance.

## PART 2

## What Can Go Wrong – And Why

Reveals how hormones may be responsible for depression, anxiety, unexplained crying, overreaction to events and other emotional upsets. Offers solutions that work with, not against, your hormones.

Helps you uncover hidden, hormonal causes of fatigue. Includes medical solutions and everyday strategies for restoring your energy levels.

## PART 3
# The Hormone-Balancing Programme

A Three-Phase Plan to Restore and Maintain Your Hormone Levels and Customize the Programme for Your Personal Needs

## PART 4

# Hormone Helpers

*Guidelines for safe use of herbs and nutritional supplements, with side effects to watch for when incorporating them into your hormone-balancing programme.*

*A directory of Internet health sites and other resources to help you resolve or cope with tough or puzzling problems.*

# Beyond Oestrogen

If you're like most women, no doubt you readily associate "hormones" with menstruation and adolescent mood swings. Chances are you probably also realize that diabetes, low thyroid function and stress are hormone-related. And if you're in the menopause – or about to enter it – dwindling levels of oestrogen and other hormones can trigger noticeable changes, like hot flushes or fragile bones.

Those connections are real and profound. But they're only a few of the many ways that those hormones and many others – 200, at last count – can and do affect your health. And their effects aren't always obvious.

If you're in your forties and are experiencing hot flushes, for example, you may be experiencing a thyroid imbalance, not menopause. An imbalance of the key female hormone oestrogen can stunt the performance of thyroid hormones. That can also leave you tired, with no obvious explanation for why you feel like you're walking around in first gear.

If diabetes runs in your family, you're probably well aware of the effects of poor control of insulin, the hormone responsible for good blood sugar control. But some women – and even a few doctors – are unaware of the role of oestrogen and other reproductive hormones in controlling diabetes. Progesterone – oestrogen's companion hormone – is critically linked to high blood glucose, especially in the week before menstruation.

Undergoing a major life crisis, such as a divorce, can affect your adrenal glands, throwing several key hormones out of whack, causing fatigue, memory problems and lowered immunity.

Hormones also affect your weight, shape and metabolism. Women have felt vulnerable to hormonal cravings and sluggish metabolisms for years, with little science behind their experiences. Now science is uncovering several bona fide links between hormones, hunger and fat metabolism. And in fact, taking advantage of hormones – mechanisms already in place in your molecular biology – can help you to manage your weight, shape and appetite.

Medications can be disrupting your hormone balance and affecting your health in unsuspected ways. Taking too much of a steroid drug commonly prescribed for asthma, for example, could lead to osteoporosis, normally blamed on declining levels of the female hormone oestrogen. Taking certain antidepressants, birth control pills, or hormone replacement therapy could change your need for thyroid medication.

# A Kaleidoscope of Hormones

Put it all together, and the hormones that make up your endocrine system are a kaleidoscope of powerful substances, in configurations that differ from woman to woman, as individual as fingerprints.

In many women, these hormonal influences all seem to converge in the years leading up to the menopause as female hormones dwindle, insulin-regulating hormones fail, and other hormones decline with age.

In editing this book, it became obvious to me that any woman who's earnestly interested in taking care of her health needs to take into consideration the effects of hormones – good or bad. Yet your doctor can't just give you a pill for low thyroid, a pill for diabetes, another pill for the menopause, and send you on your way. It's just not that simple. You need a plan to help you unpuzzle the hormonal influences at work and take steps to balance your hormones, using the best strategies experts have to offer.

This book shows you how. The benefits are amazing. The information in this book can help women:

- *Find the right form and dosage of hormone replacement therapy for them, with maximum benefits and minimum side effects*
- *Lose stubborn pounds by understanding all the hormonal influences that lead to weight gain in women, from thyroid hormones and insulin to digestive hormones and brain hormones*
- *Get rid of abdominal fat and flatten their stomachs*
- *Balance their hormones while they sleep*
- *Smooth out wrinkles while strengthening bones (oestrogen receptors feed the blood vessels in the skin, influencing skin structures)*
- *Clear up adult acne (which in adults is often a symptom of hormones gone awry)*
- *Relieve the debilitating aches and pains of fibromyalgia, influenced by hormones released during sleep, as well as stress hormones*
- *Stem stress-induced "cortisol overload", which suppresses the immune system, increasing vulnerability to colds and infections, increasing the risk of heart disease and high blood pressure, and raising the risk of diabetes*
- *Repair stress-induced memory loss*
- *Improve stress hormone levels during breast cancer recovery*

. . . and much, much more.

Throughout the book, you'll find step-by-step plans to jettison foods and food ingredients (like sugar and animal growth hormones) that can upset a woman's hormone balance, and add foods, herbs and supplements that restore a healthy balance.

You'll find dozens of fascinating reports on the latest scientific advancements in connections between hormone research and women's health. For example, did you know that:

- *The female hormone progesterone is linked to snoring in women*
- *Massage reduces stress hormone levels in women recovering from breast cancer, helping to speed healing*
- *"Neuro-hormones" released during sex may prevent wrinkles*
- *Attending religious services regularly helps to balance your hormones*
- *Fish, walnuts and dark green leafy vegetables blunt the body's production of hormone-like substances called prostaglandins, which regulate its response to inflammation*

The list goes on. You won't find this kind of in-depth, groundbreaking information in just any health book – or even in medical texts. We interviewed hundreds of leading experts in hormones, including researchers and clinicians (like "thyroidologists" and diabetes educators) who specialize in treating hormone imbalances. What's more, we present not only the conventional medical options but alternative treatments as well.

I'm proud of the unparalleled research that went into this book, and I feel confident that after reading it, you'll be able to take your health to the next level.

Sharon Faelten
Senior Editor

## PART ONE

# Your "Invisible" Health System

# CHAPTER 1

# Lowdown on Hormones:
## What They Are, What They Do

A hormone is
   a. *a circulating chemical that makes teenagers sullen.*
   b. *a protein-based compound that enables women to have babies that grow into sullen teenagers.*
   c. *an enzyme that raises your blood pressure when your sullen teenager comes home after curfew.*
   d. *all of the above.*

The correct answer is "all of the above". We can love them, hate them, or feel like they're out of control, but one thing is certain: you can't live without hormones. True, they rightly get some of the blame for physical discomfort and poor behaviour – such as adolescent sulking. (More on that later.) But hormones do a lot of good in our bodies, and they do lots more than most of us realize.

The word "hormone" means "to excite". And that's exactly what hormones do. They are chemical messengers secreted in tiny amounts from endocrine glands found throughout the body. You've probably heard of some of the glands, like the ovaries, the thyroid, or the adrenal glands. Altogether, you have nine major endocrine glands, including the "master gland", the hypothalamus, in the brain, and its main henchman, the pituitary. (Both secrete hormones that regulate hormone production in other glands.) Plus, we have patches of glandular tissue on organs such as the heart and intestines. Even some individual cells, such as those in the immune system, produce hormone-like substances, called parahormones. And some neurotransmitters – chemicals released by nerve or brain cells – also act as hormones.

Together, endocrine glands and tissues produce more than 200 different types of hormones.

Less solid than structural parts of our anatomy – bones or muscles – hormones are no less powerful or essential. Operating "under the radar", this seemingly invisible system is one of the three major systems that allow your body and all its various parts to communicate and function as a whole. (The other two are the nervous and the immune systems.) Hormones regulate and control, at least in part, virtually every activity in your body, and a lot of extraordinary life events as well.

When things go well – as they usually do – you go about your day totally unaware that your hormones are doing their job. And when things go wrong, any one of those 200 hormones could be out of balance.

## A Day in the Life of Your Hormones

Looking at a day in the life of your hormones gives just a glimpse of the complex workings of your endocrine system. To see just how indispensable hormones are, take a look at a fairly typical 24-hour period in the life of Mary, a hypothetical 47-year-old woman much like you.

### "Wake-Up" Hormones

Hours before she begins to stir, Mary's hormones prepare her for the day ahead. Sometime between 4 and 6 a.m. – about the time Mary's settling into that last, delicious bout of dream-laced REM sleep – her adrenal glands move into action. These small, pyramid-shaped organs atop the kidneys begin to step up their secretion of cortisol, the body's major stress hormone. Cortisol is secreted in small amounts at all times, with natural peaks and dips throughout the day. And it kicks in hard, and stays high, when a person is experiencing chronic stress such as illness.

The cortisol secreted prior to waking gently primes Mary's body for activity, slightly increasing her metabolism. She burns more calories. Her body temperature rises a bit. It's almost as though her adrenal glands get up early to stoke the fire so that she awakens already warmed up and ready to go.

Today, though, an alarm clock rouses Mary from deep sleep, and no matter how familiar its sound may be, it still sends a surge of another stress hormone, epinephrine, through her body. Also secreted by the adrenal glands, epinephrine quickens her heart rate and breathing and narrows blood

(continued on page 20)

# A Quick Tour of Your Hormone System

As you go about your day, nearly 200 hormones and hormone-like substances course silently through your body, acting as chemical messengers. Secreted by nine major endocrine glands (listed here) and other organs, hormones affect every cell in your body, helping to determine whether you are hot or cold, hungry or full, calm or stressed, alert or sleepy, and naughty or nice. Whether you are asleep or awake, hormones also build bone, regulate your menstrual cycles and direct myriad other essential functions. So keeping your hormones in balance is vital to day-to-day good health.

**Hypothalamus**  Located in your brain, this gland is Control Central for homoeostasis. Issues orders to other glands, especially the pituitary gland, regarding regulation of water balance, body temperature, biological rhythms and emotions.

**Pineal**  Melatonin, this gland's major hormone, helps set your "biological clock" for wake/sleep cycles.

**Pituitary**  This important endocrine gland secretes at least nine major hormones, including hormones that stimulate the thyroid, adrenal glands and ovaries.

**Thyroid**  Considered "Metabolism Central", this butterfly-shaped gland affects energy regulation in every cell in the body.

**Parathyroid**  Located near your thyroid, this is a major force for calcium balance in the body.

**Thymus**  A nursery for infection-fighting T-lymphocytes, this gland is active in establishing immunity when we're infants.

**Adrenal**  Under stress, this gland secretes specialized hormones that help us fight, flee – or hunker down for the duration.

**Pancreas**  Cells here produce insulin and glucagon, hormones that work together to regulate blood sugar levels.

**Ovary**  Its main hormones – oestrogen, progesterone and testosterone – give women generous hips, nurturing breasts, sex drive and, sometimes, PMS.

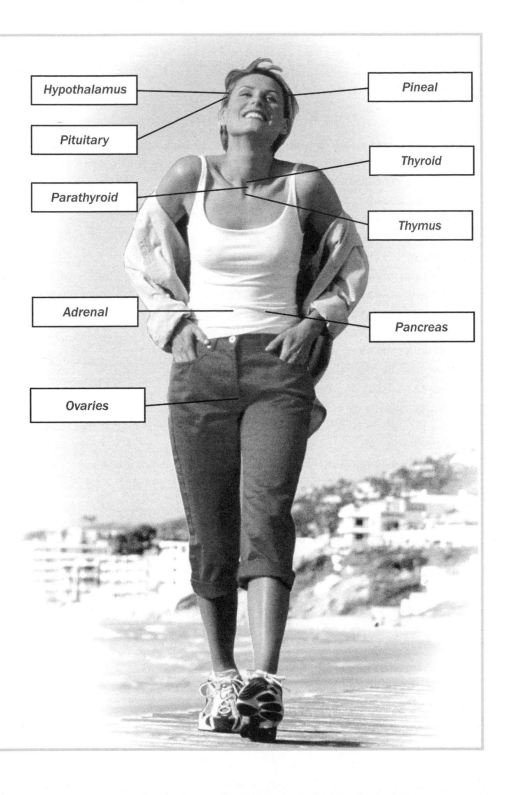

Hypothalamus

Pineal

Pituitary

Thyroid

Parathyroid

Thymus

Adrenal

Pancreas

Ovaries

vessels in her body, raising blood pressure. Without this assistance from epinephrine, in fact, Mary's blood pressure would be so low that she'd faint and fall when leaping out of bed.

## "Eat and Run" Hormones

Because she hasn't eaten for almost 10 hours, and her blood sugar (glucose) level has dropped, Mary's pancreas is secreting glycogen, a hormone that breaks down glucose stored in the liver and muscles. Once Mary eats breakfast, though, and the carbohydrates from her breakfast are broken down into glucose and sent into her bloodstream, her pancreas will switch gears and start cranking out insulin. This hormone escorts glucose from the bloodstream into cells, where it can be used to produce energy.

Hormones involved in digestion play a role here, too. Cells scattered throughout the organs of the gastrointestinal tract secrete hormones that increase intestinal mobility and secretions, causing the gallbladder to release stored bile and regulate local bloodflow. So Mary's stomach and small intestine are churning and gurgling nicely by the time she leaves the house.

Her commute to work – a 45-minute drive along a busy dual carriageway – is no picnic. So Mary brings along tapes of music that she finds soothing. The music helps her stay calm, allowing her to consciously suppress the surges of stress hormones that would otherwise occur when she gets upset about being stuck in traffic or carved up. Since these stress hormones also interfere with proper digestion, the musical distraction also helps Mary's digestive tract do its job better.

Just before lunch, Mary heads to the company gym; she and a colleague are trying to lose weight. She hops on the treadmill and runs for half an hour, covering about 4 miles. Her cortisol and epinephrine peak in response to the exertion, sending her heart rate and respiration soaring, and allowing her to sweat to cool down.

Mary feels great. Towards the end of her run, her body will have started producing feel-good hormones called endorphins, which will elevate her mood for the rest of the afternoon and dampen any little aches and pains her run has produced.

While she's running, Mary's heart, too, has produced a hormone. In response to the increase in blood pressure, which stretches her atria, the two upper chambers of her heart, specialized cardiac cells secrete atrial natriuretic peptide. This hormone signals the kidneys to increase their production of salty urine. It also inhibits the adrenal glands, which secrete a hormone called aldosterone. Aldosterone helps to maintain blood pressure by "supervising" fluid flow in the kidneys. End result: Mary has to urinate when she's finished running.

## Bone-Builder Hormones

After her run, Mary's blood sugar and insulin are low again (though still normal). She's hungry, and she eats a turkey sandwich on wholemeal bread and an apple. Within 20 minutes, her blood sugar and insulin are slowly rising. She eats sitting out in the sun, still in her gym shorts and a T-shirt. It's a clear, cool day, and soon her sun-exposed skin starts to make a hormone, cholecalciferol, an inactive form of vitamin D that is converted to vitamin D in the body. Vitamin D helps the body use calcium.

During the afternoon, Mary's blood calcium level starts to drop a bit. That triggers patches of tissue in her thyroid gland, called the parathyroid, to secrete parathyroid hormone. This hormone breaks down bone to release its calcium into the blood. Luckily, Mary decides to have yoghurt as a snack at around 3 p.m., and soon after that, the calcium she has digested reaches her bloodstream and has compensated for the calcium lost from bone. Her parathyroid is now releasing calcitonin, a hormone that facilitates the deposit of calcium into bones.

## Female Hormones

Just about the time she is wrapping things up for the day, Mary has a hot flush. Blood surges to the surface of the skin on her chest, neck and head, her heart rate and breathing quicken slightly, and she starts to sweat.

No one knows exactly what triggers hot flushes, but they are associated with the hormonal changes that occur before and during the menopause. These changes somehow stimulate the part of the brain that controls body temperature, throwing off its usually fine-tuned control. Hot flushes are synchronized with core temperature – deep inside the body. If you're most active during the day – a 9-to-5 worker like Mary – late afternoon and early evening are prime times for hot flushes.

Luckily, in just a few minutes the flush is over. It's no big deal. Mary works with other women her same age, 45 to 55 years old or so, and they all make friendly jokes about "power surges". At 47, Mary feels she's too young for hormone replacement therapy, often prescribed for menopausal symptoms. Still, she makes a mental note to ask her gynaecologist at her next appointment just what kinds of treatments might be available. She also

decides to drive home with the top down on her car. That'll cool her down
– and make her feel young.

## Energy and Metabolism Drivers

The drive home does cool Mary down, perhaps a bit too much. Her thyroid
gland has been pretty much steady during the day, secreting the hormones
that regulate metabolism – that is, energy production – in every cell in her
body. Even though Mary closes the window and turns the heat on, this late-
March evening turns rather cold, and she starts to shiver. Her thyroid gland
immediately senses the drop in body temperature and gets to work, secreting more of its hormones, which boost her metabolic rate and generate
internal warmth.

## Love and Intimacy Hormones

When she gets home, Mary gets warmed up even more. Her husband
reminds her that it's the anniversary of the exact date they first met, 25 years
earlier. She'd forgotten, and he surprises her with a big bouquet of daf-
fodils and airline tickets for a trip to Paris, where they'd met as exchange students. They make love, and afterwards, Mary's body has produced a mix of
hormones – cortisol and epinephrine, in response to the physical exertion
of sex, the same feel-good endorphins released during exercise, and a hormone called oxytocin, triggered during orgasm.

Oxytocin is better known for its role in inducing uterine contractions during labour. But this potent peptide also plays a role in sexual arousal and
orgasm and is responsible for the feeling of satisfaction that we all get from
good sex. And in non-sexual relationships, oxytocin is thought to promote
nurturing and affectionate behaviour. So it's sometimes called the "cuddle
hormone".

## Sleepy Time Hormones

About 9 p.m., some 14 hours after getting up, Mary's tiny, pinecone-shaped
pineal gland, an organ that hangs from a chamber in her brain, starts to secrete
melatonin. This light-sensitive hormone helps regulate the body's internal
clock, a part of the brain that has been programmed for aeons to help "day-
active mammals" like us function in accord with the earth's 24-hour
day/night cycle.

A rise in melatonin signals night-time, and in humans it may set the
course for other biochemical changes that eventually lead to sleep. But

melatonin is no sleeping pill. Animals that are most active at night, such as hamsters, have the same sharp increase in melatonin at dusk. So in all animals, humans included, changing melatonin levels may be a means by which day-and-night cycles impose their own rhythm on many body functions, such as temperature, sleep, appetite – and hormones.

## The Ultimate Multitaskers

How do hormones "know" where to go and what to do?

Usually, hormones travel through the bloodstream until they reach their targets – cells that can interact with them. If you think of a hormone as a key that travels throughout the body until it finds a lock to fit into, then the lock is a receptor site on a cell. When the hormone "key" enters its receptor "lock", it sets off a process that activates the cell's genetic material to do a specific action. The cell has been sent a work order it can't ignore: make this protein, secrete this enzyme, grow and divide.

Every type of hormone is a different key, and every type of cell has different locks, so it's possible for a hormone to have different effects on different cells. Oestrogen, for example, promotes cell growth in a woman's breasts, uterus and vagina. So a woman past menopause might take replacement oestrogen, or use an oestrogen cream, to keep the tissue in her vagina from becoming painfully thin and dry. But oestrogen acts differently in other cells of the body. In the cardiovascular system, for instance, it does duty as an antioxidant and opens the electrical channels that let blood vessels relax. That function may explain some of its effects in the blood vessels and in the brain and its potential in reducing the risk of Alzheimer's and heart disease.

Oestrogen also reduces the rate at which calcium is broken down from bone. That's why oestrogen replacement may protect women from osteoporosis. And it's why researchers are trying to create oestrogen derivatives that are helpful to bone but do not stimulate breast or uterine cells, says Rhoda Cobin, M.D., associate professor of medicine at the New York University Mount Sinai Medical Center in New York City. "Some of the most intense research in the field of endocrinology is looking to develop hormone-like drugs that provide the benefit of the hormone without potentially harmful side effects," she says.

In addition to vital daily functions, hormones help to orchestrate major physical changes in our bodies – puberty, menstruation, pregnancy and childbirth, and the menopause.

## Puberty Revisited

Take puberty, the period in our lives when we morph from girls to women. The hormonal changes that culminate in sexual maturity start years before any of the physical changes become obvious, sometimes as young as 7 or 8 in girls – this is early, but still normal. It's triggered by the hypothalamus, the master gland.

"No one knows exactly what makes the hypothalamus decide it's time to grow up, but genetics, nutrition, body fat and changes in neural pathways in the brain may all play a role," says Alan Jay Cohen, M.D., clinical associate professor of medicine at the University of Tennessee and medical director of the Endocrine Clinic in Memphis.

First, the adrenal glands start making a weak version of sex hormones, which cause some changes like the appearance of sparse pubic hair, pimples and body odour. At the same time, girls start a growth spurt governed by growth hormone, which is secreted by the pituitary gland.

A bit later, the pituitary gland begins to release gonadotropins, hormones that stimulate the production of sex hormones from the ovaries or testes. These hormones tend to "pulse" at first, mostly at night, and it may take some time for them to settle into an adult pattern. By the time these hormones settle down, a girl will have had her first menstrual period. (In the United Kingdom, the average age at onset is 12 years, 10 months; in the United States it is 12 years, 8 months.)

In addition to maintaining the monthly menstrual cycle, female hormones such as oestrogen broaden the pelvis, cause breasts to bud, add fat to hips and thighs, and mould the brain to a female identity.

In males, skyrocketing levels of testosterone add impressive amounts of muscle and bone, deepen the voice and put hair on the chest. Hormonal upheavals can contribute to acne, more commonly in boys but also in girls. And as for teenage angst, "hormones play a role in the roller coaster of emotions and how kids are able to handle those emotions," Dr. Cohen says. Sullenness, angry outbursts and tearful bouts can all be expected, but serious mental disturbances also can become apparent during this time, and deserve attention, Dr. Cohen says. "Suicide rates go up in both boys and girls." Seek professional help if your child shows signs of any of the following: substance abuse, changes in sleeping and/or eating habits, defiance of authority (including truancy, theft and/or vandalism), frequent outbursts of anger, or a prolonged negative mood that may be accompanied by poor appetite or thoughts of death.

## Getting Ready for Baby (or Not)

A mix of hormones orchestrate a woman's monthly menstrual cycle, giving females a 4- to 5-day window of opportunity each month to become pregnant. Low oestrogen levels at the beginning of a monthly cycle signal the hypothalamus to nudge the pituitary gland to secrete hormones that stimulate the ovaries. This includes follicle-stimulating hormone (FSH), which causes an egg-containing follicle in an ovary to "ripen" during the first 2 weeks of the menstrual cycle. The pituitary also secretes luteinizing hormone (LH), which causes the ripe egg to be released around midcycle. Both these hormones begin to drop off after that.

The ripening follicle secretes oestrogen in increasing amounts, and the oestrogen causes the lining of the uterus to grow and thicken. After the egg is released, the follicle changes in structure and function. It's now called the corpus luteum, and it secretes decreasing amounts of oestrogen and more progesterone. But after a few weeks, the corpus luteum begins to

### THE HORMONE CONNECTION
## MORNING SICKNESS? IT'S A GIRL!

Throughout history, people have tried to predict the sex of their offspring. Even Hippocrates got in on it – he noted that a woman carrying a female foetus is more likely to have a pale face, while a woman carrying a male foetus has a healthier tone to her skin.

It turns out Hippocrates could be right, if that pale face is related to losing your breakfast. Swedish researchers have found a slightly higher than normal ratio of female-to-male births in women admitted to the hospital with severe morning sickness (though this research has yet to be confirmed elsewhere).

The nausea and vomiting is caused by hormones generated during early pregnancy. One in particular – human chorionic gonadotropin, produced by the placenta – may be the main culprit. Female foetuses stimulate the production of more of this hormone than do male foetuses.

Top remedies for morning sickness? Experts suggest that you drink ginger tea, use lemons – both their smell and their taste can squelch nausea – and drink no more than 60 ml (2 fl oz) of fluid at a time (but drink frequently). And eat "solid liquids", such as watermelon or grapes, which stay down better.

degenerate, and declining hormone levels lead to menstruation, the shedding of the uterine lining. When hormone levels get low enough, the hypothalamus kicks into action and the cycle starts again.

If you become pregnant, hormones secreted by the developing embryo and, later, the placenta help keep the pregnancy on track. Late in pregnancy, the placenta also produces a hormone, relaxin, that causes pelvic ligaments to relax and the pelvis to widen and become more flexible. This increased mobility eases birth passage, but you may develop a waddling gait in the meantime.

When it's time for the baby to be born, a mix of hormones and events initiate labour. Oestrogen rises to a very high level in the blood, and this seems to sensitize the muscles of the uterus to another hormone, oxytocin, which causes the uterine contractions of labour (it may initially cause weak, irregular contractions, sometimes called false labour). As birth nears, cells of the foetus release oxytocin, which in turn acts on the placenta, causing it to release prostaglandins, also powerful uterine muscle stimulants. As labour contractions become more frequent and vigorous, the hypothalamus gets involved. It sends a signal to the pituitary to release more oxytocin, which causes greater contractile force of the uterus, and leads to the release of even more oxytocin. As blood levels of oxytocin rise, the expulsive contractions of labour gain momentum and finally end in birth. Phew!

## Retirement Planning for Your Ovaries

As we age, production of some hormones wanes. In women, the most dramatic drop-off is in sex hormones, as our ovary function gradually winds down. At the age of 30, there are still some 100,000 potential eggs in the ovaries; by the age of 50, there may be as few as 3 potential eggs left. The pituitary gland senses the accompanying drop in oestrogen levels and, so, signals for more ovary action with escalating levels of follicle-stimulating hormone and luteinizing hormone.

The ovaries continue to produce some oestrogen after menopause – how much and for how long varies from woman to woman – but eventually they cease to function. However, the adrenal glands continue to secrete small amounts of sex hormones throughout a woman's life. Still, dropping oestrogen levels affect many aspects of a woman's health, including atrophy of the reproductive organs, gradual thinning of the skin, loss of bone mass and slowly rising cholesterol levels, says P. J. Palumbo, M.D., chairman of the department of internal medicine at the Mayo Clinic Scottsdale in Arizona, and editor-in-chief of *Endocrine Practice*.

There is no equivalent of the menopause in men. While ageing men do have a steady decline in testosterone secretion and take longer to recover potency after orgasm, it seems a man's ability to produce viable sperm is unending. Healthy men are able to father children well into their eighties. However, with ageing there is a noticeable difference in the speed of sperm. Sperm of a young man can usually make it up the uterine tubes in 20 to 50 minutes. Those of a 75-year-old may take 2½ days for the same trip.

## Making Up for What's Missing

If your pancreas secretes too little insulin, you can get more of what you need by pill or injection, as insulin supplements. The same applies if your thyroid makes too little thyroxine. No surprise, then, that hormone replacement therapy – some combination of oestrogen, progesterone and testosterone – has emerged as standard therapy for low levels of reproductive hormones at menopause.

The problem is, the replacement – or even enhancement – of hormones can raise some risks, especially of cancer, Dr. Palumbo says. "Oestrogen replacement, for instance, can help maintain strong bones and may help reduce the incidence of other common age-related health problems." But oestrogen can also slightly increase a woman's risk of breast cancer. As more and more hormone replacement therapies become available (some even over the counter), it's important to know both the benefits and risks and to weigh them carefully.

Throughout this book, you'll learn more about what happens when your body produces too much (or too little) of various hormones. And you'll learn why it's important to keep your hormones in balance – starting with the next chapter.

# CHAPTER 2

# The Importance of Balance

So often, women talk about "hormones from hell". But every hormone has a purpose, and for the most part our hormones do exactly what they're designed to do: keep us healthy and functioning well. When our endocrine glands are producing the right blends of hormones, in the right amounts, at the right time, we feel fine. If they don't, we start to have problems.

Take epinephrine and norepinephrine – two major stress hormones – for example. And as unnerving as some of those stress hormones may be, we want them on our side when the spaghetti hits the fan. True, they can raise our blood pressure by constricting blood vessels. But they also help keep us from going into shock if we're rapidly losing blood. Another, longer-acting stress hormone, cortisol, helps to reduce inflammation in the body. In fact, synthetic versions of this hormone (hydrocortisone, for example) are sometimes used to treat inflammatory conditions such as rheumatoid arthritis. But in large amounts, cortisol suppresses immunity. That may be one reason people who are under long-term stress are more likely to get sick than people who lead more placid lives.

The "negatives" of these hormones aren't side effects; the hormones are doing exactly what they're supposed to be doing. Still, for one reason or another, the situation is not healthy. The key is balance.

## Your Brain, the Hormone Supervisor

Luckily, a series of checks and balances helps to keep the hormone system operating smoothly, so it's always returning to a steady internal state called homoeostasis.

In such a system, "hormone secretion is triggered by some internal or external stimulus," says Geoffrey Redmond, M.D., director of the Hormone Center of New York in New York City. "The stimulus can be just about anything – food, cold, stress, physical activity." As hormone levels rise, they affect various organs and inhibit further hormone release. As a result, blood levels of many hormones vary only within a narrow, "desirable" range.

The factors that turn hormones "on" or "off" may be modified, as needed, by the nervous system, Dr. Redmond says. Without this safeguard, endocrine activity would be strictly mechanical, much like a household thermostat. A thermostat can maintain the air temperature in your house at or around its set level. But it can't sense that your friend visiting from Florida feels cold at that temperature, and reset itself accordingly. You must make that adjustment. But the nervous system itself can override normal endocrine controls as needed to maintain homoeostasis.

Blood sugar regulation is a perfect example of how this delicate balance works. Insulin and several other hormones normally keep blood sugar levels within a range of 60 to 100 milligrams of glucose per 100 millilitres of blood. However, if you're suddenly subjected to severe stress – say, a thug knocks you down and snatches your handbag – your hypothalamus and sympathetic (fight-or-flight) nervous system centres are strongly activated, which in turn prompts your blood sugar level to rise. This ensures that your body cells will have sufficient fuel for more vigorous activity that might be called for (like running away!).

The hypothalamus, the body's "master" gland, is involved in maintaining homoeostasis in many ways. It is a part of the brain that receives and integrates signals from many parts of the body. It gets physical signals that allow it to monitor and help regulate such vital functions as water balance and thirst, body temperature and heart rate. Part of the hypothalamus acts as the body's internal clock, regulating biological rhythms such as wake/sleep cycles and sex drive. And it gets messages from our emotional, or limbic, brain. End result: sooner or later the hypothalamus "gets word" about just about everything that goes on in your body, including your thoughts and feelings. And then the hypothalamus can act on these messages by calling on the pituitary gland, its main henchman, to actually do what's needed.

The pituitary gland, which clings to the brain on a stalk, like a pea, secretes nine hormones involved in regulating hormone production in the other glands around the body, including major players like the thyroid and adrenal glands. Some of these hormones prompt the release of other hormones, while others inhibit release.

## Your Internal Thermostat

A properly working thyroid gland serves as yet another clear-cut example of this delicately balanced regulatory pathway. To stimulate the thyroid (a butterfly-shaped gland that wraps around the trachea), the hypothalamus gland secretes thyroid-releasing hormone. This hormone, in turn, stimulates the pituitary gland to secrete thyroid-stimulating hormone. It's this hormone, then, that stimulates the thyroid gland to release its thyroid hormones.

In turn, rising blood levels of thyroid hormones inhibit the pathway between the hypothalamus and the pituitary – reducing the secretion of thyroid-stimulating hormone. The thyroid puts out less thyroid hormone, and its blood level drops. As that happens, the hypothalamus and pituitary glands are once again roused to send a hormone message to the thyroid to crank up production. "The pathway allows input from all over the body," Dr. Redmond says. "For instance, it means that when your body's core temperature drops, your hypothalamus gets the signal and can in turn signal the thyroid gland to up production, increasing metabolism and, so, increasing body temperature."

If all works well, you're completely unaware of the complex interplay between those hormones. Without those hormonal interactions, though, your body temperature would fluctuate wildly. Instead, your hormones keep your body at a steady 37°C (98.6°F) or so, whether you step outside in cold weather or step outside on a blisteringly hot day.

## When Hormones Get out of Whack

Most hormone levels normally vary throughout a day, a month and a lifetime, depending on the internal and external stimuli, which, as we mentioned earlier, can be just about anything – food, water, cold, heat, or your body's own internal clock.

But sometimes hormones can get out of balance, for a number of reasons. "Simple changes in routine, like jet lag or missing a meal, can throw us off temporarily," says Dr. Redmond. Other, ongoing changes – chronic stress, illness, environmental toxins and even some prescription drugs – also can upset hormonal balance. Symptoms depend on which endocrine glands are malfunctioning.

Sometimes symptoms of hormonal imbalance develop relatively quickly, says Dr. Redmond. More often, though, they come on fairly gradually. "By the time someone is diagnosed, she can often look back over a year or two and see that something has not been quite right for some time," he says.

That's often the case for women with thyroid gland problems, for instance. Both overactivity and underactivity of the gland can cause metabolic disturbances that get increasingly worse over time. Low thyroid can result from an autoimmune disease, where the body attacks its own tissue. It can also result from a diet too low in iodine, a nutrient needed to convert the main thyroid hormones to their active form. The symptoms of a metabolic slow-down – feeling tired, chilled, mentally sluggish, constipated – slowly snow-ball until there's no doubt something is wrong.

If the thyroid gland is overactive, on the other hand, you'll feel hot and sweat a lot, have a rapid and sometimes irregular heartbeat; you'll be jumpy, nervous and lose weight. If fluid accumulates behind the eyeball, as it sometimes does, your eyes will bulge out.

Such was the case with President George Bush Snr.'s wife, Barbara, diagnosed with thyroid problems in the 1990s. Her bulging eyeballs were the clue to her problem.

## What Hormone Research Can Do for You

Due to myriad new discoveries in chemistry and biology, the study of hormone imbalances – endocrinology – has grown rapidly in the past 50 years. For researchers, these are exciting, fruitful times. For women, it means access to new breakthroughs that may improve their quality (and sometimes quantity) of life. It may also mean that, if they want, women can participate in clinical trials for promising treatments still being tested.

Yet in the quest for fine-tuning our hormone levels, women need to be aware that newly released drugs may produce unforeseen side effects. Again, the key is striking a balance – embracing new discoveries and discussing what they mean to you as an individual, considering the risks versus the benefits. The Hormone-Balancing Programme, Part 3 of this book, will help you restore balance, according to your individual needs.

But first, Part 2 will explain what can go wrong and why.

The most obvious way to determine whether your hormones are out of balance is to measure them, then replace what's missing or make other changes to restore balance. Think of diabetes: you may be monitoring your own blood glucose level, or your doctor may be measuring your blood glucose for you, then recommending ways to keep your blood sugar level on an even keel – by losing weight, changing your diet and possibly replacing insulin by pill or injection, if necessary.

Advances in technology, including improvements in hormone tests, allow researchers to accurately measure extremely small amounts of hormones and to track those substances by noninvasive means as they move throughout the body, including in the brain. This allows the researchers to detect the tiny amounts of hormones normally secreted and to see how a hormone acts in a body, what tissues it targets, where it activates cells in the brain. New technology allows researchers to make three-dimensional images of receptor sites on cell membranes, and then to make a molecular "key" that fits the image like a lock.

"Basic knowledge of hormones and how they work has grown by leaps and bounds, and at the same time, researchers are finding ways to make practical use of that knowledge," says Steven Petak, M.D., member of the Texas Institute for Reproductive Medicine and Endocrinology in Houston and chairman of the American Association of Clinical Endocrinologists' Reproductive Medicine Committee.

Most hormones have had their chemical structure defined and can be synthesized in the laboratory and used as hormone replacement therapy. The most common examples are insulin, thyroid hormones and the female hormones oestrogen and progesterone. Other, less well-known hormone replacement therapies include follicle-stimulating hormone, luteinizing hormone, testosterone, parathyroid hormone and growth hormone.

Hormone replacement isn't necessarily the only answer. Certain drugs can be used to dampen the overactivity of a gland and neutralize or suppress excessive amounts of a hormone. Less often, overactive sections of glands may need to be removed (although drug therapy makes that less likely). And look forward to the day when you can get a transplant of cells, or even whole endocrine organs, Dr. Petak says. Researchers at the University of California, San Diego, have developed an "immortal" line of human pancreatic islet cells, which make insulin, and are successfully growing them in the laboratory, hoping the cells will be available for transplantation one day. And donor islet cells have been transplanted, with apparent success, into several people with diabetes in the US.

Highlights of what hormone research has to offer women include the following:

**Insulin sensitizers.** Some people with diabetes are insulin resistant – that is, the cells in their bodies resist allowing insulin to escort glucose inside the cell. Drugs called insulin sensitizers, such as metformin (Glucophage), reduce insulin resistance. "They amplify the effects of insulin," says Richard Dickey, M.D., past president of the American

### THE HORMONE ZONE

# FOODS THAT FIGHT OR FAN INFLAMMATION

When your body is assaulted by injury, stress, toxins, or sunlight, your cells produce hormone-like substances, collectively called eicosanoids. Manufactured from fat, these biochemicals – such as prostaglandins, leukotrienes and thromboxanes – ramp up to fight the assault. In the process, they create inflammation – redness, heat, pain and swelling.

A certain degree of inflammation is helpful when you're hurt – it seals off the inflamed area and ultimately promotes healing in your body. But eicosanoids are definitely unwelcome in some situations, such as when you have rheumatoid arthritis, inflammatory bowel disease, asthma, or severe menstrual cramps, in which inflammation is already present. Inflammation is also linked with heart disease, some types of cancers, even Alzheimer's disease.

The kinds of fats you eat determine the amount of inflammation generated in your body. Omega-6 fatty acids lead to increases in inflammatory prostaglandins, and omega-3 fatty acids lead to decreases.

If you eat foods high in omega-6 fatty acids, "your body produces very potent eicosanoids that amplify inflammation," says Artemis Simopoulos, M.D., director of the Center for Genetics, Nutrition, and Health in Washington, D.C., and author of *The Omega Diet*.

On the other hand, if you eat omega-3 fatty acids, your body produces less potent prostaglandins, resulting in milder symptoms of inflammation and less pain and swelling.

If you're experiencing any kind of inflammation, aiming for a diet that maximizes foods that are high in omega-3s while minimizing foods that are high in omega-6s can help keep you in the Hormone Zone and put a lid on runaway inflammation.

**FOODS TO ADD**
- Flaxseed, rapeseed and walnut oils

- Fatty fish (such as sardines, mackerel, salmon, tuna and herring)

- Fish oil capsules

- Dark green leafy vegetables

**FOODS TO SUBTRACT**
- Polyunsaturated vegetable oils such as corn and soya oil and products made from these oils, such as margarine, crackers and baked goods

- Beef, poultry and pork that are fed mostly corn or soya beans

Association of Clinical Endocrinologists, now in private practice in North Carolina. This means either that individuals with insulin-resistant diabetes can make better use of the insulin their bodies make or that they can use a lower dose of insulin.

"That's good either way, because high levels of insulin create all sorts of other problems," Dr. Dickey says. (Even with such "wonder drugs", losing weight is the safest way to reduce insulin resistance, he adds.)

**SERMs (selective estrogen receptor modulators).** Informally referred to as "designer oestrogens", these laboratory-concocted molecules can bind to the same receptor sites on cell membranes as the female hormone oestrogen. "Researchers are hopeful that SERMs will have some of the beneficial effects of oestrogen and fewer of oestrogen's undesirable effects," Dr. Petak says. For instance, raloxifene (Evista) – one of the three SERMs currently FDA-approved – works nearly as well as oestrogen to maintain bone density after the menopause. But unlike oestrogen, it doesn't seem to promote cell growth in breast or uterine tissue. In fact, studies are under way to determine whether raloxifene helps to *reduce* the risk of breast cancer. Another SERM, tamoxifen (Nolvadex), is already used for that purpose.

"Raloxifene is a potential choice for women with low bone density who won't or can't take oestrogen and do not have breast cancer or deep venous thrombosis," Dr. Petak says.

This new "receptor modulator" technology is likely to also be used to design drugs that have oestrogen-like effects on blood vessels and the central nervous system.

**Testosterone supplements for women.** Researchers have long known that testosterone, the main male sex hormone, is what helps men maintain muscle, sex drive and general vitality. Now they're finding out that it has a similar important role in women. "The few, small studies done so far have looked mostly at sex drive, general mood and body composition – quality-of-life issues – and the results have been mostly positive," says Adrian Dobs, M.D., associate professor of endocrinology and metabolism at Johns Hopkins University School of Medicine in Baltimore.

In her own research, Dr. Dobs found that postmenopausal women taking oestrogen who also took testosterone had significant changes in body composition. They had an average of 2 per cent to 4 per cent reduction in body fat and 4 per cent to 6 per cent increase in muscle mass. So they were leaner for their weight.

By contrast, oestrogen alone yielded slight increases in both fat and muscle.

"The trick is to determine which women benefit from getting supplemental testosterone, and to determine a safe dose," Dr. Dobs says.

Although much further research needs to be done, testosterone is most likely to be added to treatment that already includes oestrogen. Testosterone alone might be used to reduce frailty in some women who are at risk for osteoporosis but who simply cannot take oestrogen because of increased cancer risks.

**Oestrogen as a memory booster.** Women going through the menopause often comment – at least among themselves – that their brains seem more like sieves than sponges. Things once easily remembered now seem to slip through. Blame it on a lack of oestrogen. Researchers are finding that oestrogen affects the structure and function of nervous system pathways in the brain. It also seems to play an important role in memory, especially verbal "working" memory – fluency and speed of articulation, or the ability to quickly retrieve words while talking – what we call "thinking on your feet". "Oestrogen influences the neural systems for working memory in post-menopausal women," says Sally Shaywitz, M.D., a Yale University researcher who, along with colleague Bennett Shaywitz, M.D., is involved in brain-hormone studies.

Research also suggests that both oestrogen and testosterone may help to protect against Alzheimer's disease.

## What Alternative Medicine Has to Offer

Alternative medicine has seen its "breakthroughs" – although less spectacular – in hormone treatments as well. Research is confirming what alternative doctors have long suspected – that biochemically identical forms of hormones, especially of progesterone, produce fewer side effects than forms that are not biochemically identical. Emerging evidence also suggests that phyto-oestrogens – plant forms of oestrogen that are found in soya, flaxseed and red clover – can alleviate both hormone excess and hormone deficiency.

Because they are weak oestrogens, phyto-oestrogens can block oestrogen receptor sites on cells, denying stronger versions of the hormone a docking site. But they still have *some* oestrogen activity, so they can help alleviate symptoms of hormone deficiency. Researchers are investigating phyto-oestrogens as "natural" versions of SERMs. Some of these are already on the market for the relief of hot flushes. Others, such as ipriflavone (OsteoPro), are thought to reduce the risk of osteoporosis.

## PART TWO

# What Can Go Wrong – And Why

# CHAPTER 3

# Don't Let Your Moods Control Your Life

Greeting cards, poets and child artists may still portray the heart as the feeling centre of the body, but we know that the true seat of emotions is the brain.

Scientists can now use computerized imaging techniques to watch different parts of the brain light up like a Christmas tree when any of the five sense organs are stimulated, as these sensations register in distinct areas of the brain. Two almond structures on either side of your brain called the amygdala will flash when fear or anger is registered, while another area – the nucleus accumbens – will glimmer with pleasure, happiness and comfort. These organs make up what's known as the limbic system – the feeling centre between your ears.

Emotional information also scoots around the brain to the memory and cognition areas, which adds the element of reason as well as more nuances to moods. Then, in a joint effort, the endocrine (hormone) and nervous systems shuttle the message to your organs, which produce the physiological reactions we associate with feelings – "butterflies" in the stomach, "fluttering" of the heart, a flushed face, or sweaty palms.

We are creatures of balance. Even when negative messages come through, most of your hormones and other hormone-like biochemicals are designed to restore a content, calm state. This chapter will explore the latest findings in the fields of neuroscience, endocrinology and psychiatry in order to show how you can influence your biochemistry to sustain positive moods and what you can do to help correct the chemical imbalances that lead to negative moods.

# The Feminine Side of Moods

Just as our reproductive capacities bring forth the pride of "becoming a woman", the awe-inspiring experience of giving birth, and the satisfaction of calling ourselves grandmothers, the life-giving power in our ovaries is not without its trade-off.

When C. Neill Epperson, M.D., assistant professor of psychiatry and obstetrician gynaecologist at Yale University, and co-researchers reviewed extensive medical research, they found that an increased risk of mood disturbances in a woman's life correlated with major reproductive events – when hormones are fluctuating after giving birth, going into the menopause, or before menstruation.

In fact, of the millions of adults each year who struggle with the sadness, hopeless feelings and angst of major depression, around two-thirds are women. Women also make up more than half of those who endure the irritability, extreme nervousness and constant fear associated with major anxiety disorders.

That's not to say women are biologically flawed. Economic and social hardships unique to women contribute to these sobering statistics. Compared with men, significantly more women live in poverty and have been victims of physical abuse, sexual abuse and sexual harassment. Even the minor day-to-day stresses of being a caretaker – male or female – can disrupt the system-controlling, mood-regulating hormones.

Nevertheless, the first question to ask if you develop a mood disorder is whether your female hormones are involved. "Major depression and other mood disorders are twice as common in women than men, and the emotional distress is most likely to take place during changes associated with reproductive function," says Carol Shively, Ph.D., professor of pathology and psychology at Wake Forest University School of Medicine in Winston-Salem, North Carolina.

Just how reproductive hormones contribute to our mood milieu has never been clear. The focus has been largely on oestrogen being sort of a chemical upper with progesterone being a natural downer, explains Peter Schmidt, M.D., senior researcher at the Behavioral Endocrinology Branch of the National Institute of Mental Health (NIMH) in Bethesda, Maryland. But then Dr. Schmidt and his NIMH colleagues conducted groundbreaking research showing that the real issue seems to be that a certain percentage of the female population have a nervous system that is more affected than usual by the intense high and low spikes of oestrogen and progesterone.

(continued on page 42)

## WHAT'S GOING ON?

If your moods are getting too negative or unpredictable for comfort, take this quiz to help you narrow down what's keeping you on an emotional roller coaster.

**1. Are you a new mother who feels hopeless, uncharacteristically anxious, or unable to care for your baby?**
While four out of five new mothers experience mild "baby blues", symptoms usually fade in the first 2 weeks after delivery. If your low mood lingers and declines, you could have postnatal depression. (See chapter 9 for more information.)

**2. Do you work a late shift or feel particularly sluggish and blue in the winter months?**
Hormone imbalances from inadequate exposure to sunlight can lead to seasonal affective disorder (SAD). If you can't get daylight for 1 hour a day, use a commercial light box to mimic the sun.

**3. Do you experience fluctuating periods of extreme elation and reckless behaviour, followed by a "crash" into states of sadness and hopelessness?**
You should be evaluated by a family doctor or psychiatrist for bipolar disorder (also known as manic-depressive illness).

**4. Is there a history of thyroid disease or another autoimmune condition (such as rheumatoid arthritis or lupus) in your family? Do you have anxiety or depression accompanied by extreme fatigue or hyperactivity, sensitivity to temperatures, or unexplained weight loss or weight gain?**
A malfunctioning thyroid gland could be at the root of your mood problems. (See "Thyroid: The Hidden Weight/Mood Connection" on page 105 for details.)

**5. Are you on a high-protein weight-loss diet?**
High-protein diets – that is, diets deriving 60 per cent or more of their calories from protein – may deny you the amount of carbohydrates that your nervous system needs to create the mood-regulating chemical serotonin. If you get anxious or depressed on a high-protein plan, experiment with including more carbohydrates in your diet and see if you feel better. Or work with a trained nutritionist to revise your eating plan.

**6. Do you take birth control pills or medication such as steroids, antihypertensives (blood-pressure-lowering drugs) or cardiac drugs, anticonvulsants, or sedatives?**

Numerous prescription or over-the-counter drugs are suspected of causing mood changes. Because oral contraceptives are combinations of varying amounts of oestrogen and progestin, they can cause depression in women susceptible to changes in hormone levels. Work closely with your doctor to resolve any side effects by altering your dosage or drug choice. If changing your oral contraceptive doesn't help, consider a non-hormonal form of birth control.

**7. Are you exposed to heavy metals (such as lead paint or copper in corroded water pipes) or industrial chemicals such as cleaning agents or solvents? Does weakness, memory loss, or muscle aches accompany your depression symptoms?**
Ask your doctor for a blood analysis. If toxic contamination shows up, make the changes to avoid the offending substance, such as switching to environmentally friendly cleansers and getting adequate ventilation when cleaning, and start a detoxification programme with your doctor at once.

**8. Do you smoke or are you trying to quit smoking?**
In some women, nicotine from either cigarettes or nicotine-replacement products, such as gum or patches, triggers feelings of depression or anxiety. Unfortunately, quitting can also bring on a depressive episode in some women. If you have a history of psychiatric illness and are trying to quit, check in regularly with your doctor until you have adjusted to withdrawal, and consider antidepressant medication or other forms of therapy to ease the transition.

"In much the same way that people have a predisposition to other psychological conditions, some women seem to be born with this increased biological vulnerability to their female hormone shifts," says Louann Brizendine, M.D., director of the Women's Mood and Hormone Clinic at Langley Porter Psychiatric Institute of the University of California, San Francisco. "In fact, it's common to see a woman develop mood disturbances just like her sister, mother and grandmother did several years after the onset of puberty, or after childbirth."

While genetics play an important role in all major mood disorders, experts stress that taking care of emotional and physical health can keep anxiety and depression from being triggered.

"Think of PMS and other mood disturbances the same way you think of allergies or migraine headaches. You need to learn what situations set your emotions off, and do everything possible to avoid them. Sometimes it's a matter of changing your lifestyle, your diet or attitude, and, when it's still not manageable, coming to terms with taking medication to correct your biochemistry," says Jean Endicott, Ph.D., chief of the department of research, assessment and training at New York State Psychiatric Institute, as well as director of the premenstrual evaluation unit at Columbia-Presbyterian Medical Center, both in New York City.

## Navigating Rocky Menstrual Cycles

Most women have learned to live with mild bouts of irritability, anger and mood swings, but for a few, the erratic behaviour has brutal consequences. "Some women tell me they've lost jobs or that they can't keep a boyfriend because of their premenstrual behaviour," Dr. Endicott says.

Fortunately, we have come a long, liberating way from the days of talking about the "curse of Eve" in hushed tones or being told that PMS was our wild imagination. Most large general hospitals actually have clinics where psychiatrists and women's health experts can help with the problem, says Dr. Brizendine.

It is now recognized that the mood component of PMS can be so severe that it warrants the diagnosis of premenstrual dysphoric disorder (PMDD). As with regular PMS, women with PMDD usually experience a whole range of physical symptoms, such as bloating, headaches, or fatigue. But they also experience, with the intensity of major depression, downcast mood, anxiety, decreased interest in activities and marked changes in behaviour. These symptoms all but disappear shortly after the start of the menstrual period and don't return until after ovulation.

To know whether you have PMDD, and how severe, you need to keep a symptom diary every day for 2 months, noting any mood disturbances as well as other symptoms of PMDD and, of course, when your period starts and ends, says Dr. Endicott.

The leading treatment for unmanageable PMDD is a selective serotonin reuptake inhibitor (SSRI) antidepressant medication, such as fluoxetine (Prozac). Fluoxetine was approved for the treatment of PMDD relatively recently. It may be prescribed to be taken only during the 10- to 14-day luteal phase of your menstrual cycle, rather than daily, and the dosage is often lower than you would take for major depression. If an antidepressant drug does not work, PMDD can be controlled by medication that will stop the hormone changes that cause severe premenstrual problems.

The first line of action, however, is to make changes in your lifestyle. These changes can be so powerful that they are sometimes enough to stop even major PMS or PMDD, says Dr. Endicott. Here is what works for some women at her clinic.

**Learn your pattern.** Look at your symptom diary. If your symptoms always start 8 days before your period, mark those days in red on your calendar. "Just seeing your distress-prone days coming up gets you mentally prepared," says Dr. Endicott. When you have an explanation for your atypical behaviour, it allows you to be patient when you slip up, rather than increasing tension with self-criticism.

**Lie low at work.** Companies in some Asian countries, including Japan, allot 2 sick days a month for menstrual difficulties. We're not likely to go that far. But you can still try to plan around predictable shifts in your disposition. "Many women report that they can get their project-related work done just fine when they're premenstrual; it's interaction with others that causes problems," says Dr. Endicott. "If you can control work flow, try to save premenstrual days for paperwork or reading. If you have to attend a meeting during this time, remind yourself to listen rather than be vocal since you may regret what you say when you're not 'yourself'."

**Communicate discreetly.** You don't have to announce to the world that you have premenstrual distress. Simply let others know you "just don't feel well today" so others – even Year 2s, if you're a primary school teacher – can cut you some slack. If you're a manager with an assistant who schedules your appointments, and you feel comfortable saying so, let him or her know that it's not a good week for you to deal with stressful confrontations.

**Involve your family.** You can be a lot more open with family than with colleagues. Tell them up front not to take it personally if you are irritable in the next few days. If you have severe PMS, arrange to see your doctor with your partner and/or family at a longer appointment than usual. You may be asked to attend a "Well Woman" clinic (see "On the Web & Other Resources" on page 58). Many women report that their families experience great relief when they learn that Mum's moodiness has a biological cause and, like any other illness, is treatable.

**Be bold in the best part of the month.** If you have big decisions to make

---

THE HORMONE CONNECTION

# THE PMS DEFENCE: AN EXCUSE FOR MURDER?

The criminal record of a barmaid with the surname of Craddock was as long as your arm. In addition to serving 30 sentences for theft, arson and assault, the barmaid is on record for stalking an officer and, once, for throwing bricks through a window. In 1980, she murdered a colleague. Her manslaughter murder trial pointed out the common denominator of her deviance: Craddock struck when she was premenstrual.

According to Craddock's officially worded plea, PMS "turned her into a raging animal each month and forced her to act out of character". Her sentence was mitigated to probation provided she took hormone medication.

Other PMS'd-out women have been fully acquitted of criminal charges for various offences, from shoplifting charges to reckless driving. One woman – a doctor – failed a breathalyser test and violently resisted arrest, but was let off.

In more than one trial, Katharina Dalton, M.D., who helped make PMS a household term, offered testimony that severe cases of PMS can cause temporary insanity. But more commonly, menstrual difficulties have been used as (1) "plea of diminished responsibility" (which in legal terms means that a person was unable to exercise control or use her moral judgement because of an abnormality of the mind) or (2) "automatism defence" (usually used for seizures, reflexes and other instances when the mind and the body act out of accordance).

Acquittals or no, recognizing severe PMS and taking steps to controlling it could have saved those women – and everyone around them – a lot of trouble.

– say, a job change, a breakup, or a property venture – and you have control over when they take place, make them on days 6 to 10 of your cycle. Ideally, this is also the best time to schedule a party or attend a reunion or another major social event where you want to shine. On the other hand, when you know you're premenstrual, try to defer major, life-changing decisions. For example, if you get so angry at your boss or your husband that you're convinced quitting your job or getting a divorce is the only answer, wait a week – the impulse may blow over.

**Keep a lid on alcohol and coffee.** "Premenstrual moods are associated with lack of impulse control, so women who may normally have one alcoholic drink a night at other times during their cycle are prone to double or triple that amount premenstrually," says Dr. Endicott. It may also be tempting to self-medicate the internal tension with alcohol and then get carried away.

Don't fill your mug with more coffee than usual either, she adds. Caffeine may seem like a remedy for your increased premenstrual fatigue, but the anxiety kickback of more than one cup a day is never worth it.

## Menopause Isn't *Always* Hell

The Massachusetts Women's Health Study surveyed more than 2,500 women between 45 and 55 years of age for 5 years and found no increase in depression associated with the menopause. This study is just one of the many on record that show that the majority of menopausal women should expect no more than minor disturbances in their quality of life from mild emotional and physical symptoms.

Of course, not everyone sails through the change without mood problems. The minority who get depressed tend to either be women with a history of previous mental illness, or women who are having an exceptionally long period of overt perimenopausal symptoms (greater than 27 months rather than the more typical 12 months). The good news is that when these women become postmenopausal, their depressive symptoms usually abate.

If you're perimenopausal, you don't have to live with out-of-control mood problems.

**Consider hormone replacement therapy (HRT) early on.** You don't have to wait until official menopause to benefit from hormone replacement. Many gynaecologists prescribe HRT for women during perimenopause. If you are having a long, difficult perimenopause or if you are depressed during perimenopause, you may be a candidate for starting hormone replacement therapy in the perimenopause stage, says Dr. Schmidt.

When Dr. Schmidt and co-researchers at NIMH gave depressed peri-menopausal women aged 44 to 55 oestrogen replacement, 80 per cent of the women recovered after just 3 weeks – even six out of the seven women in the group who had severe depression. (To learn more about hormone replacement, see chapter 11.)

**Try different versions of hormones.** In some cases, the type of hormone replacement a woman takes to ease physical symptoms ends up actually causing emotional symptoms, like hostility and sadness. "There's a real difference between the hormones that your body makes and the forms and formulations used in hormone replacement therapy and contraceptives," says Dr. Shively. What's more, each woman's body chemistry is different. Some women react to the synthetic hormones but not the so-called natural hormones, while the opposite is true for others. So if you have problems, speak up, and ask your doctor to switch you to another form. It's not unusual to change prescriptions at least once before getting it right.

**Guard your sleep.** Perimenopause is notorious for wrecking your rest, and when sleep suffers, so do your moods. To help relieve night sweats that may be waking you up, see Night Sweats on page 304. To sleep more soundly, Jonathan Zuess, M.D., a psychiatrist in Scottsdale, Arizona, and author of *The Wisdom of Depression*, recommends taking 500 milligrams of calcium with 200 to 350 milligrams of magnesium before bed. Both are neuromuscular relaxants.

## When Stress Fuels the Fire

Not all mood changes can be traced to the effects of reproductive hormones. You don't need a book to tell you that stress plays a role in how you feel on any given day. Here's why.

In biological terms, most mood-regulating biochemicals in your body seem to have one thing in common: the LHPA axis. Think of it as a space-age travel system for your hormones. Your limbic system (the emotional centre of the brain), hypothalamus, pituitary and adrenal glands are the major airports. The neurotransmitters, like serotonin and dopamine, are the air traffic controllers that manage LHPA transactions from their watchtowers in your brain.

Your reproductive system is a shuttle airport that takes trips through the major hubs, such as the hypothalamus and the limbic system, to pick up the hormones you need for ovulation. Your thyroid gland also depends on smooth connections between the hypothalamus and pituitary glands to transport the fuel it needs to regulate your metabolism and keep your moods steady.

Stress hormones rack up the most frequent-flier miles on the "LHPA Express" because they always take round trips through the entire LHPA system.

The limbic system is an ingeniously engineered network of exchanges. The emotional charge of anger or fear when you're stressed penetrates the limbic system and then is relayed down to the hypothalamus, which in turn sends corticotropin-releasing hormone (CRH) over to the pituitary glands. When the pituitary receives its hormonal cargo, it sends another load of hormones to the adrenal glands, which then squirt out cortisol and other stress-responsive hormones. The last connection is perhaps the most important because when the cortisol is shuttled back up to the brain, it tells the hypothalamus to turn down its CRH production.

Every system, however, has its breaking point. Unmanaged stress in your life is like overbooking more flights than even the ingenious "LHPA Express" can process efficiently. In such a case, from your ovaries and thyroid to your brain itself, mood-regulating biochemical connections all over your system will be missed – particularly the one that turns down your cortisol and CRH production.

The longer your cortisol or CRH is elevated, the likelier it is that you're headed for a major mood crash. And remember the air traffic controller neurotransmitters? They may get so overwhelmed that they quit under the unbearable conditions. Neurotransmitters are too important to your mood-regulating system to put in jeopardy, warns Owen Wolkowitz, M.D., a cortisol researcher and professor of psychiatry at the University of California, San Francisco.

In fact, the most well-established clinical marker behind major depression and serious anxiety conditions like obsessive-compulsive disorder and eating disorders is a deficiency of some neurotransmitters such as serotonin.

## Prevent a Crash

The most obvious way to avoid "system overload" is to get out of the situations that made you irritable or hostile in the first place. That's where Phase 2 of the Hormone-Balancing Programme comes in. See page 275 to discover ways to manage the stress brought on by your job and home and to learn about relaxation techniques that enhance your natural stress-balancing mechanisms.

It's also essential to manage *internal* tensions. Although to someone else your life may appear to be going fine, minor fears and disappointments may

(continued on page 50)

*Escape from* **HORMONE HELL**

# SHE WISHES SHE WEREN'T SO EMOTIONAL

**Q:** All my life people have been calling me hypersensitive, moody, eccentric, overintense and even neurotic. I'm told it's not normal to get freaked-out for days over a scary movie, a disturbing world event, or a bad dream. And even though I'm an adult with kids of my own, I still cry at the drop of a hat – whether my sisters hurt my feelings when they don't include me on a shopping trip, or I'm deeply moved by the beauty of the sunrise while driving to work. As if my own deep feelings weren't disruptive enough, when other people are in a nasty mood or if someone has something really great happen to them, I end up getting distracted, too.

It's really exhausting to be affected by everyone else's emotions. My supervisors usually praise my creative ideas, but I don't think I get as many promotions as other people because I have the reputation as being "too sensitive". How can I stop being so vulnerable to my moods – or at least not let other people know what I'm feeling?

Elaine N. Aron, Ph.D., a San Francisco–based psychologist and author of the books *The Highly Sensitive Person* and *The Highly Sensitive Person in Love*, responds: it clearly sounds like you are among the 15 to 20 per cent of the population with a unique biology that causes them to notice more subtleties and process information more deeply. Take it from me: there's nothing defective about being a highly sensitive person, or HSP. Instead, reframe your trait for yourself and others to appreciate it as an *asset* and as the *gift* that it is.

The truth is, you're in a position of emotional leadership. So many people can't give themselves permission to cry and are totally repressed by a culture that has hang-ups about expressing love. You have a liberation others don't. When people remark negatively about your sensitivity, respond with gentle humour and reframe their perception. A great response is "Oh, many people like my being sensitive – how is it a problem for you?"

In addition to creativity, you probably have excellent attention to detail, show exceptional consideration to others and take a well-planned, complex approach to a project rather than mindlessly diving in. In professional situations, point out those assets.

Never feel guilty or flawed for being the way you are. Your colleagues and family are so fortunate to have a person in their lives in tune with the deeper dimensions of life.

That said, you may feel more emotionally grounded if you're careful not to get overcome by stimuli. That means avoiding overarousal while not overcompensating by protecting yourself to the point where you're restless or bored from lack of stimulation.

To do that, give yourself enough downtime. Ideally, that means 8 to 10 hours a day in bed. If you can, let yourself spend 2 hours involved in quiet activities, like meditation, or simply pottering. And try to get 1 hour of outdoor exercise daily. Take 1 day a week completely off, and aim for a total of 1 month of holiday a year that includes travel.

Next, get into what I call "the umbrella walk" mindset. Think of how a closed umbrella gathers a lot of water in every crease, but when it is up, you can better deflect the stuff coming at you. Remind yourself before you leave the house to "bring your umbrella" – a reminder that are you aren't *receiving* all the time. This visualization exercise is especially important on days that you are not feeling so great. With your umbrella opened, you can go to the shop with the attitude that you are not interested in everything in it and what everyone else is up to. Instead, you stay focused on your mission. It also means deciding ahead of time what your policies are on responding to salespeople and homeless people so you don't have to decide in each case you encounter.

I also recommend always carrying a protein snack like an energy bar with you since overarousal can deplete your blood sugar. You may respond more dramatically to caffeine and medication, so always use the most minimal amounts of these possible.

become so embellished in your mind over time that they cause constant tension in your psyche, says Carol Boulware, Ph.D., a psychotherapist in Santa Monica, California. With severe anxiety or post-traumatic stress disorder, you may also be haunted by the memory of a single catastrophic event.

"All too often, people erase the memory of troubling events from their conscious minds, but the experience can still produce the biochemical response to fear, as it remains in your subconscious," says Dr. Boulware. Trying to forget the discomfort may have been your best way of coping at the time but, years later, can show up as panic attacks and elevated stress hormones as the memory lives on in your subconscious, she says. If you experience panic, phobias and other anxious states, make an appointment to be evaluated by a doctor or therapist. Deep-seated issues may take extensive talk therapy to undo, so the sooner you start on the road to progress, the better, says Dr. Boulware. You may be helped by some anti-anxiety medication to help manage your reactions while you do the work.

Not only can chronic internal or external tension lead to anxiety disorders, but researchers like Dr. Wolkowitz have preliminary evidence that it may lay the hormonal groundwork for major depression – since it appears that half of all people with major depression have elevated cortisol levels.

Stress affects more than your moods; it affects your bones, your heart and even your memory. Women with chronically elevated cortisol have lower bone mineral density than women with normal cortisol and may have a higher heart disease risk. More sobering is a study from the Washington University School of Medicine in St. Louis that found that chronically elevated cortisol seems to cause part of the brain, the hippocampus, to shrink in depressed women. The women in the study who had undergone major depressive episodes had on average 10 per cent smaller volume in this learning and memory brain structure than the brains of emotionally healthy women.

The point is, it's essential to honour your emotions and take care of external and internal tension before it starts to overstimulate your mood-regulating system, says Dr. Wolkowitz. Fortunately, there is much you can do to enhance your built-in biochemical balancing mechanisms.

## Control Your Contentedness

Respecting that little things can get under you skin and upset your hormone balance may make the difference between going through life as a slightly agitated person and being a contented person.

If you had a "breakdown" in the past or have a family history of psychiatric illness, paying attention to even seemingly minor things may be the difference between setting off a genetic tendency to a major psychiatric event and beating the odds.

**Heed your personal "mood climate".** To care for your emotional well-being, slow down and pay attention to the subtle messages that your five senses are bringing in, says Dr. Zuess. For example, did you know that the secretion of many hormones follows a rhythmic daily cycle that appears to be governed by the pineal gland in your brain?

When the pineal gland secretes melatonin, it not only regulates sleep but also stimulates the brain's production of the important mood-regulating neurotransmitter serotonin. The secretion of a certain, basic amount of cortisol also follows a rhythmic daily cycle. If less than that amount is produced, you feel lethargic; if it's overproduced, you feel nervous tension. The best way to keep these cyclic hormones on track is to keep your schedule on track – in other words, sticking to regular times for sleeping, eating and exercise keeps your mind and your chemistry in harmony, says Dr. Zuess.

**Follow nature's light patterns.** The release of hormones in your pineal gland is regulated by the nerve impulses that are sent by your retinas in response to light, says Dr. Zuess. In other words, living by the earth's natural cycle of light and darkness keeps your serotonin and cortisol at their proper levels.

You may not be willing to go to bed soon after twilight, but you can keep on the minimal number of lights that you need at night, and use dimmer switches to create a more natural night-time. At the same time, take every opportunity to bathe yourself with daylight for at least an hour a day – including early-morning walks and more outdoor hobbies like gardening. If you can't get outside, Dr. Zuess recommends spending an hour a day next to a commercial light box that has full-spectrum bulbs to mimic natural light's signals to your pineal gland.

**Avoid electromagnetic fields when possible.** Frequent prolonged exposure to magnetic fields upsets the pineal gland's regulation of melatonin and serotonin, according to Dr. Zuess. That means it's ideal to avoid living or working close to large electric installations or high-voltage lines. And because electromagnetic fields grow exponentially stronger as you move closer to them, Dr. Zuess says it's also best to stay at least 3 metres away from electric appliances. Using a blow dryer or blender for a few minutes isn't so much of a problem. But because you spend close to half of your life in bed, he recommends making sure your electric alarm clock and television are opposite your bed in your bedroom. Or use a battery-powered clock. Get rid of electric blankets, too, advises Dr. Zuess.

**Meditate to calm your brain chemistry.** Meditation gives you a solid sense of your inner being, which will naturally develop more sensory awareness. From a biochemical perspective, it may help lower cortisol while potentially raising the good-mood hormones DHEA and testosterone. You'll need to research which form of meditation appeals to you, and don't get intimidated thinking your practise has to be as sophisticated as Buddhist chanting or Christian mysticism.

Dr. Zuess offers a beginner mediation you can do right away: sit comfortably and focus on the most distant sounds you can hear, such as traffic on the street. Then very gradually take in slightly closer sounds, such as your cat's walking across the floor in the other room. Next, concentrate on sounds within the room, such as the hum of an air conditioner or heater. Then focus on the sounds of your own body. First listen to your breathing, and, finally, try to hear your own heart beating. This is one of many simple meditations that will introduce you to the soothing sensation of being centred in your body.

**Help yourself adjust to changes.** It's a scientific fact that in all species, including the human animal, unfamiliar surroundings release the hormones associated with anxiety. If you are changing your job or living situation, the brain's limbic system can be overwhelmed by so much new stimuli, says Elaine N. Aron, Ph.D., a San Francisco-based psychologist and author of the books *The Highly Sensitive Person* and *The Highly Sensitive Person in Love.*

How do you ease the transition? Think about the kinds of things you would do for your cat if you had to move. Would you talk to your cat soothingly and transfer some familiar objects into its new environment? Likewise, be gentle and patient with yourself, says Dr. Aron. Tell yourself that you don't have to *like* the change at first. To get more quickly settled in, it may help to hang up old pictures right away and burn your favourite aromatherapy candle, she says.

**Get organized.** Some people are more overtly bothered than others by disarray – but on a subtle, subconscious level, even your teenage son is probably agitated by piles of "unfinished business", runaway socks and worktops full of unwashed dishes. If a woman is vulnerable to the shift of her reproductive hormones, a chaotic environment can really set off her agitation. Do whatever it takes to get organized. That may mean you'll have to actually schedule time in your week for housekeeping, delegate chores, or accept that you need to hire some help.

## People-to-People Contact Fosters Healthy Moods

How you stand in relation to others also influences the biology of your moods. Dr. Shively studied the hormonal effects of social status on primates whose endocrine systems were remarkably similar to female humans – down to the approximately 28-day menstrual cycles. Female monkeys categorized as having low social status were treated aggressively by the other primates and weren't included in the usual monkey affections, like sitting together or grooming. Unlike other females, low-status females showed signs of anxiety by looking around nervously and sat in slumped postures typical of depression.

Blood tests confirmed that that the low-social-status females had disturbances of both the hypothalamic–pituitary–adrenal axis and the hypothalamic–pituitary–ovarian axis. In other words, the systems that govern the mood-regulating hormones as well as the reproductive hormones had gone off track.

Dr. Shively's research confirms the importance of fostering healthy relationships in order to keep our biochemistry in balance. At the same time, Dr. Boulware points out the need to take care of our relationships with *ourselves*. "Negative self-image can sabotage a woman's sense of well-being," she stresses. In fact, Dr. Boulware sees negative self-image as a major trait associated with the generalized anxiety disorder so many women come to her to treat.

To enhance your standing with others and yourself – and improve your moods:

**Put "people connections" on your schedule.** People are gregarious, social beings and not happy unless they are intimate with other human beings. When we get too swept up in the pace of our lives, we become isolated from our sources of social support, says Dr. Shively. Being so deliberate about social engagements may seem silly, but these days, unless you schedule in dates with friends as you would dentist and doctor appointments, they won't happen. Chances are, your friends' schedules are as filled up as yours, so scheduling time together – even if it's months in advance – is the only way you're going to see one another.

**Put limits on technology.** In order to be healthy, we have to stop sacrificing social support for our highly technologized society, says Dr. Shively. "Turn off the television, turn off the computer and call someone to go for a walk. Instead of bringing work home at night, try to go for coffee with someone. These seem like really simple ideas, but they are big challenges these days."

**Reassess your hobbies.** Get rid of any "extracurricular activities" that make demands on your time and energy but don't lead to close, warm, intimate relationships, says Dr. Shively. "If volunteering to be the Cub Scout mum means that you see other Cub Scout mums and get to laugh together and be supportive of each other, then it's a great activity. But if being the Cub Scout mum is just another obligation to race around for on weeknights, stop doing it."

**Fall in love – it's good for your chemistry.** "People who have a secure love relationship in their lives are generally calm and emotionally resilient," says Dr. Zuess. In fact, a cascade of good-mood hormones follows the stages of meeting and settling down with that special someone.

The initial infatuation floods your system with dopamine, norepinephrine and phenylethylamine, a biochemical concoction chemically similar to amphetamines. As time passes, the natural opiates wear off, but feelings of more mature, levelheaded love are supported by endorphins acting in the brain to induce the sensation of contentment. In addition, the "bonding hormone", oxytocin, also comes into play, providing the emotional charge that makes you glow when you hold your mate's hand after 50 years.

**Find out what's holding you back from intimacy.** Do you worry excessively that your partner won't stay with you or doesn't really love you? On the other hand, are you uneasy being close with others or prefer not to depend on others? Either tendency could be a sign of what psychologists call an insecure attachment style. Insecure attachment could have elevated your cortisol and adrenaline as early as infancy and may still be causing stress on your chemistry and your psyche.

"Some cases of insecure attachment style can take years of careful therapy to resolve," says Dr. Aron. "But reflecting on your fears as realistically as possible will start your progress." If you are fearful of meeting new people, for instance, you can be more conscious about not assuming they will reject you. If you are preoccupied with a fear of letting go of people, your task is trusting that people will come back to you.

## Nutritional "Mood Maintenance"

You may already be taking vitamins and minerals to protect yourself against the flu or other physical health problems. But they can also protect against psychological illness. So can a diet centred on vegetables and whole grains. People who eat a vegetarian-style diet tend to be healthier overall, physically *and* emotionally, says Dr. Zuess.

"On the other hand, any kind of nutritional deficiency can produce mood disorders," he says. "For example, extremely low levels of B vitamins – especially folate – has landed people with stays in psychiatric hospitals. If you suffer from unexplained anxiety and sadness, it's reasonable to ask your doctor to do a blood test of your nutrient levels."

**Take basic supplements in the morning and evening.** A standard multivitamin/mineral can help you avoid the even minor nutritional deficiencies that can contribute to a mood disorder. "Supplements formulated to be taken in divided doses keep your nutrient levels most even," advises Dr. Zuess.

Because $B_{12}$ naturally occurs in only animal sources, if you're a vegetarian you may need to take an additional supplement of 500 to 1000 micrograms. Make sure your supplement also contains at least 5 milligrams of the all-important $B_6$. Both of these B vitamins are involved in the production of brain neurotransmitters and are essential for every organ system.

Don't go overboard, however, by trying to take much more than your RDA, listed on the label. "Megadoses of vitamins A and D and calcium can actually *cause* depression," Dr. Zuess adds.

**Boost your amino acids.** Because your brain's neurotransmitters are made of amino acids, the right mix of these protein elements will encourage your brain to keep your serotonin and dopamine levels even, says Dr. Zuess. They are abundant in normal food and in the UK doctors are not convinced that people with a normal genetic make-up will benefit from taking extra amino acids. (If you are deficient in them you will know about it from birth.) However, there are quite a few amino acids available in supplement form (the two most recognized to reduce mood disorders are DL-phenylalanine and L-tyrosine) and if you do want to take them they are widely available in health food shops. Don't take amino acids, however, if you are already taking an antidepressant drug, have high blood pressure, or have a history of panic attacks.

**Eat fish.** If your hormones are out of balance, it's all the more important to keep your prostaglandins *in* balance. Essential fatty acids found in certain fish – such as tuna, salmon, trout or herring – are used by the body to make prostaglandins, which are important substances for regulating a number of systems in the body, and which are typically imbalanced in people with major depression. Adding one or more servings of fish to your diet every day can help restore this balance. If you are a total vegetarian, the next-best essential fatty acid source is 2 tablespoons or 5 to 10 grams of flaxseed oil each day, according to Dr. Zuess.

# The Hormonal Side of Depression

Everyone feels blue from time to time, but when your low moods are so severe that they prevent you from going about your day-to-day activities, it's time to get medical help. It's also worth getting evaluated if you think you have dysthymia – a chronic low-grade depression where you can still drag yourself to work or school but you are so robbed of the usual energy, enthusiasm, or enjoyment that your quality of life is seriously compromised. Of course, if you feel suicidal, go to your nearest casualty department or call your doctor at once.

These are the signs that a minor mood disturbance has spiralled into clinical depression.

- *Loss of interest in hobbies, sex and other pleasurable activities*
- *Persistent anxious, sad, or "empty" mood*
- *Feelings of hopelessness, helplessness, guilt, or worthlessness*
- *Unexplained fatigue*
- *Changes in appetite and weight*
- *Unexplained, untreatable physical symptoms such as chronic pain, headaches and digestive disorders*
- *Inability to sleep well or sleeping too much*
- *Difficulty concentrating, remembering, or making decisions*
- *Preoccupation with death*
- *Withdrawal from friends and family*

If you have several of these depressive symptoms for more than 2 weeks, pick up the phone and make an appointment with your doctor or a psychiatrist. Expect your doctor to give you a complete physical and run blood tests to check for underlying causes.

If you're diagnosed with depression, work closely with your doctor or psychiatrist to personalize your treatment plan, says Dr. Zuess. For severe depression, your doctor may immediately start you on antidepressant drugs, to increase the levels of mood-regulating, hormone-like neurotransmitters in your blood.

The three major categories of antidepressants are selective serotonin reuptake inhibitors (SSRIs), monoamine oxidase inhibitors (MAOIs) and tricyclics. Since the SSRIs have the fewest side effects, you will most likely start with fluoxetine (Prozac), sertraline (Lustial), or another drug from this category. Each SSRI has slightly different characteristics, so you may need to try a few before you find the one that works best with your chemistry. You won't know for 4 to 8 weeks whether they are really working since SSRIs take that long to create their full effect in the brain.

Depression tends to run in families, so tell your doctor if another family member has success with a particular drug since it's likely to work on your chemical imbalances, too, says Dr. Endicott.

All antidepressants have about a 65 per cent success rate. "But don't ever accept medication as the sole treatment being offered," Dr. Zuess emphasizes. "Think of medication as something to fall back on when you're literally too depressed for counselling and other forms of therapy to work."

## Taking Action Helps to Normalize Hormones

According to the American Psychological Association, therapy that has an "action plan" for depression can increase chances of recovery significantly.

"Any intervention that increases someone's sense of control over her life will help normalize stress hormone output," says Dr. Wolkowitz.

Your healing programme should be tailored towards correcting whatever vulnerability you have, so you need to do some soul-searching to find what led up to a major depression in the first place, says Dr. Zuess. "The deeper you get to the root of the problem, the best chance you have in complete remission and avoiding a reoccurrence," he says.

Painful as it may be, ask yourself what's missing in your life, he says. Is forgiveness, self-acceptance, career satisfaction, or spiritual enlightenment remiss? "If you listen, your body is crying for transformation of some kind."

The first step is asking your family, friends and doctor to refer you to a counsellor who will help you examine your inner psychological conflicts. You may have to sample a few different styles of therapy before you find the one that answers your needs, and sometimes this requires interviewing a variety of potential counsellors, too, says Dr. Zuess. A good counsellor should provide hope, insight, information and loving support.

Here are some other steps that get you on your way to deep and permanent emotional healing.

**Call on your faith.** "Accept that prayer or spiritual rituals won't feel as good as when you were more well, although they will do you more good than ever, even if you are just going through the motions," says Dr. Aron. "In other words, you may have to pray even when you don't believe in God, but that may be the time that you most need to pray."

Even if you don't practise a formal form of religion, don't overlook what soul-enriching experiences you already have in your life, like reading novels, practising yoga, stargazing, lighting candles at dinner, or volunteer

## ON THE WEB & Other Resources

If you're experiencing mood problems, the following resources may help you control your moods before they control your life.

The main mental health charity in the UK is MIND (the National Association for Mental Health). Its Web site has all the information needed to access resources for women needing help with depression, anxiety and panic disorders as well as more serious psychiatric problems such as schizophrenia and manic depression.

**MIND** *www.mind.org.uk*
15–19 Broadway, London E15 4BQ
Tel: 0845 766 0163

**SANE** *www.sane.org.uk*
1st Floor, Cityside House, 40 Adler Street,
London E1 1EE
Tel: 0845 767 8000

FOR COUPLES IN TROUBLE:
**Relate** *www.relate.org.uk*
Herbert Gray College, Little Church Street,
Rugby, Warwickshire CV21 3AP
Tel: 01788 573 241

**The Association for Postnatal Illness**
*www.apni.org.uk*
145 Dawes Road, Fulham,
London SW6 7EB
Tel: 0207 386 0868

**No Panic** *www.no-panic.co.uk*
The National Phobics Society,
339 Stretford Road, Hulme, Manchester
M15 4ZY
Tel: 0808 8080545

FOR SCHIZOPHRENIA:
**Rethink** E-mail: *advice@rethink.org*
30 Tabernacle Street, London EC2A 4DD
Tel: 0208 974 6814

**The Manic Depression Fellowship**
E-mail: *mdf@mdf.org.uk*
21 St Georges Road,
London SE1 6ES
Tel: 0207 793 2600

FOR ACUTE DEPRESSION:
**The Samaritans**
*www.samaritans.org.uk*
E-mail: *jo@samaritans.org*
Tel: 08457 909090

**The Mental Health Foundation**
*www.mhf.org.uk*
7th Floor, 83 Victoria Street,
London SWIH OHW
Tel: 0207 802 0300

The British Medical Association (BMA) also provides direct help in the form of Family Health booklets and advice through general practitioner services.

**British Medical Association**
*www.bma.org.uk*
Tavistock Square,
London WC1H 9JP
Tel: 08459 200169

FOR SCOTLAND:
The Scottish Mental Health Foundation
E-mail: *scotland@mhf.org.uk*
5th Floor, Merchant's House, 30 George
Square, Glasgow G2 1EG
Tel: 0141 572 0125

**The Scottish Association for Mental Health**
E-mail: *www.samh.org.uk*
Cumbrae House, 15 Carlton Crescent,
Glasgow G9 9JP
Tel: 0141 568 7000

work. Try to make these activities more central in your life than ever.

**Releasing of painful memories.** Eye movement desensitization and reprocessing (EMDR) is a new psychotherapy technique used by practitioners to resolve anxiety and depression of all kinds, including the haunting memories of serious abuse and post-traumatic stress disorder. EMDR therapy uses eye movements or tactile stimulation to relieve emotional distress by stimulating certain parts of the brain to signal the release of emotionally "trapped" experiences, then to process it so that memories remain but no longer create the same anxiety and emotional upset as before, explains Dr. Boulware, who is a certified EMDR practitioner.

"Processing even the most difficult memories with EMDR can be achieved in a fraction of the time it would have taken with traditional therapy," she says. Only psychotherapists and other mental health professionals are eligible to receive training in this highly specialized technique. For information on locating a licensed EMDR practitioner, contact The EMDR Association, PO Box 32283, London W5 3YB, UK, or visit its Web site at www.emdr.com.

**Work with your dreams.** Dreaming is a special mode of the brain designed for intense problem solving, says Dr. Zuess. In fact, depressed people tend to spend more time dreaming – it's a self-healing instinct. To make use of dreams, he suggests you reflect on a specific problem before going to sleep.

"There's no such thing as a universal symbol in a dream – your work is to uncover what the unique metaphors and imagery mean to you," says Dr. Aron. "When you awake from a dream, repeat the story back to yourself," she adds. Write down on one side of a piece of paper a word for every detail, and on the other, your associations with it. Try to make a statement incorporating all the details. If that doesn't help you find meaning, continue the story in your imagination based on the details and setting in your dream, Dr. Aron suggests. If you feel overwhelmed by images or feelings, especially those of sadness or anxiety, you should seek the help of a qualified psychotherapist.

**Take an active role in emotional healing.** It's well-established that regular aerobic exercise is as effective as antidepressant drugs in helping you recover from depression. Better yet, researchers in the department of psychiatry and behavioural sciences at Duke University Medical Center in Durham, North Carolina, found that regular exercisers had significantly less chance of relapse than those taking antidepressants.

To maximize the mood-stabilizing benefits of exercise, make fitness playful. If it gives you a real inward chuckle to toss a plastic disk through the air with your friends, for example, add some Frisbee fun to your schedule. To laugh when you sweat gives you an even better chance of lowering cortisol levels and boosting painkilling chemicals, says Dr. Zuess. Doing the chicken dance or the monster mash every morning with your kids is the right idea. If wearing your flamingo socks gives you extra jauntiness at the gym, make sure you wear them.

# CHAPTER 4

# You Don't Have to Feel Tired All the Time

Fatigue is the number-one reason women consult their doctors. Most don't need elaborate tests to figure out why they're tired. Many simply have too much to do and not enough time to do it. Others don't get enough sleep. Some are overweight and get too little exercise. A rare few are underweight or exercise too much.

All those causes can be fixed.

Other women are tired due to chronic stress at home or at work (or both). Still others take medication that keeps them functioning in low gear. Or eating on the run leaves them short on vitamins or minerals essential to high-energy living. Or they've just had a new baby.

If you've ruled out those causes and still feel like you have a permanent case of jet lag, though, the problem could be hormonal – especially if you have other, seemingly unrelated health complaints, such as hair loss, poor memory, constipation and brittle nails. In particular, you may have an underactive or overactive thyroid gland.

Chronic stress, nutritional deficiencies, medications and pregnancy can disrupt hormone levels and lead to fatigue.

"A thyroid condition can be tricky to pin down because many other illnesses cause the same symptoms. But when enough specific cognitive, emotional and physical symptoms come together, they can suggest a thyroid problem," says Paul Ladenson, M.D., professor of medicine, pathology and oncology and director of the division of endocrinology at Johns Hopkins University in Baltimore and board member of the Thyroid Foundation of America.

(continued on page 64)

## WHAT'S GOING ON?

An underactive or overactive thyroid isn't the only possible hormonal explanation for fatigue. This quiz can help you and your doctor rule out (or deal with) other endocrine changes at play.

**1. Did your fatigue start mysteriously and suddenly, after a severe flu-like illness?**
You may have chronic fatigue syndrome. (For details, see page 383.)

**2. Have you recently undergone a major life stress – divorce, loss of a loved one, job change, or financial difficulty?**
A crisis in life can mean a crisis in your adrenal glands, which throw levels of cortisol, adrenaline and dehydroepiandrosterone (DHEA) out of whack. Over time, your thyroid can go haywire in a chain reaction. Follow Phases 1 and 2 of the Hormone-Balancing Programme. (See pages 258 and 275.)

**3. Do you have difficulty getting a good night of sleep?**
Your pineal gland may be neglecting to signal your brain to rest. Dimming the lights and pulling down the shades may help trigger your pineal gland to secrete melatonin later in the evening as you prepare for sleep. But if you snore, you may have sleep apnoea, a disorder linked to an underactive thyroid. (See Snoring on page 443.) Plain old insomnia, on the other hand, could signal an overactive thyroid.

**4. Do you feel tired, anxious and mentally foggy, especially between meals? Does it get significantly better when you eat?**
Thyroid imbalance can cause symptoms similar to those of hypoglycaemia, or low blood sugar – notably, weakness, trembling and mental confusion. Only blood tests can determine if the problem is poorly controlled glucose levels or disruptive thyroid hormones. If you have glucose imbalances or diabetes, you are at higher risk for thyroid disease, so you still need a thyroid test annually. (For more information, see chapter 13.)

**5. Did your moods start to plummet when you first started to feel lethargic? Have you felt blue for more than 2 weeks or lost interest in things you normally enjoy?**
Clinical depression can truly make you feel washed-out and has other symptoms similar to thyroid disease. And if you're being treated for clinical depression now, your medication may be suppressing your thyroid.

**6. Do you have unbearable menstrual cramps and heavy bleeding along with weariness?**

Losing iron via menstrual flow can leave you feeling exhausted. (See chapter 7.) But your gynaecologist will need to rule out endometriosis, uterine cysts and thyroid disease.

**7. If you tire easily, do you also have an irregular period, irritability, weight gain and dry nose? Do you often feel clammy and sweaty?**

If you're in your late forties, you could be entering the menopause. But a sweaty feeling similar to hot flushes could also be a sneaky sign of thyroid dysfunction. A thyroid test can help sort it out.

**8. Do you have no energy for sex, or are you just not in the mood?**

Your oestrogen, progesterone and other sex hormone levels may be fizzling, even if you're premenopausal. Replacing oestrogen can help. (See chapter 11.) But if you have a hidden thyroid condition, which is marked by low sexual desire, taking reproductive hormones can make your thyroid condition worse.

**9. Do you feel run-down and seem to catch a lot more colds and other bugs than everyone around you?**

If your thyroid gland is underactive, your immune system isn't up to par and you're more vulnerable to viral infections. Get a complete physical and a thyroid test.

**10. Are you being treated for hypothyroidism or hyperthyroidism but still feel tired all the time?**

Get your levels retested. In your first year of treatment, you should be retested approximately every 1 to 2 months until your levels stabilize. After that, you still need to be retested at least once a year. If your levels are in range but you still feel like you're going through life in low gear, ask your doctor to try $T_3/T_4$ combination therapy.

If you're often exhausted and have other mysterious health complaints, you owe it to yourself to get checked out for an underlying thyroid imbalance or other medical causes. After diet and genetics, thyroid disease is the most common contributing cause of high cholesterol. Left untreated, it can increase your risk of heart attack, stroke, osteoporosis, cancer and depression. Yet more than half the people with thyroid disease – most of them women – have never been diagnosed.

Preventing stroke and heart disease is a stellar reason to be tested and treated for even mild forms of hypothyroidism, says Raphael Kellman, M.D., founder and director of the Kellman Center for Progressive Medicine in New

# Is Your Thyroid Underactive – Or Overactive?

Many people swing between *hypothyroidism* and the less common *hyperthyroidism* within the first 6 weeks of treatment. If that happens, your doctor will need to adjust your medication. (Some symptoms, like mood swings, occur in both states.) This checklist can help you listen to body changes that call for an adjustment.

"Report any lingering or new symptoms to your doctor so you can get your dosage adjusted or rule out another medical condition," says Sheldon Rubenfeld, M.D., clinical professor of endocrinology at Baylor College of Medicine in Houston, founding chairman of the Thyroid Society for Education and Research, and author of *Could It Be My Thyroid?*

**HYPOTHYROIDISM**
- Difficulty getting up in the morning, needing to sleep longer
- General drowsiness
- Sensitivity to cold
- Slow reflexes
- Depression
- Apathy; loss of enthusiasm
- Mood swings
- Difficulty concentrating
- Impaired memory
- Sluggish thinking ("brain fog")
- Headaches
- Loss of interest in sex
- Dry skin; dry eyes
- Brittle hair and nails
- Prematurely grey hair or hair loss
- Hearing loss
- Visual disturbances or hallucinations
- Extreme menstrual pain; heavy bleeding
- Milky discharge from breasts
- Constipation

York City and author of *Eat with Your Brain, Think with Your Gut.*

This crash course on your thyroid gland and how it works will help you collaborate with your doctor to sort things out, restore your energy and protect your health.

## Your Metabolic Motor

Your thyroid is a butterfly-shaped gland in your neck that affects every cell in the body by producing hormones used for metabolism, growth, nerves, muscles and circulation. Essentially the thyroid tells the body how fast to work and use energy.

- Slow heart rate
- Abnormally low or elevated blood pressure
- High blood cholesterol
- Shortness of breath
- Goitre (swelling) or nodules in throat
- Hoarseness; sore throat
- Diminished appetite
- Unexplained weight gain
- Sensitivity to sugar
- Muscle and joint pain
- Increased infections
- Raynaud's phenomenon, carpal tunnel syndrome and other nerve conditions

**HYPERTHYROIDISM**

- Protruding eyes
- Insomnia
- Exhaustion following hyperactivity
- Sensitivity to heat; sweating
- Jitters; hand tremors
- Anxiety; mania

- Apathy; loss of enthusiasm
- Mood swings
- Difficulty concentrating
- Impaired memory
- Racing thoughts, sometimes irrational
- Increase or decrease in sex drive
- Puffy face, especially under eyes
- Visual disturbances or hallucinations
- Fewer or lighter menstrual periods
- Diarrhoea; increased bowel movements
- Racing pulse; heart palpitations
- Elevated blood pressure
- Osteoporosis
- Shortness of breath
- Goitre (swelling) or nodules in throat
- Insatiable hunger
- Unexplained weight loss
- Muscle and joint pain

Certain autoimmune diseases can attack this "metabolic motor", causing myriad complaints, along with fatigue. In a case of mistaken identity, your immune system sends out antibodies – the fighter proteins usually reserved for clobbering viruses and other threats – to sabotage healthy tissues.

In Hashimoto's disease, the leading cause of hypothyroidism (underactive thyroid), an "antithyroid" antibody preys on your thyroid gland. In its weakened state, the thyroid cannot produce enough thyroid hormones. In Graves' disease, the leading cause of hyperthyroidism (overactive thyroid), other antibodies force your thyroid gland into overdrive.

Science has few definitive explanations as to why autoimmune attacks occur, but they seem to be genetic.

Even if your thyroid gland is healthy, problems with one of the many biological processes needed to keep your hormone levels stable can cause trouble.

The main hormone secreted by the thyroid gland is thyroxine (known as $T_4$). It is essentially a prehormone, bound to protein, and remains in storage until acted upon by enzymes and converted to the active hormone, triiodothyronine (known as $T_3$). To work up to par, each organ needs precisely the right amount of $T_3$ at a perfectly controlled rate.

Even if your gland makes enough $T_4$, certain medications, nutritional deficiencies, stress, smoking, other illnesses and even imbalances of other hormones (such as oestrogen) can stunt the conversion of $T_4$ to $T_3$ and deprive your organs of this much-needed thyroid hormone.

"When that happens, you feel like you're walking around in low gear all the time," says Dr. Kellman. What's more, everything from your gastrointestinal system to your reproductive system will work poorly, which will wear on your energy level, your concentration and your mood. "Even mild hypothyroidism will create subtle deficiencies that lead to a self-perpetuating fatigue," says Dr. Kellman.

You might also feel remarkably tired from too *much* thyroid hormone, or hyperthyroidism. But it's a different kind of fatigue. Instead of your feeling understimulated and sleepy, your metabolism is so revved up that you end up with symptoms like insomnia and anxiety and feel hot and sweaty, all of which often add up to feeling drained, says Dr. Ladenson.

## Should You Ask for a Thyroid Test?

You can't tell for sure if you have a thyroid problem without a doctor's help. But these questions can help determine if you should get your thyroid checked.

*Have you or anyone in your family ever been diagnosed with*

*Hashimoto's or Graves' disease or other autoimmune diseases, such as pernicious anaemia, vitiligo, diabetes mellitus, systemic lupus, rheumatoid arthritis, Addison's disease, or premature menopause?* If so, experts say you should have your thyroid levels checked annually.

*Are you pregnant or planning to become pregnant, or have you recently given birth?* "Fertility is profoundly affected by thyroid hormone levels," says Ken Blanchard, M.D., Ph.D., an endocrinologist in Newton Lower Falls, Massachusetts. And after pregnancy, women may be diagnosed with postnatal thyroiditis – an inflammation of the thyroid gland in the postnatal period. These women tend to cycle between hypothyroidism and hyperthyroidism, says Dr. Blanchard. So you need to be carefully screened prior to conception and during pregnancy, and also in the postnatal period.

*Are you 50 or older and postmenopausal?* One out of five post-menopausal women has thyroid disease. So experts recommend that all women be screened annually once they reach 50.

*Do you have high LDL blood cholesterol, high triglyceride levels, or both?* "If an underactive thyroid is the cause of your elevated LDL and triglycerides, taking thyroid replacement could reverse or lessen the problem," says Dr. Ladenson.

*Are you taking amiodarone (Cordarone), carbamazepine (Tegretol), cholestyramine, colestipol (Colestid), lithium (Camcolit, Liskonum, Priadel or Li-Liquid), phenytoin (Epanutin), rifampicin (Rifadin), steroids, a sustained serotonin reuptake inhibitor (SSRI), an antidepressant such as Prozac, or sucralfate (Antepsin)?* Any of these medications can induce abnormal thyroid levels. For example, hypothyroidism occurs in half of those taking lithium (Priadel), a drug for bipolar disorder. You may need to increase your thyroid replacement or have an alternative prescribed.

*Do you smoke?* Cigarettes contain chemical compounds that can impair thyroid hormones, and smoking may contribute to autoimmune attacks on the thyroid. Research shows that smokers have a much higher rate of Graves' disease than nonsmokers.

## Which Test Do You Need?

Your doctor has not one but five tests available to help determine if you have a thyroid problem and, if so, what kind.

**TSH.** This clever test takes advantage of the body's wisdom to send out thyroid-stimulating hormone (TSH), chemical messages from the pituitary gland telling the thyroid gland to produce more or less hormone, depending on your needs. Therefore, if your thyroid hormone levels are lower than normal, your TSH will be higher than normal in an attempt to stimulate your thyroid. If the pituitary senses an overload of thyroid hormone, it sends less TSH to the thyroid gland in an attempt to turn down the heat, so to speak.

Criteria vary, but generally a TSH higher than 5 mIU/ml (milli international units per millilitre) usually indicates hypothyroidism, and a TSH below 0.1 indicates hyperthyroidism.

**Free T$_4$ and T$_3$.** To fine-tune your diagnosis and treatment, your doctor may need to measure the actual amount of the thyroid hormone in your blood that is available to your tissues and cells to use. As you might expect, a below normal level of these thyroid hormones confirms an underactive thyroid and a higher-than-normal level indicates hyperthyroidism. Your doctor will tailor thyroid replacement drugs depending on how far your hormone levels stray from the optimal range. Comparing this test to the TSH will also reveal if you may have a rare form of thyroid dysfunction caused by your pituitary gland.

"Make sure you have *free* levels of T$_4$ and T$_3$ measured – what your tissues and cells are actually using – not the outdated serum T$_4$ test, T$_3$ uptake, total T$_4$, or total T$_3$, which only shows the level of hormones bound together with protein in the blood for storage," says John Vlok Dommisse, M.D., a physician who specializes in nutritional and metabolic medicine in Tucson.

**TRH.** Testing for thyrotropin-releasing hormone (TRH) is not standard practice, but may be asked for by a specialist. If your TSH is near the higher end of normal – say, from 1.5 to 5 – indicating mild hypothyroidism, this test can back up the decision to treat the problem.

Unlike the other 5-minutes-or-less blood tests, the TRH takes up to a half an hour, and is a relatively expensive test to run. "It's well worth the effort," says Dr. Kellman. "I've seen the lives of hundreds of people turned around just because this one test finally got them the treatment they needed after years of unresolved fatigue and other mysterious complaints."

**Antibody screening.** This is optional and will confirm if Hashimoto's or Graves' disease has caused your thyroid dysfunction.

Your doctor will also check for lumps in your neck. In Graves' disease or Hashimoto's disease, your thyroid sometimes swells in reaction to the autoimmune assaults; it looks like an overgrowth in your neck and is called a goitre. In some cases, a small growth called a nodule may appear on the thyroid gland. Goitres and nodules usually disappear during treatment for underactive or overactive thyroid. If they don't, they may be due to another cause and will be surgically removed.

## If Your Thyroid Is Overactive

Temporary or mild hyperthyroidism can be controlled with antithyroid medication, to suppress overactivity. If you have a related condition, such as eye disease, your doctor may suggest surgery to relieve the eye inflammation. For atrial fibrillation (irregular heartbeat), your doctor may prescribe a blood thinner, like warfarin, to help prevent strokes and blood clots. If you have advanced Graves' disease, you can take a radioactive iodine solution or have surgery to disable the gland. Either way, you would then need to take thyroid replacement medication for the rest of your life, just as with treatment for hypothyroidism.

## If Your Thyroid Is Underactive

The conventional drug for hypothyroidism is levothyroxine (Thyroxine), the synthetic version of thyroxine hormone ($T_4$) produced by your thyroid.

As an alternative or complement to levothyroxine, some doctors prescribe triiodothyronine ($T_3$), available in synthetic (such as Tertroxin) or natural form (such as Armour in the US). Doctors who use $T_3$ believe that when only $T_4$ is used, too many things can prevent the medication's saturation of cells at the deepest level. "After all, $T_3$ is responsible for 90 per cent of thyroid action in the body," explains Dr. Dommisse.

## Work with Your Doctor

If you're like many women who are accurately diagnosed with a thyroid condition, taking a pill may be all that's needed to feel better than you have in years.

"It sounds too good to be true, but it's simply a matter of entering a productive partnership with a caring, capable doctor, getting on the right medication at the right dose, and monitoring your progress," says Dr. Blanchard. Some pointers:

**Ask for your records.** "There's no reason why you shouldn't ask your doctor for personal copies of all screenings," says Mary Shomon, author of *Living Well with Hypothyroidism: What Your Doctor Doesn't Tell You . . . That You Need to Know*. Then, if you switch doctors, rather than waiting for reports from other doctor's offices, your practitioner can quickly see your history and make the most well-informed and efficient decisions. You'll also be able to keep track of any changes in your condition and identify what works best for you. "Follow what's going on, so you can ask the right questions and discuss options with your doctor," says Shomon.

**If you hate needles, you could ask for a saliva test.** Regularly getting

*Escape from* **HORMONE HELL**

# SHE'S RIGHT – THE TEST IS WRONG

**Q:** When I read an article in a women's magazine about how hypothyroidism makes you feel overwhelmingly tired, the symptoms sounded just like me. I always felt worn down and moody around my menstrual period. But now a "fog" seems to haunt me 7 days a week, all month long. Not only do I feel physically drained, but my brain is sluggish, too – I can't remember names or stay focused in meetings. I'm cold all the time, and my husband is tired of seeing me come to bed in flannel pajamas and socks. And with the 10 pounds I've put on over the past winter, the last thing I'm interested in is lovemaking.

Even though I follow a low-fat diet, my total cholesterol has shot up to more than 200 over the past year. When I finally convinced my family doctor to perform a TSH test to evaluate my thyroid, he said my levels were normal. He just told me to wear more sweaters and get more sleep!

If I don't find an answer soon, I'm going to lose my job, my husband – and my mind. Help!

Raphael Kellman, M.D., founder and director of the Kellman Center for Progressive Medicine in New York City, and author of *Eat with Your Brain, Think with Your Gut*, replies: you're caught in what some alternative health doctors call "the tyranny of the TSH test". The results may be normal compared to other people. But they're abnormal for *you*.

Your symptoms are much more revealing than an isolated lab report and point to an underactive thyroid, or hypothyroidism. Provided other illnesses have been ruled out, a low dose of thyroid replacement medicine could give you relief.

I'd also recommend steps to help your body heal itself. You should be checked for nutritional imbalances and digestive function. I recommend you phase out from your diet refined carbohydrates, such as white bread, pasta and pastries. Because the adrenal glands affect the thyroid, your adrenal function should be tested. A supplement of DHEA, taken temporarily, could also help.

It sounds as though you could also do with some help managing stress and depression. So I'd advise seeing a psychotherapist and an acupuncturist. Taking care of deeper spiritual and emotional issues will support your recovery by taking additional stress off your body.

With proper treatment, you won't need those "extra blankets" any longer.

your hormone levels checked is a reality of living with thyroid disease. That's a lot of needle pricks. More and more American doctors use saliva tests, which are painless, convenient and – some say – more accurate (though, as with blood tests, cost and quality vary from lab to lab), although they are rarely done in the UK. Basically, you spit into a tube and send it off to a lab. "I find it faster, cheaper and more sensitive," says Joseph Mercola, D.O., medical director of the Optimal Wellness Center in Schaumburg, Illinois.

**If you're not getting better, see a specialist.** Your family doctor is qualified to treat basic thyroid disease. If your practitioner takes you seriously and uses current treatment options, you're in good hands. But if you have a unique problem or aren't getting any better, don't feel obliged to stay with the doctor who first diagnosed you. Ask to see an endocrinologist, who has more specialized training in hormonal conditions. Some focus specifically on thyroid conditions. (To find one, see "On the Web & Other Resources" on page 77.)

**Consider the combination therapy.** If you don't feel up to par after you've been treated with $T_4$, your thyroid tests have come back normal, and your doctor has ruled out other illness, you can still get your groove back. Adjusting the amount of $T_4$ you take and adding $T_3$, the more active form of the two thyroid hormones, may help. "Combining the two thyroid hormones is the most cutting-edge treatment available for hypothyroidism," says Dr. Dommisse.

Researchers examined the physical, emotional and mental performance of 33 men and women with hypothyroidism. The researchers gave the patients their regular replacement, containing $T_4$, for 5 weeks, then measured how the same people felt on 5 weeks of $T_3/T_4$ combination replacement. Twenty people preferred the combination therapy – they were more energetic, were better able to concentrate and felt better overall.

"People who take $T_4$ alone might not even know that they are only operating at a 50 to 75 per cent state of wellness, while on the $T_3/T_4$ combination therapy, they shoot up to 90 or 100 per cent," says Dr. Blanchard. "The difference is amazing."

**Take your pills every day, ideally at the same time.** "In order for hundreds of bodily functions to work up to par, your body relies on a stable level of thyroid hormone in your bloodstream," says Dr. Kellman. So, to prevent energy and mood changes, avoid missing a dose, especially if you are taking $T_3$. And be careful not to take a double dose by accident since too much of the hormone can cause stress on your heart and, if done habitually, could lead to osteoporosis. To ensure regular dosages, use a pillbox with a section for every day of the week. If you take more than one pill a day, use a container with morning and evening sections.

**Take your thyroid pills 1 hour after or 2 hours before other pills.** Certain foods and nutritional supplements interfere with your body's absorption of thyroid replacement. When researchers at UCLA School of Medicine gave calcium for 3 months to 20 people with hypothyroidism who took thyroxine (the most common thyroid replacement drug), more than half had significantly reduced hormone levels. When they stopped taking calcium, their thyroid levels returned to normal. "By all means, continue taking your calcium, but don't take it less than 1 hour after or 2 hours before your thyroid replacement," says Sheldon Rubenfeld, M.D., clinical professor of

---

### THE HORMONE CONNECTION
# A HEALTHY THYROID MEANS SMARTER BABIES

When it comes to having a whizz-kid for a son or daughter, good genes and the right schools will only get you so far. Research suggests you also need good hormones.

Before you start reading Shakespeare to the budding genius in your womb, ask for a thyroid test. when researchers in Scarborough, Maine, compared the IQs of children of mums with normal thyroid function to children born to mothers with untreated hypothyroidism, children in the second group scored an average of 7 points lower.

In fact, 7-to 9-year old participants who were born to untreated hypothyroid mums scored lower on all 15 of the tests evaluating attention, language, visual motor performance, reading, and school problems. What's more, the children of mothers getting proper treatment for hypothyroidism were just as intelligent as those with mums with normal thyroid status.

We have known for years that hypothyroidism during pregnancy can cause birth defects like cretinism and mental retardation, but this new research shows that even mild hypothyroidism could result in slight cognitive disadvantages, comments Ken Blanchard, M.D., Ph.D., an endocrinologist in Newton Lower Falls, Massachusetts, who specialises in treating hypothyroidism.

if you have hypothyroidism, you'll need as much as 50 per cent more thyroid hormone replacement medicine during pregnancy. Don't double up on your own. Do make sure your dosage is adjusted as needed.

endocrinology at Baylor College of Medicine in Houston, founding chairman of the Thyroid Society for Education and Research, and author of *Could It Be My Thyroid?*

Iron supplements and dietary fibre also can block absorption of thyroid replacement medication. So make it a general practice to take *any* food 2 hours before or 1 hour after your thyroid dose, says Dr. Rubenfeld.

**Tell your doctor if you're considering birth control pills or HRT containing oestrogen.** If you have hypothyroidism, taking oestrogen may increase your thyroid replacement requirements. Get a baseline of your thyroid levels just before you start birth control or hormone replacement therapy (HRT), and then get another test 2 months later. Don't be surprised if your doctor ups your thyroid dose.

**Get yearly checkups.** You can't expect to simply call your doctor and get thyroid refills over the phone indefinitely. Your hormone requirements will probably change over time. In addition to changes in the thyroid gland itself, pregnancy, stress, other medication and even ageing can affect how much thyroid medication you need – more or less. Don't let more than a year slip between surgery visits, even if you're feeling fine. And see your doctor right away if you have symptoms – with a 2-month follow-up whenever your dosage changes. To stay on track, set up the following year's appointment at each checkup.

## Your Personal Hormone-Balancing Programme

If your thyroid is low but still functioning, some simple lifestyle changes may enable you to reduce or phase out pills altogether, with your doctor's supervision. Even if you have to take replacement permanently, these additional steps can lower your risks for other autoimmune diseases and avoid complications of thyroid deficiency.

**Buy reverse osmosis water.** "I think heavy metal toxicity is one of the reasons why there is such an upsurge of hypothyroidism," says Dr. Dommisse. "Tap water and even spring water are often a source of high copper levels, which can compound the hypothyroid symptoms of fatigue and dull memory," he explains. "Reverse osmosis removes unhealthful heavy metals from water without removing beneficial minerals like magnesium and potassium." You can buy a reverse osmosis water system from most speciality water system suppliers. At a pinch, go for distilled water – all the minerals have been removed, but at least the potential toxins, too, are gone.

**Switch to nonfluoride toothpaste, avoid fluoride dental procedures and steer clear of unfiltered tap water.** Reams of research written over the past 80 years document fluoride's dubious affects on the thyroid. "Proper iodine levels are essential to manufacture the right amount of thyroid hormones, and we know that fluoride impairs iodine levels. In fact, fluoride has been included in antithyroid medication deliberately to suppress an overactive

---

### THE HORMONE ZONE
# REGULATE YOUR THYROID WITH FOOD

For years, people with goitre were warned against eating cabbage, kale, nuts and other foods high in "goitrogens", plant substances that interfere with the manufacture of thyroid hormones. And they were encouraged to use iodized salt. Now experts know that the links between diet and thyroid balance aren't so simple.

"Since vegetables are the foundation of any healing diet – including one to restore thyroid balance – you don't want to avoid these foods completely," says Carol Roberts, M.D., the founder and medical director of Wellness Works in Brandon, Florida, and the editor of the American Holistic Medical Association's newsletter. "Just don't eat huge quantities. Also, cooking might neutralize goitrogens," she says.

Soya is also a goitrogen. In addition, because it acts like oestrogen in the body, in excess it can disrupt hormone balance and interfere with your absorption of thyroid pills.

Yet soya has documented benefits – it helps to keep your cholesterol down and maintain strong bones, both key concerns of women with thyroid dysfunction. So, again, the key is moderation.

As for iodine, your body needs this mineral to process thyroid into its active state for tissues and organs to use. Excess iodine, however, will overwhelm the thyroid and either push it into the hyperactive state or burn it out completely, says Sheldon Rubenfeld, M.D., clinical professor of endocrinology at Baylor College of Medicine in Houston, founding chairman of the Thyroid Society for Education and Research, and author of *Could It Be My Thyroid?* "So there's no need to go out of your way to buy iodine-enriching products like algae and kelp," he adds. "Everyone gets plenty of iodine from iodized salt, seafood and baked goods we routinely consume," says Ken Blanchard, M.D., Ph.D., an endocrinologist in Newton Lower Falls, Massachusetts.

The key for staying in "the zone" for thyroid balance is a diverse variety of vegetables and protein, moderate intake of whole grains, with fewer refined and processed foods.

thyroid," explains Dr. Mercola.

**Ask for mercury-free fillings.** We can't always avoid inhaling or digesting random heavy metals in the environment, but why deliberately place a potential toxin just inches from your thyroid gland? "I've found that one of

### FOODS TO ADD

- Cooked soya food products, but no more than three servings a week
- Wheat germ, brewer's yeast, Brazil nuts and other foods high in selenium, a trace mineral integral to the enzyme that converts thyroxine ($T_4$) to its active form ($T_3$)
- Dark green leafy vegetables and colourful produce (supply antioxidant vitamins and minerals needed for thyroid health)
- Olive and other vegetable oils (for the monounsaturated fats your thyroid needs to function properly)
- Deep-sea fish, such as mackerel, shark, halibut, tuna, herring, sardines and cod (contain essential fatty acids and some iodine)
- Spices like basil, ginger, cumin and coriander (help digestion)
- Onions and garlic (may improve impaired immunity and help lower cholesterol related to thyroid function)
- Up to 1 milligram of iodized salt (get at least 150 micrograms of iodine a day)

### FOODS TO SUBTRACT

- Excessive amounts of goitrogenic foods: soya, kale, turnips, cabbage, peanuts, pine nuts, radishes, mustard and peaches
- Foods high in saturated fats (your body is less efficient at burning fat when your thyroid is underactive)
- Fried foods (free radicals created in frying can inhibit impaired metabolism)
- Sugary foods, white-flour baked goods, cereals and potatoes (blood sugar fluctuations they trigger can lower energy, concentration and mood)
- Caffeine (too much can contribute to anxiety and irregular heart rate which are associated with thyroid dysfunction)
- The herb thyme in excessive amounts (may reduce thyroid activity); only small amounts of thyme should be used, as seasoning
- High-iodine foods (kelp, seaweed, algae, salt); limit to 500 micrograms of iodine a day

the more common causes of hypothyroidism is mercury toxicity from silver fillings," says Dr. Mercola, who has treated more than 2000 people with thyroid dysfunction. It can be expensive to get mercury fillings removed, so your best bet is to avoid them in the first place by asking your dentist for a synthetic composite alternative when you have a cavity. If you do have a mouthful of metal and are concerned, ask your doctor to test you for mercury toxicity, says Dr. Mercola.

**Go organic.** "One theory says that autoimmune disorders like Hashimoto's or Graves' disease represent an attack on the body by a dysfunctional immune system deranged by toxins," says Carol Roberts, M.D., the founder and medical director of Wellness Works in Brandon, Florida, and the editor of the American Holistic Medical Association's newsletter. "If so, a diet based on organic produce accompanied by organic and free-range meat is better than food raised on chemical fertilizers, pesticides, herbicides – not to mention animals injected with growth hormones that can confuse your already malfunctioning endocrine system."

## Make Time for Yourself

"One common trait I've seen among women I've treated for hypothyroidism is that they think they exist to make other people happy," says Dr. Roberts. "I haven't decided whether this is the *result* of being hypothyroid or if it's the *cause*, but these women are so caught up with other people's needs that they are out of touch with their own higher mission in life – they don't even remember they have one." If this sounds like you, take these steps to regain your identity.

**Meditate every morning.** Build a door of potential in your mind, says Dr. Roberts. Stand in front of it, and then open it and greet what's on the other side. You may soon find, when you really listen to yourself, that it's time for a career change or that you have to start saying no more often, she says.

**Cultivate creativity.** "I find that in women with hypothyroidism, more than their thyroid hormones are suppressed – they are usually holding back their creative force and are stuck thinking too much with the left side of their brains," says Dr. Roberts. "Whether you are looking at it from a spiritual perspective or as a way to de-stress your adrenal gland, restoring your intrinsically joyful, artistic nature is necessary to fully recover from thyroid dysfunction."

"Try new things, indulge in silly, simple fun, and be a little more adventuresome," says Dr. Roberts. Experiment with whatever helps you step out of constrained mode, and rediscover yourself. Wear a new colour, paint your house, sample new foods. Take a course in something you always wanted to explore or in something completely off-the-wall to which you feel drawn, says Dr. Roberts. "Through this self-discovery process, it's imperative to give yourself permission to make mistakes," she adds.

**Take up yoga.** "Yoga in general will foster the self-growth and deep physical restoration necessary for a full recovery, but the poses that increase bloodflow to your neck specifically tone your thyroid gland," says Kathleen H. Fry, M.D., an holistic physician and gynaecologist in Scottsdale, Arizona, and the president of the American Holistic Medical Association.

"I encourage women to develop a daily yoga practice with a certified yoga instructor, but they can start reaping benefits immediately by practising the 'cat' and 'cow' postures on their own," she says.

*The cat:* Begin by balancing evenly on all fours, with your hands placed

## ON THE WEB & Other Resources

To learn more about the latest tests and treatment for underactive or overactive thyroid glands, contact:

**The Thyroid Society for Education and Research**
7515 South Main Street
Suite 545
Houston, TX 77030
(800) THYROID (849-7643)
*www.the-thyroid-society.org*
*help@the-thyroid-society.org*

**The British Thyroid Foundation**
PO Box 97, Clifford, Wetherby, West Yorkshire LS23 6XD
Tel: 0808 808 3555

FOR FAMILY HEALTH BOOKLETS:
**British Medical Association**
*www.bma.org.uk*
Tel: 08459 200 169
Tavistock Square,
London WC1H 9JP

FOR INFORMATION ON THYROID EYE DISEASE:
**Brenda Johnstone**
E-mail: *tedassn@eclipse.co.uk*
Tel: 01797 222338
*www.rnib.org.uk/info/thyroid.htm*
Thyroid Eye Disease, Solstice, Sea Road, Winchelsea Beach, East Sussex, TN36 4LH

OTHER SOURCES
**NHS Direct Helpline**
Tel: 0845 4647

*How to Cope Successfully With Thyroid Problems*
Dr Tom Smith
Published by Wellhouse, 2001

For further reassurance and information contact your GP.

directly under your shoulders and your hips directly over your knees. Slowly exhale and pull your abdomen up into your body by tucking in your chin towards your sternum and curling your tailbone in towards your torso. Exhale completely. *The cow:* Inhale as you slowly sway your back and raise your chin toward the ceiling.

Alternate between the cat and cow for 1 minute at your own, steady pace.

**Enlist a partner in motion.** Aerobic activity is the key to fully taking charge of your health again. Whether it's walking your dog around the block or walking your kid to the bus, get some form of exercise, preferably with someone who will encourage you to do it every day, says Dr. Roberts.

The increased bloodflow and oxygen surging through your system will enliven you with the mental alertness, more sustained energy and higher-quality sleep that your system has been craving for so long.

Other suggestions: sign up for a kayaking course with a friend, or schedule a dancing date with your husband every Friday night. Mix up your daily workout with everything from walking, swimming and biking to exuberant housecleaning and ambitious leaf raking.

Work your way up to hitting a sustained, increased heart rate for 30 to 60 minutes, 4 to 6 days a week, accompanied by warmup and cooldown stretches.

"If you are new to aerobic activity, remember that it gets easier after the first 6 weeks. Lean on your partner to get you through that time, and you'll probably come back for more," Dr. Roberts says.

**Get to bed by 10 p.m.** Because a thyroid disorder can make you feel sluggish all over, it's more important than ever to get the highest quality sleep possible. Aim for a full 8 hours, but more important, turn in around 10 o'clock at night, when your body's "regeneration-repair phase" kicks in.

Prime sleep time is well before midnight. "I believe that every minute of sleep before midnight is equal to 10 minutes afterwards," says Dr. Mercola.

"There's a reason why secretions of melatonin (your 'drowsy' hormone) are released around 8 or 9 p.m. – your body's inner wisdom is signalling that it's time to start getting ready for bed," adds Nancy Lonsdorf, M.D., an Ayurvedic medicine specialist.

"Lots of fatigued people get marvellous improvements if all they do is turn in by 10 o'clock. Your quality of life is too high a price to pay for catching the 11 o'clock news," says Dr. Mercola.

Equally important for reducing sluggishness is to get up by 6 a.m., says Dr. Lonsdorf. This increases alertness and energy during the day and helps avoid that "hungover" feeling that begs for a morning cup of coffee, she adds.

# CHAPTER 5

# Remember Everything Better

**W**hy is it that sometimes we can deliver a well-prepared presentation flawlessly, without any hesitation, and at other times our minds go completely blank when we are just searching for a simple word for an everyday object?

Even more puzzling: why can your teenager recall the lyrics to every CD ever recorded but can't remember that you told her 15 minutes ago to clean up her room?

Like fertility, blood sugar and moods, memory, too, is flexible and ever-changing, often in response to hormones.

"I was taught to think of memory like it was a fixed thing, like IQ," says John W. Newcomer, M.D., associate professor of psychiatry at Washington University School of Medicine in St. Louis. "Now we understand that memory function can vary in response to changing hormone levels", he adds.

Some women notice memory lapses at midlife, especially at the menopause, says John C. Morris, M.D., Friedman professor of neurology at Washington University School of Medicine in St. Louis. Forgetting conversations, names of people you know, or even where you put your car keys often causes women to worry that they may be starting to develop Alzheimer's disease.

However, these memory lapses may result simply from "information overload" rather than the beginnings of Alzheimer's, says Dr. Morris. Or they may be the result of hormonal fluctuations caused by perimenopause, menopause, or even stress.

## WHAT'S GOING ON?

Is your forgetfulness related to hormones – or something else? This quick quiz can help you determine if oestrogen, insulin, or stress hormones are affecting your memory.

**1. Have you been temporarily "blanking" on information you've known by heart for years, such as your phone number or the town where your dearest friend lives? Same goes with remembering information you've just read moments ago.**
If you're in your forties or fifties, or if you've had a hysterectomy and aren't taking hormone replacement therapy (HRT), you may be feeling the subtle effects of oestrogen decline. Oestrogen not only helps the brain create new connections; it may also protect old ones. When our oestrogen levels fluctuate, as they do in midlife, it briefly may affect our long-term memory.

**2. Have you started to fumble when you play sports like tennis or work with garden tools around the house? Do you goof up doing everyday things like making coffee in the morning or using the fax machine at work?**
Oestrogen not only influences and protects our cognitive abilities; it's also involved in motor skills, which means we may notice changes in our physical abilities when levels vary.

**3. Do your mind and mouth seem to be "on different pages" lately as you find yourself saying one word when you were thinking of something entirely different?**
Oestrogen is particularly important for verbal memory, which is often affected as we approach and go through the menopause.

**4. Have you felt like you're becoming absentminded, forgetting things you've just done?**
When we're distracted and forgetful, oestrogen deficiency may be to blame: this hormone activates neurotransmitters that help us focus and remember what we're doing.

**5. Are you currently taking hormone replacement therapy that includes oestrogen?**
If you're experiencing troubling memory problems while taking HRT, talk to your doctor. It may be a sign you need your prescription adjusted.

**6. Are you diabetic? Does diabetes run in your family?**
Insulin resistance – a hormonal disruption in glucose regulation – can interfere
with memory in various, complex ways. With too little glucose, memory suffers.
Controlling blood sugar may improve memory.

**7. Have you recently had surgery?**
The physical and emotional stress of an operation boosts levels of cortisol, a
stress hormone that at high amounts may temporarily interfere with memory,
although animal research suggests women may not be as affected by stress as
men.

**8. Are you having trouble with tasks that involve planning and organization, such as
packing for a trip?**
The normal memory changes that come with age and hormone fluctuations
generally don't affect our ability to make "executive decisions" that require
drawing on information from multiple sources (such as weather reports, scheduled
activities and the clothes in our wardrobe to pack for a weekend in the country) to
complete. This could be a sign of depression or other mental disorders.

**9. Do your memory problems come and go?**
Unlike Alzheimer's, which is a progressive disease, hormonal memory problems at
midlife happen irregularly and unexpectedly.

**10. Are memory problems preventing you from living your life?**
Upsetting as they are, hormone-related memory failures tend to be brief, as we
sooner or later remember the name, face, or task we were trying to recall. If
memory problems are affecting multiple aspects of your life in major ways,
preventing you from doing your hobbies or your job, however, talk to your doctor to
identify other, non-hormonal causes.

# Making Memories

Creating a memory – whether it's a mental snapshot of your daughter's wedding or how to bake chocolate cake from scratch – is an amazing and complicated process involving multiple regions and chemicals in the brain. Like the footsteps of a child in search of a lost mitten, the path to remembering crisscrosses all over our brain, stopping here, resting there, until a memory is made.

It begins in an area of the brain known as the prefrontal cortex, the outer layer of our brain, located near our forehead. When we're in the middle of creating a short-term memory – a new neighbour's name, a grocery list, deciding on a computer password – life gets very busy for the prefrontal cortex. It bustles with energy, gathering the data we need from the immediate moment (such as the pronunciation of a name), adding it to stored information and putting it in context.

To store information for the long haul, the experience must travel to the hippocampus, where it's consolidated in a process called long-term potentiation. The hippocampus is a seahorse-shaped structure located in between the temple areas (above the ears), deep in the middle of the brain. It plays a critical role in forming new memories.

But all memories aren't created equal, explains James L. McGaugh, Ph.D., director of the Center for the Neurobiology of Learning and Memory at the University of California, Irvine. While some experiences remain fuzzy, you may remember other moments with photographic and emotional clarity – the birth of your first child, for example, your husband's marriage proposal, or your son's graduation. That's because emotionally exciting events cause the release of hormones such as cortisol and norepinephrine. Those in turn activate a brain structure known as the amygdala, which causes changes in the hippocampus, creating a sharp and intense memory.

Other hormones and neurotransmitters, too, support memory, by regulating our sleep (through melatonin) or boosting our mood (with serotonin) so we can learn and retain information.

# Oestrogen: The Memory Defender

The female hormone oestrogen helps women's hearts and bones. But it's also essential for our brains in various ways.

**Oestrogen develops the brain.** This female hormone spurs the growth of glial cells, which act as "nursemaid" intermediaries between our blood

*Escape from* **HORMONE HELL**

# FORGETFULNESS HAS HER WORRIED ABOUT ALZHEIMER'S

**Q:** I've always had a sharp memory. Phone numbers, presentations, fascinating facts – I remembered them all. But now that I've hit the menopause, I often forget where I put things. Sometimes I go blank on names. Or I make stupid mistakes. Is forgetfulness going to get even worse as I get older? I'm really worried that I'm getting Alzheimer's disease. Isn't that incurable? What can I do to keep my mind clear?

John W. Newcomer, M.D., associate professor of psychiatry at Washington University School of Medicine in St. Louis, replies: there's much more to Alzheimer's than occasional forgetfulness. It involves a steady, progressive mental decline with personality changes and other cognitive problems. In contrast, some women experience a decline in memory function as a result of the oestrogen decline associated with the menopause. The brain is a target for many hormones, including oestrogen and one of the brain functions exquisitely regulated by hormones is memory.

Taking oestrogen may help boost your memory. Canadian studies have found changes in cognitive functioning in younger women across their menstrual cycles. Among postmenopausal women, such as you, those on oestrogen have performed better on memory tests than women who weren't on oestrogen. That improvement can make a real difference in recall.

Bear in mind, though, that oestrogen acts not just on the brain but all over the body. So if you're considering oestrogen replacement, your doctor may advise against taking oestrogen if your mother had breast cancer that was oestrogen receptor positive, which would increase your breast cancer risk.

If memory problems are your only concern, think about what's happening in your life. If you're under a lot of stress – someone close to you has died or you've recently had an operation – your levels of cortisol, a powerful stress hormone which also affects memory, could be high. So before considering oestrogen therapy, try taking steps to deal with stress. That may be all you need to cure forgetfulness.

supply and our neurons, providing energy to the brain as well as affecting the neurons themselves. This happens during foetal development, infancy, puberty and pregnancy. Thanks to oestrogen, they grow more dendritic spines (spiky outgrowths that look like "thorns on a rosebush," says Craig H. Kinsley, Ph.D., associate professor of neuroscience at the University of Richmond in Virginia), creating more connections for processing information.

**Oestrogen keeps our brains working normally.** "It influences neural activity in areas in the brain that are important for learning and memory," says Victoria Luine, Ph.D., distinguished professor of psychology at Hunter College in New York City. "In doing so, it enhances activity of neurotransmitters like norepinephrine and acetylcholine that promote memory." Acetylcholine, which helps us learn, concentrate and recall information, is often deficient in people with Alzheimer's. Norepinephrine increases blood-flow to the brain and makes us more alert. The body's synthesis of norepinephrine also produces dopamine, yet another neurotransmitter, which helps us recall events, facts, faces and more.

**Oestrogen protects the brain.** It prevents the creation of beta amyloid plaques, "dead spots" in the brain associated with Alzheimer's. It also may reduce inflammation and even serve as an antioxidant, fighting off the free radicals that attack brain cells.

"Lots of neurons in the brain are responsive to oestrogen," says Dominique Toran-Allerand, M.D., Sc.D., professor of anatomy and cell biology and neurology at Columbia University in New York City. "If you deprive the brain of oestrogen, those neurons will suffer. And many neurons in the brain are related to cognitive function. That's why the loss of oestrogen at menopause can have profound effects on cognition." We get forgetful. We can't concentrate. We feel mentally fuzzy. We transpose words in conversation. And we begin to wonder what in the world could be wrong with us.

Still, absentmindedness and memory problems aren't necessarily symptoms of early Alzheimer's but instead may be a direct result of the oestrogen fluctuations we experience at midlife, says Claire Warga, Ph.D., a research neuropsychologist in Brooklyn, in her book *Menopause and the Mind*. Even before we hit perimenopause, fluctuations in oestrogen levels may affect both our verbal and spatial ability. For example, when women ovulate, their oestrogen levels are at their highest, potentially boosting verbal skills at that time.

# A Welcome Bonus from HRT

Many experts see promise in hormone replacement therapy (HRT) as a means of helping to prevent or lessen memory problems associated with ageing. Using neuroimaging technology, researchers at the US National Institute on Aging recently found evidence that the brains of postmenopausal women who received oestrogen replacement therapy aged differently and had significantly greater bloodflow to areas of the brain involved in memory than the brains of women who did not receive hormone replacement. This suggests that hormone replacement may lower susceptibility to changes associated with Alzheimer's.

"This is the first study comparing brain ageing in women who receive oestrogen to women who do not receive oestrogen," says lead author Pauline Maki, M.D., investigator at the Laboratory of Personality and Cognition at the National Institute on Aging in Bethesda, Maryland.

Oestrogen also may protect us against Alzheimer's, according to Dr. Warga, reducing our risk of getting the disease by as much as 60 per cent. However, the question of whether oestrogen replacement therapy actually prevents Alzheimer's disease is controversial, according to Dr. Morris. Although circumstantial evidence suggests a protective effect, he says, no study has shown directly that oestrogen stops Alzheimer's from developing. Dr. Morris also believes that there is no benefit in giving oestrogen to women who already have Alzheimer's. He warns against taking oestrogen solely to prevent Alzheimer's.

"The data isn't strong enough to support a protective role for oestrogen, particularly given its risks," he says.

But if you've decided to take oestrogen for other reasons, then memory enhancement could be a welcome bonus.

# How's Your Blood Sugar?

Oestrogen isn't the only hormone associated with memory. Surprisingly, one of the best predictors of remaining sharp as a tack as you age is blood sugar.

Glucose regulation – or how your body manages your blood sugar – is beginning to emerge as a critical influence on our brains as we age, says Suzanne Craft, Ph.D., associate professor of psychiatry at the University of Washington and director of the Geriatric Research, Education and Clinical Center at the Puget Sound Veterans Administration Medical Center, both in Seattle.

That's because glucose is the essential energy source for our brains. Without it, we cannot learn or remember information. And since the brain neither makes nor stores glucose, it relies on – what else? – glucose obtained from the body. Glucose, in turn, is regulated by insulin, a hormone secreted by the pancreas. The result? "Insulin can modulate memory," Dr. Craft says.

Researchers suspect insulin may do this by:

- *Providing glucose, or energy, to areas of the brain involved in memory*
- *Producing, as a by-product, the neurotransmitter acetylcholine, which is essential in memory*
- *Increasing brain activity involved in long-term potentiation – that is, making new connections in the hippocampus*
- *Boosting levels of the neurotransmitter norepinephrine, which increases attention and therefore may improve learning and memory*
- *Opposing the effects of cortisol, a stress hormone that interferes with memory retrieval if we are under sustained stress (although in small doses it enhances memory)*

## THE HORMONE CONNECTION
# HAVE A BABY – IT MAKES YOU SMARTER

Trying to convince your kids that Mum indeed *does* know best? Science will back you up.

"Motherhood is an amazing time for the female brain," says Craig H. Kinsley, Ph.D., associate professor of neuroscience at the University of Richmond in Virginia. He studied how quickly mother rats completed a maze and found food, compared to non-mother rats. Like a human mother, who races through the grocery shop, trying to remember what she needs and where to find it while impatient teenagers wait in the car, the mother rats beat the others rats hands down.

One reason for the mother rats' superior spatial memory and speed: hormones.

"In rodents, the hormonal events of pregnancy appear to rework the female brain in ways that facilitate learning and memory – perhaps for the rest of the female's lifetime," Dr. Kinsley says. Nerve connections flourish, thanks to increased oestrogen and progesterone. And the more connections we have, the better our power to think, process information and remember.

At last: a scientific explanation for motherly multitasking.

These processes are disrupted in people with insulin resistance, commonly associated with type 2 diabetes and, increasingly, Alzheimer's. When you're insulin resistant, you need more insulin to have the same effects on your body, so your pancreas produces more insulin. But the more insulin circulating in your body, the less sensitive you become to it. At the same time, the high insulin spurs an increase in the stress hormone cortisol, which at high levels impairs memory. It's a bad situation for the brain. With too much stress hormone and not enough glucose for energy, memory suffers.

Yet for many, insulin resistance is easily avoidable – with two simple fixes, says Dr. Craft.

**Take a 20-minute walk three times a week.** Exercise improves your body's usage of glucose and insulin, protecting you against insulin resistance. If you're already having insulin problems, exercise can help resensitize your body to the hormone, improving your memory.

**Choose foods high in fibre and complex carbohydrates and low in refined sugars and, especially, fat.** "The fastest way to get type 2 diabetes is not by eating sugar but by eating fats," Dr. Craft says.

"Women need to be making these changes in their forties," she says. See chapter 13 for more advice on preventing or controlling diabetes.

## Remember to Relax

Cortisol isn't the only stress hormone that affects memory. Coursing through our minds and bodies, cortisol, epinephrine (also known as adrenaline) and norepinephrine fire up our brains and call our muscles to attention. Under stress, our hearts beat faster. Our breaths get shorter. Physically and mentally, we feel like we're in overdrive. These same hormonal responses may either sharpen or dull memory.

Take, for example, a frightening or embarrassing situation, like a car accident or awkward workplace encounter. Chances are, you can recall the event in great detail. That's because stress hormones, like cortisol, seek to protect us from future harm by creating a powerful memory of this risky, stressful event so we can avoid it or make better choices.

Unfortunately, cortisol levels surge when we anticipate a stressful event like a job interview, hindering memory and temporarily preventing us from retrieving data stored in our brains. So we "freeze up," says Dr. McGaugh.

If your cortisol levels are high for a prolonged period of time – say, in response to a major stressor, such as a death of a close family member – your memory will suffer. Prolonged production of cortisol interferes with insulin's transport of glucose into the brain. Without this essential energy, our brain cells falter. It may even interfere with our brains' process of turning short-term memory into long-term memory, says Dr. Newcomer.

Stress-induced memory problems aren't permanent. Once cortisol levels drop to normal, memory returns. Follow strategies to reduce stress outlined in Phase 2 of the Hormone-Balancing Programme on page 275.

## Tune Up Your Memory with Herbs and Vitamins

Here's what to try. Be patient. Supplements may take as long as three months to work, says Liz Sutherland, N.D., a naturopathic physician with the National College of Naturopathic Medicine's Natural Health Sciences Research Clinic in Lake Oswego, Oregon.

**Ginkgo.** This herb potentially boosts memory in two ways: by increasing blood circulation, which helps the brain, and by preventing the hippocampus from shrinking. Until recently, most herbal experts agreed that ginkgo was useful only for modestly improving mental function of people with mild Alzheimer's disease. But a new English study indicates that it may have broader memory-boosting ability – and may be helpful if your forgetfulness is due to plain old information overload.

"We now have proof positive that ginkgo can boost memory in healthy young people," says Douglas Schar, Dip.Phyt., M.C.P.P., a medical herbalist who practises in London and Washington, D.C.

Try 80 milligrams of ginkgo extract (read the label; the product should contain 24 per cent ginkgo flavonglycosides) three times daily, says Dr. Sutherland. And she advises not taking ginkgo for 3 weeks before or after surgery because it's a blood thinner.

**Phosphatidylserine (PS).** A protein similar to lecithin, a natural substance found in foods and also in the brain, phosphatidylserine is thought to improve memory by activating neurotransmitters like epinephrine, norepinephrine, serotonin and dopamine. Dr. Sutherland recommends 100 milligrams of PS three times a day. PS is available in the UK but usually in combination with other products.

**Siberian ginseng.** Feeling stressed and forgetful? Try Siberan ginseng (*Eleutherococcus senticocus*). "Ginseng will help memory by supporting the function of the adrenal gland, thereby helping with stress management," explains Dr. Sutherland, who suggests taking 100 to 200 milligrams a day.

**B vitamins.** Known individually as thiamin, riboflavin, niacin, pantothenic acid, $B_6$, folic acid and $B_{12}$, B vitamins support memory in countless ways. They help the body produce neurotransmitters. They improve circulation. They help cells make energy. They optimize the functioning of the adrenal glands, helping us respond appropriately to stress that might otherwise cause memory lapses, according to Dr. Sutherland. Look for a B-complex supplement containing at least 100 per cent of the RDA of the vitamins listed above.

**Vitamin E.** When we don't get enough of this antioxidant, one of several naturally occurring substances that prevent cellular damage, our nerves – and memory – may suffer. Dr. Sutherland suggests taking 400 IU a day.

## More Ways to Sharpen Your Brain

Memory aids can do only so much if your brain is on overload. "Midlife women just have too much to keep track of," says Carolyn Adams-Price, Ph.D., associate professor of psychology at Mississippi State University in Starkville. "You're not only thinking about your concerns; you're also keeping track of what your children and mother-in-law need to do." Hormonal fluctuations don't help matters.

Here are some other ways to get back into balance and crank up your memory – naturally.

**Prioritize sleep.** "My wife says women don't have time to sleep," says Allen Hobson, M.D., associate professor of neurology at Harvard Medical School and specialist in the neurophysiology of sleep and mental performance. "But the brain needs sleep to perform adequately – when you're asleep, it works on information you've gathered." When you're sleep-deprived, he explains, your hippocampus, the brain structure responsible for transforming short-term into long-term memory, actually shrinks. Aim for at least 8 hours a night.

**Use your nose.** Scents can help us remember. Studies have indicated that students who sniffed peppermint, ammonia, chocolate, or even perfume while studying were able to recall the information better if the same smell was repeated to "cue" their brains to retrieve that information when needed.

**Get musical.** Listening to soft instrumental music you enjoy may lower your cortisol levels, relaxing you, says Norman M. Weinberger, Ph.D., editor of the *MuSICA Research Notes* newsletter (www.musica.uci.edu), executive director of the International Foundation for Music Research, and a professor of neurobiology and behaviour at the University of California, Irvine.

# CHAPTER 6

# Reach the Weight You Want

Taking the Pill made me put on 2½ kilos (5 pounds)."
"I was always able to control my weight . . . until I hit the menopause."
"I've been so stressed about losing my job, my eating is out of control."
"After I had a hysterectomy, I put on 13 kilos (2 stone)."
"Everyone in my family is overweight – it's hereditary."

Whether due to oral contraceptives, the menopause, stress, a hysterectomy, or plain old heredity, changes in hormone levels influence your weight, your shape, even your appetite.

Take appetite, for instance. Peptides, proteins and mood-regulating neurotransmitters constantly run messages back and forth between your cells, organs and gastrointestinal tract and your brain to get instructions on whether it's time to start eating. And if it is time to eat, hormones influence which foods you choose, how much you eat, how fast or slow you process it and whether to store or burn fat.

Women have felt vulnerable to hormonal cravings and sluggish metabolisms for years, with little to prove it but instinct. Now science is uncovering several bona fide links between hormones, hunger and fat metabolism. It seems that lately every time you open a medical journal, you see that scientists have discovered either a new hormone or new relationships between old hormones that end up affecting your waistline.

Taking advantage of hormones – mechanisms already in place in your molecular biology – can help you to manage your weight, shape and appetite. What follows is a hormone-harmonizing plan, based on the latest data, designed to get you to the weight you want for the rest of your life.

## It All Starts at Secondary School

You probably began to suspect that hormones play a role in your body shape about the time you first started to use lipstick and develop an interest in boys. At puberty, oestrogen receptors in your hips, thighs, buttocks and breasts woke up and lured your pubescent fat their way. Don't hate them. It's the fat stores in those areas that make the rewards of breastfeeding possible when we later decide to have children and that historically protected mother and baby during times of starvation.

Not all women have an hourglass silhouette. But oestrogen makes all women more prone to fat storage in these areas, whether we are interested in child rearing or not.

When reproductive hormones decline at menopause and a woman no longer needs the extra fat-fuel storage for child rearing, fat takes up residence in her abdominal area. Even if she weighs the same, wearing a belly-baring bikini becomes less of an option now more than ever.

Why the shift from hip- to stomach-oriented fat? For starters, after the menopause you have higher levels of androgen hormones (so-called male hormones typically present in women in small amounts). And men – the androgen-based beings that they are – are genetically predisposed to store fat particularly in their abdominal area.

But a much more interesting – and, well, feminine – theory is that when you approach the menopause, your abdomen becomes a production site for alternative oestrogen in order to compensate for your ovaries, which are going into retirement. These factories, naturally, need to bring fuel – in the form of fat – to their site, which takes up extra storage space in your middle.

Now is not the time to try to starve away your rerouted curves. Whether you're hourglass-shaped or apple-shaped at midlife, some fat is normal and necessary. Fat is precious bubble wrap for your organs, keeping them safe and warm. Your body takes the utmost care to manage the foods you supply it with by storing some away for when you don't get enough. Fat even helps regulate your hormones.

Being underweight, on the other hand, puts you at risk for early menopause, osteoporosis and even depression, says Larrian Gillespie, M.D., author of *The Menopause Diet*.

## Size Up Your Weight

How do you know if you've crossed the line from having "healthy curves" to too much avoirdupois? Body mass index (BMI) can give you a ballpark of what's healthy for your age, height and gender. A ratio of your weight to

(continued on page 94)

## WHAT'S GOING ON?

**Not sure why you can't reach the weight you want? Take this quiz to help determine if there's something you've overlooked.**

**1. How much do you really eat?**
Multiply your weight in pounds by 15. If you want just to maintain that weight, you must eat no more than that number of calories a day, in addition to regular exercise. To actually lose weight, you need approximately 20 per cent fewer calories than that, in addition to regular exercise. Example: 145 pounds x 15 = 2175 calories – 435 calories (or 20 per cent) = 1740 calories (daily need).

**2. Are you still not losing weight, no matter how much you diet?**
Very low calorie diets (800 to 1200 calories per day) can actually slow your metabolic rate, which means you burn less fat and actually sabotage your weight-loss efforts. Not to mention, with any extreme diet, it's nearly impossible to maintain loss even if you are successful.

**3. Does obesity run in your family?**
You may be genetically resistant to leptin, a hormone that controls appetite and fat storage. You could have also inherited susceptibility to medical conditions that can lead to obesity. So-called fat genes are rare, though. More than likely you've inherited lifestyle habits (like a high-fat diet and lack of exercise). And that's good news since you can change your habits, not your genes.

**4. How much exercise do you get, really?**
It's not possible to lose weight, or even maintain your current weight (not to mention current health in general), without physical activity – especially if you're approaching or passing through menopause. Any activity is better than none, but it's best to work up to 30 to 60 minutes of activity a day, at increasing levels of intensity.

**5. Do you take antidepressants or corticosteroids?**
Either type of drug could be contributing to weight gain. It's mainly the older brands of antidepressants like imipramine (Tofranil) and amitriptyline (Triptafen) that cause you to gain. You may have better luck with another class of antidepressant.

Unfortunately, there are few alternatives to cortisone and prednisolone, but you could ask your doctor to experiment with a lower dosage or every-other-day use.

**6. Do you wake yourself with snoring? Does your husband tell you that you seem to sometimes stop breathing or have laboured breathing while you sleep?**
Sleep apnoea is a condition caused by progesterone's affecting the epiglottis – the spoon-shaped cartilage that guards the air passageway to the throat. In addition to preventing you from getting a good night of sleep, the lack of oxygen that sleep apnoea causes may disrupt your hormones enough to cause weight gain or prevent weight loss. If you have the symptoms above, see your family doctor or a sleep specialist.

**7. Do you attribute weight gain to water retention?**
If it's fluid retention, you will probably notice that your ankles are swollen and your hands and abdomen are puffy. See chapter 7 for managing water weight that plagues you during your monthly cycle. It could be related to excessive salt intake or a heart, kidney, or liver condition. You should ask your doctor about lifestyle changes and medication that may help.

**8. In addition to being overweight, do you have heat or cold sensitivity, suffer chronic fatigue, or experience difficulty concentrating?**
Your thyroid may be out of balance. (See chapter 4 for more information.)

**9. Is weight gain concentrated in your abdominal area? Do you also experience anxiety, fertility problems, or low resistance to colds and infections?**
Ask your doctor to evaluate you for Cushing's syndrome, a rare endocrine disorder involving excessive production of the hormone cortisol. Abdominal weight gain may also be a sign of polycystic ovary syndrome (discussed on page 150).

height expressed in numbers from 19 to 40-plus, BMI has replaced the old Height-Weight charts of years ago as an indicator of what constitutes a healthy weight.

The average BMI is 25, with 26 to 30 considered mildly overweight, and 31 to 40 considered obese. Over 40, and you are seriously obese. Obesity puts women at higher risk for developing heart disease, diabetes and breast cancer. In contrast, a lower BMI considerably increases your chances for living a long, healthy life.

---

THE HORMONE CONNECTION

## IS FAT AN ENDOCRINE GLAND?

In the past, science thought of fat as a holding area for excess fuel. Dieters have always considered fat a nuisance. One of these two points of view has changed.

"Adipose tissue – what we call fat – is hardly just an inert storage depot. It's actually an endocrine organ," says Sheila Collins, Ph.D., a molecular biologist who studies fat cell metabolism at Duke University Medical Center in Durham, North Carolina.

Granted, it's hard to regard the masses jiggling under your arms or padding your seat as a respectable hormone machine. After all, it's not poised in one logical place – like, say, your ovaries. But when you consider what fat *does*, there's no doubt that it holds a place in the endocrine world.

Like a conventional endocrine gland, fat actually produces hormones and hormone-like substances, and even has receptors to receive messages from hormones. Fat's most famous product is leptin, which gave fat its new image when leptin was discovered, in 1995.

Fat tissue also pumps out hormone-like immune system agents called cytokines. Some of these cytokines are the same as the ones that assist your mighty immune cells in destroying threats like viruses, bacteria and tumours. Others have a darker role of contributing to type 2 diabetes and inflammatory conditions.

This blubbery endocrine gland also interacts with your reproductive hormones to make you fertile. And at menopause it's your fat cells that produce a modified version of oestrogen when your ovaries slow down.

"We are just at the tip of understanding these sorts of things," says Dr. Collins. "But what we're sure of is that fat is incredibly biologically active."

To calculate your BMI:
1. Multiply your height in inches by .0254, then square it (multiply the result by itself).
2. Divide your weight in pounds by 2.2 to get kilograms.
3. Divide number 2 by number 1.

You should also measure your middle because abdominal fat has its own, separate set of risks. Since this fat wraps around the organs deep in your abdomen, it has an easier route to get artery-clogging cholesterol to your heart. In fact, women who gain weight mostly in the abdomen have a higher risk for developing heart disease than those with weight in their legs.

Abdominal fat also puts you at risk for arthritis, irritable bowel syndrome, gallstones, kidney stones, incontinence and kidney failure.

Measuring your middle is just another method to track your weight. Before reading the tape measure, ensure that the tape is snug but does not compress the skin. Women with a waist circumference measurement greater than 88 cm (35 inches) are in the high-risk group for obesity.

## Control Your Blood Sugar to Control Your Weight

While many hormones affect the way you store or release fat, insulin is the most well known and usually the most manageable. "In weight loss and weight control, your first goal should be to keep insulin levels from getting too high since insulin clearly promotes fat storage," says Geoffrey Redmond, M.D., author of *The Good News about Women's Hormones*.

"Insulin can also cause you to overeat when it goes up too high – usually because the body's response to its own insulin has become sluggish," says Dr. Redmond. You can read about blood sugar control in more detail in chapter 13. But for the purposes of weight control, here's a crash course.

Any carbohydrates in the food you eat are absorbed by your small intestine and sent into your bloodstream as glucose. When glucose in your blood reaches a certain level, your pancreas releases the processor hormone, insulin, to move glucose out of your blood and into your cells. Insulin will send some glucose immediately to the cells of your brain and other organs, and ushers what is not needed as fuel into storage. When enough blood sugar has been processed by insulin, your pancreas will send out the hormone glucagon to "turn down" insulin.

While it's running the sugar show, insulin stimulates an enzyme called lipoprotein lipase (LPL), which essentially "unzips" the entrance door to fat cells and uses them like a laundry bag for lipids (fat "filler"). Think of a laundry sack: when it's empty, the sack can be folded inconspicuously in your pocket; when it's loaded, you can't close the boot on it. Fat cells similarly can expand and collapse a great deal – in biologists' terms, holding between 100 picolitres and 1000 picolitres of lipid when stuffed to the max.

The more insulin there is around, the more your adipose cells (fat) pack in; then you end up hiding under tracksuit bottoms. In fact, women's "laundry bags" can be stuffed even more than men's.

## *Escape from* HORMONE HELL
# SHE'S IN A QUANDARY OVER PMS-INDUCED BINGES

**Q: Between out-of-control cravings and 2½ kg (5 pounds) of extra water weight, premenstrual changes leave me hiding under oversize clothes once a month. The bloating goes away when my period is over, but I'm worried that monthly PMS-related chocolate and biscuit binges are going to make me huge. I've read that taking birth control pills can help cravings and bloating, but friends of mine who went on the Pill claim that they put on at least 2½ kg (5 pounds). What should I do?**

Pamela Peeke, M.P.H., M.D., assistant clinical professor of medicine at the University of Maryland School of Medicine in Baltimore and author of *Fight Fat after Forty*, responds: first, realize that it's normal to experience bloating and food cravings around the time of your period. The menstrual cycle delivers a double whammy of two different hormone groups increasing at the same time – sex hormones (oestrogen and progesterone) and stress hormones (cortisol and adrenaline). Some say the hormone-like chemical serotonin also fluctuates with your monthly cycle. These changes drive up appetite and prompt you to eat the kinds of foods that increase your insulin levels; higher insulin levels, in turn, cause bloating.

You're never going to be able to eliminate cravings and bloating, but there's a lot you can do to minimize them. Acknowledge what your body is going through, and be sure to take care of yourself a little differently than you do the rest of the month.

Eating more protein when you have PMS can help prevent wild cravings because it gives you an exquisite sense of satisfaction. I don't mean eat loads of meat. Instead, work

But before giving your skinny jeans away, keep in mind that your pancreas sends out glucagon, which stimulates LPL's opponent, hormone sensitive lipase (HSL). This enzyme empowers glucagon to lock up the top zip of fat cells so nothing else can be stuffed in, and, heroically, unzips a side pouch in your cells that lets the laundry tumble out. Glucagon then burns up fatty acids, the by-product of this process – a far heart-healthier alternative to insulin, which turns most of it into cholesterol, which is then incorporated into cells throughout the body.

protein, like an egg or a tin of beans, into your breakfast, lunch, dinner and snacks, and accompany it with high-quality complex carbohydrates like wholemeal toast or brown rice.

On the other hand, if you give in to cravings for sweet foods and simple carbohydrates, like baked goods, they'll raise your insulin levels and only make your appetite more voracious in the long run. Most of all, avoid white starches since they are directly linked to bloating. That means save potato crisps, tortilla chips and pasta for very occasional treats when you're not having your period.

Research shows that taking calcium helps to reduce PMS cravings, and I think it really works. By consuming the RDA of 1000 to 1500 milligrams of calcium every day from food and supplements, you may notice a difference. Drinking mineral water all month is an easy way to keep up levels of calcium and its helper minerals.

Next, get thyself to the gym, no matter how bad you feel. Even if you have cramps, are too bloated to wear your running shorts, and are dragging your tail, if you just stay on that treadmill (or favourite piece of equipment) for a few minutes, you will notice a miracle. The feel-good chemical endorphins your brain releases during aerobic activity are a natural anaesthetic to take away the discomfort – not to mention that the aerobic charge will dampen your appetite and help sweat off extra water weight.

As far as the Pill is concerned, you can't make any assumptions about birth control from how another woman responds to it since everyone has a different chemistry. A significant minority notice water weight, but an equally significant minority find that the Pill *reduces* bloating. You won't know how you'll react until you try it. And the lower the dose that you can take, the less likely bloating will be.

Fortunately, glucagon can stay elevated in the blood for several hours after a protein-rich meal. This gives your body plenty of time to start collapsing those fat sacks on your thighs to get you back in your skinny jeans. The trick is to avoid chasing the protein-rich meal with a high-carbohydrate treat. If you scoff down candy floss, glucagon will retreat faster than a cat in a rainstorm, leaving you no better off than before.

What this means is that unless you are a type 1 diabetic (totally dependent on an outside source of insulin), you can control whether insulin or glucagon runs the sugar show in your cells. The first step is to become familiar with foods that hike up your blood sugar (and, so, keep insulin hanging around). You'll find such so-called high glycaemic index foods listed in "A Diet for Better Blood Sugar Control" on page 242. As you might suspect, heavily sweetened and white starches are usually the worst offenders, as well as foods low in fibre, or soft and overcooked in texture. Foods like this should be avoided or eaten only occasionally.

## The Hormones Behind Your "Survivor" Appetite

"It's really quite impressive that so many of us eat different foods every day, and have different activity levels every day, but most of us maintain the same body weight despite all these variables," says Sheila Collins, Ph.D., associate professor in psychiatry and behavioural sciences at Duke University Medical Center in Durham, North Carolina. "There is a tightly controlled circuitry in our brains that regulates our food intake and how we process it."

This circuitry seems to be rooted in our ability to survive. Over the millennia, the human body has learned to maintain a safe amount of fat in case of famine, illness and other hardships where food is scarce. At the same time, an internal governor signals us to curb eating and empty fat stores when sated, enabling us to maintain a body agile enough to accomplish the work we need to do to survive.

Since our current environment is usually anything but scarce on food and doesn't require as much physical work, humans seem to be overriding many of the control mechanisms that maintain weight – and growing obese. But scientists are working overtime to learn how to manipulate the "survival techniques" that govern appetite and weight gain.

For the first time in history, scientists are mapping out the molecular chart for appetite and metabolism, says Dr. Collins. And hormones, or chemicals that interact with our hormones, are some of the missing links.

Once the whole puzzle comes together, obesity may be a thing of the past.

But even some early pieces of the puzzle can shed light today on how we can bring appetite and metabolism into the balance it was meant to have.

## Galanin: Your Fat-Seeking Stimulator

Galanin is a peptide hormone lurking in your brain's hypothalamus gland that may be to blame the next time you can't get your mind off fatty foods. When galanin is secreted in the brain, it appears to stimulate a strong appetite, particularly for fat. To put the fatty icing on the fatty cake, galanin alerts other hormones to usher the fat you eat straight to your fat stores.

Studies so far indicate that the hormone dopamine may help compensate for the effects of galanin because it inhibits the ingestion of fat and protein, which reduces body weight. It also seems that insulin and galanin play a hormonal tug-of-war, so one cannot rise when the other is high. It's not yet clear how we can take advantage of these galanin-regulating relationships. For now, committing to an eating plan that heads off out-of-control cravings, described later, can help.

Galanin isn't the only peptide that's at play when you're craving chocolate eclairs. A whole network of biological chemicals are at work, and scientists are still trying to understand how they fit together, says Pamela Peeke, M.P.H., M.D., assistant clinical professor of medicine at the University of Maryland School of Medicine in Baltimore and author of *Fight Fat after Forty*. "Most of the research on galanin is on animals – we need to find out if humans fare the same," she says.

## Neuropeptide Y (NPY): On the Hunt for Carbohydrates

Known simply as NPY, neuropeptide Y is an incredibly powerful appetite stimulant. In fact, when obesity researchers infused NPY into animals' brains, the animals ate themselves to death, says Dr. Peeke.

"It is suspected that the by-products of carbohydrates broken down in the body stimulate the production of NPY – which implies that the more carb cravings you give in to, the stronger the urge to break into a bakery after hours. As if this cycle alone weren't enough to make a bread addict out of any of us, NPY also appears to stimulate insulin – which, as we know, can increase the desire for carbohydrates," says Dr. Peeke.

Not only does NPY trigger feeding frenzies, but studies conducted on animals suggest that it has a knack for transforming the food that you eat into fat, while at the same time making sure that you hold on to the fat that you already have, says Robert E. C. Wildman, R.D., Ph.D., associate professor of nutrition at the University of Louisiana in Lafayette.

As nature would have it, NPY does not go unchallenged. Enter the hormone leptin.

## Leptin: Your Thinness Regulator

If NPY and galanin are the pitchfork-holding devils on one side of your brain taunting you to overeat, the protein hormone leptin is the halo-wearing angel on the other side cheering you on to practise moderation.

Appropriately named after the Greek word "leptos" meaning "thin", leptin

# An At-a-Glance Guide to Weight-Control Hormones

Few people realize that more than 20 different hormones and hormone-like substances influence your weight, shape, appetite and eating habits. Summarized briefly for easy reference, here are some of the major players.

**APPETITE**

**Dopamine** A brain chemical that sends sensory signals for you to start and stop eating.

**Galanin** A peptide hormone, found mostly in the hypothalamus, that encourages you to overeat fatty foods.

**Leptin** A protein hormone secreted by fat cells that reduces food intake and decreases fat stores.

**Neuropeptide Y (NPY)** A peptide hormone, secreted in the hypothalamus and the adrenal glands, that is linked to overeating, particularly carbohydrates.

**Norepinephrine** A brain chemical that can reduce food intake.

**Serotonin** A hormone-like neurotransmitter that, when adequate in supply, helps regulate the size and duration of meals.

**DIGESTION**

**Cholecystokinin** A hormone, secreted by the pancreas, that causes your gallbladder to contract, making you feel full.

**Gastrin** A hormone that signals digestive enzymes, as well as the other "gut hormones" needed for the stomach to contract.

**Motilin** A hormone that jump-starts contractions in your gastrointestinal tract.

stimulates the nerve cells that release peptide hormones known for controlling eating. It also decreases your fat stores by kicking your metabolism up a notch. In fact, this multitalented protein hormone preserves muscle mass while it melts fat – which is more than any strict calorie-restricting diet can achieve.

At the same time, leptin intercepts the release of certain appetite-stimulating peptides, NPY included.

In early trials, when a group of dieters were injected with leptin, each lost approximately 1 kg (2.2 pounds) each month for the 6 months that they took the hormone. In another experiment, one leptin-deficient person was given

## METABOLISM

**DHEA**  A hormone that helps regulate metabolism and insulin levels.

**Growth hormone**  A hormone that regulates muscle–fat ratio.

**Thyroid**  Hormones that ultimately control your body's "metabolic motor".

## BLOOD SUGAR

**Glucagon**  A hormone stimulated by proteins and secreted by the pancreas to regulate insulin.

**Insulin**  A hormone, secreted by the pancreas, that moves glucose from the bloodstream to the organs (for fuel) or to fat tissues (for storage).

## STRESS AND MOODS

**Adrenaline**  A hormone, signalled by corticotropin-releasing hormone (CRH), that raises blood pressure and heart rate.

**Beta-endorphins**  The body's natural opiates, which help you exercise through pain and also help curb appetite.

**Corticotropin-releasing hormone (CRH)**  A messenger hormone released by your hypothalamus in response to a thrilling or alarming event.

**Cortisol (also known as corticoid)**  A hormone, triggered by CRH and released from the adrenal glands, that moves fat and glucose out of storage for the body to use in a crisis.

## REPRODUCTIVE SYSTEM HORMONES

**Oestrogen**  A female hormone that's needed in adequate amounts for efficient digestion and metabolism.

**Progesterone**  A hormone, produced in your ovaries, that can contribute to a woman's rising insulin levels.

**Testosterone**  A hormone partially responsible for fat accumulation in the midriff.

leptin and lost more than 13 kg (2 stone). The person's metabolism also improved when the leptin levels were raised.

Unfortunately, obese people appear to be unable to take advantage of leptin's appetite-control features because of a possible defect in their leptin receptors.

"At first we thought obese people were low on leptin, but that's not the case," says Dr. Collins. "They just seem to become desensitized to it."

Harvard School of Public Health researchers found that people with leptin resistance could regulate their leptin levels by exercising regularly. It's also possible that you can get into the leptin protection zone by losing a few pounds, but you have to lose them very gradually.

In the case of those with true low leptin levels – which appears to be a genetic flaw – studies are under way to perfect a treatment. (For updates, see "On the Web & Other Resources" on page 109.)

## Cholecystokinin (CCK): Your Fullness Signal

When food moves out of your stomach, receptors in the small intestine notify the pancreas to release CCK, a peptide hormone needed to empty your gallbladder. Since this action essentially completes an important phase of digestion, your appetite decreases.

The brain also produces some CCK, which seems to pair up with your intestine's supply of CCK, so you feel full, push back from the table and have the rest of your meal wrapped to take home.

Cholecystokinin seems so effective at curbing appetite that the medical community is working on drugs that can trip CCK into action. But there are dozens of natural ways that you can help influence the digestive processes that curb your appetite, says Dr. Gillespie.

For example, proteins and certain saturated fatty acids stimulate the cholecystokinin response. "More specifically, we found that it takes a little less than 1 tablespoon of butter to trip off CCK, so if you have 2 tablespoons of melted butter with your steamed vegetable appetizer, you'll feel full sooner," explains Dr. Gillespie.

Cholecystokinin is just one reason to eat in a manner that fosters good digestion. A host of other gastrointestinal hormones and enzymes are also involved with the chain of events leading up to this fullness signal. Efficient digestion also has a lot to do with how you metabolize fat – whether you store it or use it for energy.

In fact, when insulin levels are high, CCK will backfire and actually make you eat more. Following food ratios recommended later in this chapter can help keep overeating in check.

## Can Stress Widen Your Middle?

Unlike most obesity experts, Dr. Peeke spends most of her research on hormones like corticotropin-releasing hormone (CRH), cortisol and adrenaline – your trio of "stress alarms". These hormones create a chain reaction that makes you eat like you just outran an elephant stampede and turns your abdominal area into a storage warehouse, she explains.

It all goes back to the fight-or-flight response you probably recall from biology lessons. If we really had to outrun a predator or defend our village, we'd appreciate the fact that in crisis, the brain releases CRH, which then triggers the adrenal gland to release adrenaline and cortisol to give us the extra pep to react swiftly.

The problem is, given the nature of stressors in the 21st-century, where confrontations with prehistoric predators are a thing of the past, fighting or fleeing isn't a typical option. "Instead, you're probably just going to 'stew and chew'. In other words, if your boss criticizes your work, and you're just sitting on your behind at your computer, suddenly the office stash of Smarties looks really good. Same goes if you get a letter from the bank saying you're overdrawn. You can't fight or flee, so you eat.

"It's a problem for several reasons," Dr. Peeke says. Cortisol automatically kicks up your appetite, prompting you to replace the very fuel it expected you to use during your crisis, whether you did or not. Under cortisol's influence, you not only want to eat huge quantities but also want to eat the very kind of food that will make you fatter since sweets and simple carbs turn into sugar more quickly in the body.

"Stress fat" is concentrated in the last place you need it: deep in your tummy. Probably as a matter of survival, the fat cells in your intra-abdominal region have more than their share of receptors for cortisol – at least twice as many as anywhere else on your body, actually. That's because intra-abdominal fat is located so close to the liver, where fat is converted to fuel (glucose) for the fight-or-flight response.

"Since we seem to put ourselves through mock disaster training several times a day, we set ourselves up for our 'fuel' to make a beeline for the belly," says Dr. Gillespie. "Chronic stress also causes insulin, another fat storage hormone, to rise. When insulin is paired with cortisol, insulin's ability to store fat and inhibit its release is only enhanced," she adds.

Stress is not the only mental state that causes you to let out your belt. Researchers in the behavioural science department of Pennsylvania State University analysed 1300 people and discovered that those with the high levels of cynicism, anger and depression in the group also had the largest amounts of abdominal fat. All those mental states are linked to elevated cortisol's contributing to increased fat storage specifically in the area of the abdomen.

"Our bodies were never meant to run hot all the time," says Dr. Peeke. "It's a matter of either developing a more stress-resilient lifestyle or watching your physical and mental health deteriorate and your weight soar."

## In the Mood for Eating

The hormone-like neurotransmitter serotonin is most commonly associated with moods. But when serotonin levels are what they should be, it also functions as a signal to make you feel sated. In fact, serotonin is a key ingredient in the popular weight-loss medication Reductil (sibutramine), originally sold as an antidepressant until researchers found that it could control appetite.

In cases of depression where serotonin levels are usually very low, you may eat uncontrollably (although depression can, for a different reason, also cause loss of appetite). In fact, recent evidence indicates that serotonin imbalance can trigger the carbohydrate-starved peptide galanin to stimulate food intake.

Voracious eating when you are experiencing depression is your body's way of self-medicating in an attempt to boost serotonin. Since plummeting oestrogen levels can bring serotonin levels down with it, loss of this appetite inhibitor also helps explain the erratic eating patterns that many women experience premenstrually, postnatally and during the menopause.

To increase serotonin, you must first eat adequate protein, which is a source of tryptophan, the amino acid needed to produce serotonin. You also need to consume enough complex carbohydrates, which get tryptophan to the brain, where serotonin can then be released, says Dr. Gillespie.

A better goal is to not get your serotonin off track to begin with. The eating plan outlined later in this chapter is designed to help you keep protein and carbohydrate levels even, which in turn will help prevent your serotonin from plummeting and disrupting your appetite. (For more on mood changes, see chapter 3.)

## Thyroid: The Hidden Weight/Mood Connection

A depressed mood may also be a tip-off to an imbalance of your metabolism-regulating thyroid gland. When your thyroid gland is overactive (hyperthyroidism), the appetite triggers in the brain are superstimulated, causing you to eat more often, which can sometimes lead to weight gain. On the other side of the doughnut, when your thyroid levels are low (hypothyroidism), an impaired metabolism means processing food less efficiently and burning off fewer calories. And since hypothyroidism often causes depression and

### THE HORMONE CONNECTION
# THE HRT MYTH

You may have heard that taking hormone replacement therapy (HRT) can cause weight gain. Not so. "Too often physicians make the mistake of assuming that the changes that come naturally with menopause and ageing are due to oestrogen therapy. Nothing could be further from the truth," says Larrian Gillespie, M.D., author of *The Menopause Diet.*

Of the 875 women who participated for 3 years in a US study known as the Postmenopausal Oestrogen/Progestin Interventions trial, those who used HRT actually put on less weight than non-users. Better yet, other studies of postmenopausal women showed that women on oestrogen therapy actually reduced the trickiest fat storage area of all, their abdominal region.

If HRT *is* sometimes to blame for weight gain, it's due to progestin in the formulations, not oestrogen, says

Dr. Gillespie. "Progestin increases insulin, which inhibits growth hormone and glucagons – both well-known fat fighters. In addition, progestins can cause fluid retention," she explains.

Dr. Gillespie prefers the combination of oestrogen with progesterone, an alternative to progestin that doesn't seem to cause weight gain in women who take it.

In short, research seems to indicate that hormone replacement may help you keep your lean body. What you should be more concerned about is maintaining excellent diet and exercise habits since for many women fitness programmes go south around the time of menopause, Dr. Gillespie says. Without a doubt, the women who exercise the least, who overconsume fat and calories, who drink alcohol and who smoke are the ones who put on the most weight.

fatigue, you are less motivated to exercise. With all these strikes against them, hypothyroid women can put on up to 13 kilos (2 stones).

Fortunately, getting treated for a thyroid disorder should get your weight back to normal. For details, see chapter 4.

## Beat the Menopause Weight-Gain Trap

A number of hormonal changes work in concert to contribute to weight gain at midlife. Growth hormone levels start to steadily drop off in your twenties. You can easily lose 3 kg (7 pounds) of lean muscle every 10 years – the equivalent of burning approximately 290 fewer calories per day by the time you reach your forties.

At the same time, the decline in oestrogen that begins around the age of 40 starts a chain reaction that compromises your digestion and decreases your tolerance for carbohydrates, says Dr. Gillespie.

At midlife, women take about 4 hours to process food, compared to the 2 hours needed previously. The extra processing time allows for more carbohydrate absorption, and more fat is stored rather than broken down and used as energy. It also raises insulin, the fat storage hormone.

In addition, women begin to develop sluggish thyroids after menopause. We also become more vulnerable to the cortisol/fat cycle.

The good news is that growing fatter is not an inevitable consequence of ageing. The Women's Healthy Lifestyle Project in the US studied 535 women expected to reach menopause between 1992 and 1999. Part of this group went about their normal lives, and another part was given a 1300-calorie diet with less than 25 per cent fat and could chose any exercise routine that used up 1000 to 1500 calories a week. After 5 years, the women who did not perform lifestyle modification put on an average of 2½ kilos (5 pounds) (which is on a par with the half a kilogram a year expected during and after menopause), while the women in the lifestyle modification group *lost* a bit of weight – suggesting that with lifestyle intervention it is possible to avoid change-of-life weight gain.

Ageing is a matter of adaptation, says Dr. Gillespie. "It's encouraging to know that women who exercise through menopause have minimal changes in weight, and there are dietary strategies that can make you beat the odds."

## A Lifestyle to Harmonize Hormones and Weight

Maintaining weight is only one reason to control negative emotions, develop a more stress-resilient lifestyle, and learn to enjoy life more. Start with these easy self-care steps designed to bring hormonal influences into harmony.

**Cry if you feel like it.** "Releasing excess emotions can release excess weight," says Christiane Northrup, M.D., author of *Women's Bodies, Women's Wisdom* and *The Wisdom of Menopause*. This is partially because the hormone cortisol, secreted in excess when you are under chronic emotional stress, causes fluid retention and weight gain, she says.

**Tackle the hardest problems early in the day.** Your trio of stress hormones (CRH, cortisol and adrenaline) peak in the morning. To take advantage of the high levels of energy and concentration they bring, plan your most challenging tasks early in the day. Otherwise you may be tempted to eat food high in sugar and other fattening quick fixes if you need to be super sharp later in the afternoon, when your stimulant hormones are on the decline.

"It's as if your tastebuds were linked to your stress hormone biorhythm – the hours between 3 p.m. and midnight are when a woman is tired, frazzled, mindless and heading for the vending machine. Watch out for frappuccino hour," says Dr. Peeke.

**Wake up with peppermint, not caffeine.** Coffee is not evil, but when consumed late in the day, it can raise your cortisol levels enough to make you want to follow it up with biscuits. Plus, enough coffee can inhibit glucagon, the insulin-regulating good guy that activates your fat-burning mechanisms, says Dr. Peeke.

"I find that the best way to rejuvenate is to rub a drop of peppermint oil into each of your temples," says Dr. Peeke. "Just be careful not to get it near your eyes. The peppermint will activate your sympathetic nervous system, and you'll quickly feel on top of things again."

**Join a choir or sing in the shower.** If you have low oxygen levels, it can promote weight gain by reducing the production of growth hormone and oestrogen. "Growth hormone and oestrogen work together to mobilize fat in your body, so get your diaphragm moving," says Dr. Gillespie. Singing has the added benefit of lowering your stress hormones, and the increased oxygen supply may also improve your insulin sensitivity, she adds.

**Sleep 8 hours or more a night.** Besides making you cranky, sleep loss can contribute to weight gain by dramatically disrupting hormones that control your eating habits and your metabolism. Researchers in the department of medicine at the University of Chicago compared the hormone levels of 11 men while they got 8 hours of sleep for several nights, followed by several nights of a mere 4 hours in bed. During the sleep-debt stage, the men's glucose clearance was impaired as much as a person with type 2 diabetes –

indicating that sleep debt could lead to insulin resistance and obesity. In all the afternoons that followed a sleep-deprived night, the men also had consistently elevated levels of cortisol – which, as you know, encourages your cells to store more fat, particularly when paired with insulin resistance. Not to mention the fact that levels of thyroid hormone, the metabolism powerhouse, were lowered during sleep deprivation.

**Don't join your husband for a beer.** Men may get beer bellies, but when women drink, they get Buddha bellies, says Dr. Gillespie.

A woman's stomach empties slower than a man's, especially when it comes to alcohol. That means that we get much higher blood alcohol levels than men from the same amount of alcohol. Not good, she says, since alcohol is associated specifically with increasing deep abdominal fat, which your lowered oestrogen is already predisposing you to store when you go through the menopause.

(Not to mention that alcohol reduces control, so after a drink or two you're more inclined to order those deep-fried potato skins with extra sour cream.)

**Keep a wellness journal.** Write down your meals, exercise and moods every day, even if you only have time for one sentence. "At the end of every week, you can look back at your entries, identify destructive patterns and prepare to avoid or better cope with those stressors the next time," says Dr. Peeke. For example, if you have a stressful encounter coming up, schedule in a walk right after the meeting, rather than anaesthetizing yourself with a bag of crisps.

## Coach Your Hormones into Shape

Lacing up your trainers is virtually a call to action for the hormones that reverse fat storage and curb eating. On the other hand, exercise squelches appetite-stimulating peptides and fat-storage mechanisms – which is probably the best reason for you to learn to like it.

"Your muscles are loaded with insulin receptors," says Dr. Northrup. "The more muscle mass you have and the more heat you generate from your muscles on a regular basis, the more efficiently you'll burn carbohydrates and body fat."

To make the time you spend sweating as efficient *and* hormone friendly as possible, follow this expert advice.

**If you're obese:** Start with breath work. The idea of balancing on those racing seats of the fitness bike may be a little daunting. But even non-exercisers can give their lungs a workout, says Dr. Gillespie.

A tai chi or yoga class is a great way to start, but you can reap immediate benefits by doing the "ha" breath every day: hold on to the back of a stable chair in case you get dizzy. Now let your belly balloon out as far as it can while you slowly inhale through your nose. On the exhale, exclaim "ha!" as you let your navel be sucked in towards your spine. Work up to doing seven ha breaths or more in a row daily. If you're tingling all over, you've increased your oxygen level – and probably toned up your abdominal muscles in the process.

**If you're moderately overweight:** Focus on steady, low-intensity exercise. You don't have to run marathons. Research indicates that people who are 20 per cent overweight can benefit from low-intensity exercise, such as walking at 2 miles per hour for 30 minutes a day for at least 5 days a week.

**If you're trying to lose your belly fat:** Pick up the pace. Thanks to your hormones, your belly is usually the first place to fill out and the last place to tone up. But it's not impossible. You need to do rigorous exercise for approximately 30 minutes a day to reduce the layers of adipose tissue (fat) wrapping around your abdominal organs. At the least, that means walking at 4 miles per hour for 30 minutes a day.

## ON THE WEB & Other Resources

For information and advice on all aspects of diet go to:
**British Dietetic Association**
*www.bda.uk.com*

To learn more about the latest American thinking on nutrition and weight loss, write to:
**American Dietetic Association**
216 West Jackson Boulevard
Chicago, IL 60606-6995
(800) 366-1655
*www.eatright.org*
*hotline@eatright.org*

For discussion of topical food issues and general food-related advice, see:
**Food Standards Agency**
*www.foodstandards.gov.uk*

**The British Medical Association** gives advice to patients with weight problems through its publishing group:
*www.bmj.com*

For science-based information on obesity, weight control and nutrition (the site offers fact sheets, biocharts and other publications as well as a list of weight loss and weight control associations and resources):
*www.niddk.nih.gov/health/nutrit/win.htm*

OTHER SOURCES
If you're struggling to maintain a healthy diet and lifestyle, getting support and information may help you reach your goal. Try looking at:
*www.weightloss.about.com*

"If you prefer tennis, you need to play several games in a row to significantly shrink your belly," says Dr. Gillespie. She also suggests adding skipping to your regular exercise, and anything else you gravitate towards that gets you breathing heavily. "And remember to warm up slowly and stretch before and after vigorous exercise," she adds.

**If you want to lose weight all over:** Lift weights. Muscles are your calorie-burning furnace, so the better you maintain them, the higher you keep your metabolic rate. "The truth is, weight training is essential for women over 40 to compensate for the decreased muscle mass from falling hormones, not to mention the best guard against osteoporosis," says Dr. Peeke. So if you hate to exercise, using weights gives you a lot of value since you actually burn extra calories for hours after you put down the weights.

If you're new to weight training, hire a personal trainer or buy 1½-, 2½- and 3½-kg (3-, 5- and 8-pound) weights and a video that will safely take you through a weight-training routine, complete with warmup and cooldown.

**If you want to maintain your current weight:** Burn 400 calories a day. That's how many calories were dropped through exercise by women who maintained a substantial weight loss for more than 3 years, according to the US National Weight Control Registry. That's also the number of calories that you need to lose to prevent the metabolism-slowing effects of declining growth hormones as you age, adds Dr. Peeke.

Some ways to make the grade: 45 minutes of digging a garden, inline skating for an hour, 1½ hours at the dance club, or 2 hours of steady housecleaning (washing windows, sweeping, mopping, vacuuming, carrying clothes baskets up stairs).

**If you want to avoid weight gain on holiday or while travelling on business:** Think ahead, and book a room with a hotel that has a gym or a pool. (That means you have to remember to pack your trainers and swimsuit.) Even if you're on a business trip, make your downtime something that's fun *and* physical. Look for opportunities like climbing the lookout tower at a scenic point, renting a bicycle – or be a *real* tourist and paddleboat in the park (who else does those things!).

## Trick Your Weight-Control Hormones with Food

The human body was designed with more mechanisms to protect you from starvation than to make you look good in your little black dress. If you eat randomly, you're more inclined to put on weight, as hormones like NPY, galanin and out-of-control insulin coax you into eating oversized portions of rich foods.

## The Hormone-Harmonizing Mini-Meal Plan

Instead of eating three big meals a day – plus random snacks – eat five or six smaller meals spaced out evenly throughout the day. Keep each meal between 250 and 350 calories.

"By eating smaller yet more frequent meals, with correct proportions of protein, fat and carbohydrate, you are directly manipulating your hormones in favour of reaching the weight you want," says Dr. Redmond.
Here's why it works.

- *You aren't as affected by fat when you don't eat it all at once. Your body can tolerate a rise in fat levels between 10 and 30 per cent and still keep insulin, glucose and corticosterone levels low, but if you eat more than 30 per cent fat at a single sitting, you end up with elevated blood sugar and more fat storage.*
- *Spreading small calorie loads throughout the course of a day will trigger growth hormone and keep its levels high. Growth hormone is a lead hormone in keeping your metabolism efficient.*
- *Regular meals (in a protein-rich plan) will keep glucagon stoked so your fat-burning furnace stays on.*
- *In what's known as the second-meal effect, the closer one small meal is to the next, the less your glucose levels will soar, which means lower insulin on a regular basis.*
- *Small meals relieve stress on your body, as evidenced by lower cortisol and cholesterol levels, making it easier for your stomach to empty.*

Some practical tips for success:

**Make your schedule sacred.** "Eating breakfast is the single greatest factor in maintaining portion control and stable hormone levels throughout the day," says Dr. Redmond. "People with 'morning anorexia' – who aren't hungry in the morning but feel hungrier as the day goes on and culminate their day with a giant and often late-night dinner – really put on the pounds."

To counteract that tendency, be sure to eat some breakfast before 9 a.m., emphasizes Dr. Peeke. That way, you can fit in five meals by 7 p.m. Calories eaten after 7 p.m. are more inclined to stick to your tummy and thighs since your metabolic rate slows down while you're sleeping. In fact, by the time you reach menopause, it's 15 per cent lower during sleep. And the later you eat complex carbohydrates, the more weight you gain, says Dr. Peeke.

**Redefine "breakfast".** Kick-starting your mini-meal plan doesn't mean grabbing a Pop Tart on the way to the bus. Instead, think fruits, vegetables – and, yes, protein. If you eat carbs, make sure they are low-glycaemic rather than high-glycaemic choices (pumpernickel or oat bran bread, instead of white

## THE HORMONE ZONE
# A HORMONE-FRIENDLY MENU PLAN

It's not only possible but *pleasurable* to master an eating plan that gets or keeps you slim while staving off weight-gain hormone effects. The following sample menu summarizes what experts recommend you eat and when in order to balance protein, carbohydrates and fats in the right proportions throughout the day.

### FOODS TO ADD

- Breakfast (before 9 a.m.): two soft-boiled eggs, vegetarian sausage, and some fresh fruit or porridge with low-fat milk and peppermint tea

- Midmorning snack (around 10 a.m.): vanilla yoghurt with cinnamon stirred in, small handful of almonds

- Lunch (around noon): hearty black bean soup, grilled chicken loaded with lettuce, tomato and mustard on wholemeal roll; or chicken stir-fry, cup of chicken broth, with some basmati rice

- Afternoon snack (around 3 p.m.): energy bar that's low in fat made specifically by nutrition companies

for women, peppermint tea to gently pep you up

- Dinner (around 7 p.m.): Caprese salad starter (tomatoes, buffalo mozzarella, basil, olive oil), grilled salmon, salad, unsweetened iced tea

### FOODS TO SUBTRACT

- Breakfast (after 9 a.m.): sugary cereal, more than one cup of coffee, or doughnuts and other white-flour baked goods

- Midmorning snack: low sugar biscuits or regular biscuits, leftover birthday cake at the office

- Lunch: cream-based soup, breaded and deep-fried chicken on white roll, bowl of potato salad, fizzy drink

- Afternoon snack: energy bars that are supersized, over 250 calories, or high (over 4 grams) in sucrose and have a fat content of 10 per cent to 20 per cent; chocolate; frappuccinos; other "quick fixes"

- Dinner (late): glass of wine, selections from bread basket, pasta main course with more wine, followed by dessert

bread or fried potatoes, for example). "In fact, considering the traditional waffle, bagel, potatoes and sugar cereals that Americans eat for breakfast, I'd almost prefer people eat dinner leftovers," says Dr. Gillespie.

**Make your midmorning and midafternoon snack as important as your main meal.** If you miss a snack, you may be overly hungry for the next meal, which causes physiological and psychological stress that disrupts your hormones for the rest of the day. During business meetings you can nibble an energy bar. When travelling, save a piece of fruit and hard-boiled egg from breakfast to supplement your main meals.

**Bypass the burger bar.** Studies show that people are 1 kilogram (2.2 pounds) heavier the day after they eat at a fast food restaurant. Chances are, the times you weaken enough to order that double cheeseburger and fries are near the end of a stressful afternoon or evening, when your cortisol and adrenaline levels have been elevated all day, disrupting normal appetite, says Dr. Peeke.

To prepare for those moments, keep an emergency stash of non-perishable food with you: dried fruit, wholewheat pretzels, small bags of nuts, low-sugar cereal biscuits, bottled water – even flip-top cans of tuna or chicken with packs of mustard to mix in (don't forget utensils and plates) for when you're really ravenous.

**Become aware of portions.** "Cup your hands in front of you. That's the size of your stomach. Now, don't eat more than that at a single meal," says Dr. Northrup.

"The toughest time to eat mini-meal portions is at restaurants", where the size of an entrée (main course) seems to grow all the time, says Dr. Gillespie. "Rather than order a meal for a giant – which is what most entrées are – I order one or two appetizers (depending on their size) as my main meal, along with steamed vegetables as a side dish. If the restaurant serves bread, ask that your salad be brought with the bread so you are more occupied with your greens than with a high-glycaemic carbohydrate," she says.

**Begin every meal with a protein starter.** "My best trick to avoid overeating at any meal, especially a restaurant, is to nibble a bit of protein 10 minutes before I eat," reveals Dr. Gillespie. Doing this sends your body the right signals not to overeat since protein stimulates the production of the appetite-regulating hormones cholecystokinin and glucagon.

At home, keep cheese in your refrigerator, or keep small packages of nuts around, so you can nibble on a bit of protein before you sit down to dine, she says.

# Protein, Fat and Carbohydrates: The Key Is Balance

According to Dr. Gillespie, the ideal mix of nutrients for any given meals is roughly 40 per cent protein calories, 25 per cent fat calories and 35 per cent carbohydrate calories. But who has the time and resources to look up five times a day the number of grams of protein, fat and carbohydrate in every mouthful you eat?

"Instead, think of your plate as the face of a clock," explains Dr. Gillespie. "Fill the section between 12 and 5 o'clock with protein, the section between 8 and 12 o'clock with low-glycaemic carbohydrates, the section between 5 and 6 o'clock with a tablespoon of fat or oil such as unsalted butter – and the little space between 6 and 7 nicely holds a fat-containing food or treat." That way, you'll stay in the right range, she says.

If you're like so many women, this is going to be more protein that you may be used to eating, and fewer carbohydrates, says Dr. Gillespie. But she says most women are "carbaholics" and benefit by better balance, especially since it compensates for the hormone-driven metabolic changes that affect your weight in your menopausal years.

**Say yes to red meat twice a week.** Red meat contains conjugated linoleic acids, which are a key factor in losing weight and building muscles – that's why you don't want to knock red meat out altogether, says Dr. Gillespie. It does contain some saturated fat, though. So choose lean cuts of meat, and limit it to twice a week.

**Buy organic or hormone-free meats.** Meat that wasn't treated with growth factors actually has a much different type of saturated fat that's easier on your body, says Dr. Gillespie. Try to get wild game, like pheasant, she says. Also, your health food shop and some supermarkets have a section for orgainic non–hormonally altered meat.

**Share your protein budget with beans.** Boosting your protein is essential, but get too much of it from animal sources, and you risk stressing your kidneys. So you should spend no more than 25 per cent of your protein budget on meat, and get the other 15 per cent with beans, says Dr. Gillespie.

"At the beginning of the week, I mix up a bean salad and try to have some available for a quick mini-meal all the time," she says. Her recipe: your own favourite proportions of red beans, chickpeas and navy beans mixed with chopped white onion, fresh coriander, jalapeño and a drizzle of olive oil.

**Don't overdo soya.** Soya is wonderful for lowering your cholesterol and reducing fat in your diet, but too much of the isoflavones in tofu and other soya products can disrupt your oestrogen and your thyroid. A general rule is to stay below 40 milligrams of isoflavones a day – that's no more than 3 tablespoons of soya powder or 45 grams (1.5 ounces) of tofu.

**After 5 p.m., turn down the carbohydrates.** Avoiding carbohydrates with dinner and afterwards will set you up for a more reasonable appetite and better sugar levels the next day. You've got four other mini-meals to munch on grains and starches, says Dr. Peeke.

**Choose cheese based on calcium content, not fat.** "Weight loss in women, especially those with hormone imbalances, improves when you consume more calcium," says Dr. Gillespie. Calcium in the cheese binds with fat to form a "soap" that prevents your body from absorbing the fat in cheese and milk. "I recommend three servings of cheese per week, about 30 grams (1 ounce) each," adds Dr. Gillespie. Women should have at least 1000 milligrams of calcium per day, she adds. So go ahead and reach for the Gruyère – 30 grams (1 ounce) of it supplies you with 287 milligrams of calcium. The same amount of Cheddar is loaded with an impressive 204 milligrams of calcium.

**Focus on the right fat.** The general rule is to minimize saturated fats, go easy on polyunsaturated fats, and try to spend most of your 25 per cent fat budget on monounsaturated fats, says Dr. Peeke.

One of the easiest ways to stay in balance is to substitute unsaturated oils for solid (saturated) cooking fats. Of the oils, extra virgin olive oil and rapeseed and peanut oils are monounsaturated options, and since olive and peanut have rich flavours, you tend to use less, says Dr. Gillespie.

**Forget fat-free foods.** Compare labels of fat-free treats to their full-fat versions, and you're likely to find that in many cases the calories of fat-free foods are actually higher. That's because sugar and high-glycaemic fillers are used to make up for the fat-based ingredients. Getting your blood sugar off track can make you fatter than if you ate the fat. So fat-free foods may work against, not with, weight-control related hormones.

"My advice," says Dr. Peeke, "is to eat biscuits, crackers and cream cheese much less often, but when you do, spend your calories on the creamier, tastier real stuff."

**Indulge wisely.** If on occasion you can't say no to a baked potato with your meal, cut it in half. Make sure you also halve the servings of rice, pasta and other starchy selections.

When it comes to dessert, you deserve an occasional indulgence, but split it with everyone at the table. Or ask for a bite-size portion, says Dr. Peeke.

Again, try to take your sweet treats before 5 o'clock, when you're less vulnerable to out-of-control proportions.

"If you eat a little more protein than you're allotted," says Dr. Gillespie, "make the next meal a little lighter on it." Conversely, if you're faced with a full-size-meal occasion, focus more on vegetables at the preceding mini-meal.

**Don't fret over minor setbacks.** "If you get momentarily off track changing dietary habits, it's not a disaster," says Dr. Collins. Just take a minute to admit that you blew it, but don't get into telling yourself you have no control or are a failure. This is a lifetime plan, so you have a lifetime to practise these better habits. Say 'today is a new day', and then do your best," she says.

# CHAPTER 7

# Rein In Menstrual Discomforts

Women have always had a kind of love-hate relationship with menstruation. We take comfort in the regularity of our cycles if they're regular, and experience varying degrees of anguish when they're not. We notice all the many different influences on their pattern. Aside from months-long sabbaticals from menstruation due to pregnancy and breast-feeding, other factors – like heartbreak, any kind of stress and even weight gain or loss – can upset hormonal balance and disturb this regularity.

Most women have some pain during the first day or two of their periods. That's normal. It's due to the uterus's production of prostaglandins and prostacyclins, biochemicals that cause muscle contractions as the uterus expels the shed lining. What's *not* normal are cramps and pain that are intense enough to interfere with normal activities and that aren't relieved by aspirin or ibuprofen, says Carol Wheeler, M.D., associate professor of medicine at Brown University School of Medicine and a reproductive endocrinologist at Women and Infant's Hospital of Rhode Island, both in Providence. See a doctor. You could have fibroid tumours, endometriosis, or even pelvic inflammatory disease, a sexually transmitted disease that needs prompt treatment.

Enough irregularity and we may come to thank the day the menopause arrives and frees us from endometriosis, fibroids, cramps, or heavy bleeding.

For the 30 or so years of your reproductive life, here's what you'll need to know about menstrual discomforts.

# Uncramp Your Style

The time-honoured medications that relieve menstrual cramps are still the ones to turn to.

**Take ibuprofen, early and often.** Ibuprofen, the standard drug approach for relieving menstrual discomfort, acts directly to reduce prostaglandins, the hormones that cause pain and cramping, Dr. Wheeler says. In several studies, ibuprofen beat aspirin and acetaminophen in relieving menstrual cramps, backache and headache. Some women also say it relieves the diarrhoea and nausea that they have during the first day or two of their periods. "The trick is to take it early, and to take enough," Dr. Wheeler says. Take 400 milligrams, with food, at the onset of pain, and then every 4 to 6 hours for the first day or two of your period, not exceeding 2400 milligrams per day.

**Try birth control pills.** Because they suppress normal hormonal cycles, oral contraceptives lighten periods and reduce cramps, Dr. Wheeler says. They are an appropriate treatment when cramps are part of irregular or heavy periods.

## WHAT'S GOING ON?

If your period is out of sync, any number of things may be throwing your cycle off schedule. To help narrow down possible causes – and get back on track – do this quiz, then see your doctor.

**1. Is there no telling when your period will show up or how long it will last, even though you were regular as clockwork until recently?**
If you're in your late thirties or forties, the hormone roller coaster of perimenopause could be to blame. But you could also have some other sort of hormonal imbalance. Best to see a doctor.

**2. Have you always had some pain with your period but notice that now it's worse than ever? Have you also started to have pain during intercourse?**
You could have endometriosis. These are two of its more common symptoms.

**3. Have your periods been heavier since you had your last child, more than a year ago? Are you also extremely tired?**
Ask your doctor to check your thyroid function. Low thyroid function is not

Any kind of birth control pill will work. Ask your doctor to prescribe the lowest dose that relieves your symptoms without causing bothersome side effects.

## The "A" List of Alternatives

There's no shortage of alternative treatments for menstrual cramps. In fact, there are so many, it may be hard to figure which to try. Herbs can provide quick relief, while dietary changes may take weeks or months to show results. Here is a selection of experts' top choices. Start with whichever option suits you best or whichever combination it takes to bring relief.

**Walk it off.** Sound too simple to work? Don't knock it until you've tried it, says Marcey Shapiro, M.D., an holistic physician and herbalist in private practice in Albany, California. Walking relieves pelvic fluid congestion, often associated with cramps. Aim for a relaxed, easy walk. Make a point to swing your hips and your arms freely so your whole body, and especially your lower back, has a chance to stretch out. If it's cold outdoors, wear a coat that

uncommon after pregnancy. Get her to check your iron status, too. Both can create a vicious circle of heavy periods and fatigue.

**4. Have you had all sorts of cramping pain just within the past month? Do you also feel as though you may have the flu?**
Ask yourself if there's any chance you could have an STD. Could your partner have brought one home unbeknownst to you? See your gynaecologist. The sooner you start on an antibiotic, the less likely you are to have lingering problems.

**5. If you've had fibroids for years, have you started lately to have back pain, pain when bearing down, even constipation? Are you considering a hysterectomy?**
It might be time to do something about your fibroids. But before you decide the "something" is a hysterectomy, consider your many other options, including alternative therapies.

comes down over your hips. Breathe freely, letting your belly expand.

**Belly breathe.** Loosen your waistband, sit upright but relaxed, and use your breath to help reduce muscle spasms, Dr. Shapiro suggests. Start by exhaling a bit longer than usual, and then breathe into your belly, allowing your diaphragm to drop and your belly to expand. This helps to improve blood-flow in your abdominal cavity and softens the abdomen, relieving pain.

---

## THE HORMONE ZONE
# A PAIN-MINIMIZING MENU FOR THAT TIME OF THE MONTH

Dietary changes to eliminate menstrual cramps and pain from endometriosis or fibroids do three things, says Allan Warshowsky, M.D., an holistic gynaecologist at Beth Israel Hospital's Continuum Center for Health and Healing in New York City. They change the types of fat you eat, thereby reducing the production of inflammation-producing prostaglandins; eliminate major sources of xeno-oestrogens, hormone-mimicking chemicals found in animal fats, pesticides and some plastics; and help your liver and bowels more efficiently eliminate hormones from your body. If you have severe endometriosis or fibroids, you may need to avoid any form of red meat or poultry, whether organically produced or not.

**FOODS TO ADD**
- Salmon, sardines, mackerel, tuna
- Ground flaxseed, up to 4 tablespoons per day
- Soya foods
- Beans and other legumes
- Broccoli, cabbage, kale, Brussels sprouts, spring greens
- Olive oil
- Walnuts, pumpkin seeds and sunflower seeds

**FOODS TO SUBTRACT**
- Red meat (unless produced without hormones, antibiotics and pesticides)
- Poultry (same as above)
- Dairy products (same as above)
- Wheat and other gluten-containing grains
- Processed foods – especially margarine, crackers, snacks and baked goods – containing hydrogenated fats (trans fatty acids)
- Refined sugar and foods containing it

**Do gentle stretches.** Focus on stretches that elongate the abdominal and lower-back muscles. You'll help the uterus relax and ease the lower-back pain that often accompanies menstrual cramping.

**Give black haw a try.** This herb relaxes the uterus so well that it is also used to prevent miscarriage and to treat false labour pains, says Dr. Shapiro. Take 1 to 2 millilitres of standardized black haw tincture, three times a day, as needed for menstrual discomforts. It can be mixed with water or juice. Severe cramps may require a teaspoon dose every ½ hour for 2 to 2½ hours. If you prefer, you can mix with water or juice the same dosage of cramp bark tincture, a chemically similar herbal cousin.

**Add magnesium and calcium.** It's important to have a proper balance of both these minerals to allow muscles to relax fully, Dr. Shapiro says. Take 500 to 600 milligrams daily of each mineral throughout the month, not just when you have cramps. To avoid a laxative effect, take the two minerals at different times of day.

**Pour on the cinnamon.** Cinnamon has "warming" properties, so it's used for cramps that are also relieved by heat. Make a tea, steeping ½ teaspoon of ground cinnamon in a cup of hot water. Ginger works the same way, and is doubly helpful if you have cramps *and* nausea.

## Getting Irregular Periods Back on Track

"Normal" periods come every 21 to 35 days and last between 3 and 7 days. There are many reasons for irregular periods, including changes in body weight, emotional stress and hormone imbalances. Irregular menstrual cycles may become the norm for a few years prior to menopause as levels of cycle-regulating hormones fluctuate, Dr. Wheeler says. Younger women who have irregular cycles may have polycystic ovary syndrome (PCOS), a problem compounded by insulin resistance and too much of the male hormone testosterone. (For details on treating PCOS, see page 150.) Women who use birth control pills have lighter and more regular periods, fewer cramps and a reduced incidence of iron deficiency.

**Boost your oestrogen levels.** "If the first half of your menstrual cycle is too short, you may ovulate soon after your period ends," Dr. Wheeler says. Eating foods that contain plant oestrogens, also referred to as phyto-oestrogens, can lengthen your cycle by up to 5 days, possibly by delaying ovulation. Try adding plant oestrogens to your diet: drink 240 ml (8 fluid ounces) of soya milk a day. Or, better yet, add plant oestrogens from a variety of sources: soya and flaxseed are the best sources.

**Pump up your progesterone.** If dietary changes that add plant oestrogens don't help your problem, you could have a shortage of progesterone, Dr. Shapiro says. "Many perimenopausal women don't ovulate, and so they don't produce adequate progesterone during the second half of their menstrual cycles." Spotting the week before your period or getting your period early can be a sign of insufficient progesterone. Your doctor can prescribe Crinone, a vaginal gel, to help. (For more details on getting more progesterone, see "Which Natural Hormone Is Right for You?" on page 209.)

**Try chasteberry.** This herb, also known as vitex, naturally raises progesterone levels by increasing levels of luteinizing hormone, which is secreted

*Escape from* **HORMONE HELL**

## SHE'S SO BLOATED, SHE CAN'T ZIP UP HER TROUSERS

**Q: For the past 3 or 4 years, I've been getting so bloated premenstrually that I can't fit into my trousers. My rings, bra – even my shoes – are tight. I wake up puffy. I tried over-the-counter diuretics, and they helped initially, but now it seems my body has become dependent on them. Plus, I also have headaches and feel tired premenstrually. Are there any nondrug options I can try?**

Allen Warshwosky, M.D., a holistic gynaecologist and director of the Women's Program at Beth Israel Hospital's Continuum Center for Health and Healing in New York City and a founding member of the American Board of Holistic Medicine, replies: over time, diuretics can make a fluid retention problem worse because they deplete your body of minerals that help maintain proper fluid balance.

For quick relief, use a diuretic herb. Both dandelion leaf and corn silk are safe and effective diuretics. They can be used as tea or tincture, up to three times a day, for the 3 or 4 days when your bloating is at its worst.

Next, add magnesium and $B_6$. Both affect the body's handling of aldosterone, a hormone that causes the kidneys to retain sodium and, so, fluid. Take 400 to 500 milligrams a day of magnesium, and 50 to 100 milligrams of a $B_6$ supplement, twice a day. It's best to do this throughout your menstrual cycle, not just when you have bloating. Over time, you may be able to reduce the dosage of vitamin $B_6$ to 25 to 50 milligrams per day in the first half of your menstrual cycle, as a maintenance dose.

Ask your doctor about taking

by the pituitary gland and stimulates the ovaries to release progesterone. "I might use vitex for irregular or short periods if a woman is also having some warming trends, or even some early hot flushes, because it is a nice, cooling herb," Dr. Shapiro says. You can try chasteberry on your own – it's available from health food shops. But don't use it if you have PCOS. It can make that condition worse. Chasteberry can be used instead of progesterone. "I rarely use both of them together," Dr. Shapiro says. The usual dosage is either 40 drops of standardized extract, taken once a day or up to three times a day in water or juice, or 500-milligram capsules once or twice a day – but follow the directions on the package if you are dosing yourself.

progesterone, a reproductive system hormone that influences aldosterone regulation in the body. Use a progesterone cream that contains at least 400 milligrams of progesterone per ounce, and rub in ¼ to ½ teaspoon, twice a day, during the second half of your menstrual cycle – usually from day 15 to day 28, if you have regular cycles.

If you have problems with yeast overgrowth, use the herb chasteberry (also called vitex) instead. This herb raises progesterone levels naturally. Note that chasteberry may counteract the effectiveness of birth control pills and should not be taken if you are pregnant. Take a daily dose of 40 drops of tincture of standardized extract during the 2 weeks prior to menstruation. The drops can be taken straight, mixed with water or juice, or added to hot water to make a tea.

It's also a good idea to stay off sweets. Increased insulin levels as a result of a high-carbohydrate load cause the body to conserve salt and fluid.

The same kinds of dietary changes that reduce menstrual pain and cramps can help reduce bloating. If you have headaches and fatigue, you may also have an accumulation of toxins that your liver isn't able to metabolize and excrete. Instead of individual supplements, you can use a supplement formula that includes B vitamins, such as $B_6$, $B_{12}$, the related compounds choline and inositol; vitamin C; magnesium; herbs such as milk thistle and dandelion root; and amino acids such as methionine and cysteine.

# Help for Heavy Periods

When it comes to menstrual flow, what constitutes "heavy" can be hard to quantify. "If you soak a pad an hour for 2 hours in a row, that's a lot of bleeding," says Dr. Wheeler. "It you have to get up several times during the night to change pads because you're bleeding so much, that, too, is heavy. Those are barometers I use." Any change to heavier bleeding, even if it is a gradual change, should be brought to your doctor's attention, she adds.

**Get your iron levels checked.** Heavy bleeding can cause iron deficiency. But the opposite is also true: iron deficiency can cause heavier-than-normal menstrual bleeding, creating a vicious circle that must be stopped, Dr. Shapiro says. If your periods are heavy – and especially if you feel tired and weak, with shortness of breath and trouble concentrating – see your doctor. Iron deficiency is easy to detect and treat.

If you're truly anaemic, your doctor may initially prescribe large amounts of iron – usually in a form called ferrous sulphate. To avoid stomach upset and constipation, some doctors use a more readily absorbed form – iron succinate or iron fumarate –  in small doses several times a day. Some use liver extract, a cholesterol-free liquid that contains other nutrients also needed to rebuild blood – such as vitamins $B_6$ and $B_{12}$, folic acid, riboflavin, copper, vitamin C and protein. "This approach often resolves anaemia better than simply using iron," Dr. Shapiro says.

**While you're at it, consider getting your thyroid gland checked.** An out-of-whack thyroid gland can trigger heavy periods and irregular cycles. Additional symptoms: fatigue, cold hands and feet and dry skin. Ask your doctor for a thyroid-stimulating hormone (TSH) test. Iron deficiency interferes with proper thyroid function. Iron is needed to incorporate iodine into molecules of thyroxine to activate this major thyroid hormone. "Correcting an iron deficiency may also iron out your thyroid problems," Dr. Shapiro says.

If your doctor has ruled out a serious underlying cause for heavy flow, here's what you can try.

**Yarrow.** An astringent, this herb contains tannins, compounds that constrict blood vessels. "Yarrow is very helpful for excessive menstrual bleeding," Dr. Shapiro says. Taken for several days before the menstrual cycle begins, it serves to lessen the flow and prevent the problem of cyclic haemorrhaging. Taken during a heavy period, it can reduce flow. Make a strong tea, using about a teaspoon of yarrow tincture per cup of hot water, Dr. Shapiro recommends. Take up to three cups of tea a day.

**Red raspberry leaf.** Red raspberry leaf tea is considered a "uterine tonic",

Dr. Shapiro says. "It helps the uterus to contract fully when it needs to do that, and also to relax fully." It's used during pregnancy to prepare the uterus for labour, and can be used for menstrual pain and cramps or for heavy flow. Drink one to two cups of tea a day, throughout the month. (Use 2 tablespoons of dried leaf to 480 ml (16 fluid ounces) of water, and steep, covered, for 10 to 20 minutes.)

**Dang gui.** In China, dang gui (or dong quai) is a classic blood tonic, used to restore balance in a woman's reproductive system by toning the muscle tissue of the uterus, nourishing the blood and stimulating healthy circulation.

"Use it between periods, in the middle of the month, not while you are bleeding, since it is a uterine stimulant and can increase bleeding if taken during menstruation," Dr. Shapiro says.

The Chinese simply add a few pieces of pressed dang gui root, available from health food shops, to chicken or vegetable soup. You can also take it as a tincture (20 to 40 drops up to three times a day) or capsules (500 to 600 milligrams up to six times a day). Dang gui is not currently available as a standardized extract.

## Put an End to Endometriosis

Endometriosis occurs when tissue similar to the inside lining of the uterus, the endometrium, is found outside the uterus, in the abdominal cavity and even elsewhere in the body. In these abnormal locations, endometrial cells attach to other tissues and grow in response to hormones. They secrete prostaglandins and oestradiol, the most potent form of oestrogen, which fuel their growth even more. Pain, the main symptom of endometriosis, comes from the inflammation and fluid generated by the implanted tissue, says Richard Mabray, M.D., a gynaecologist in private practice in Victoria, Texas, with a special interest in endometriosis. (Because ibuprofen and aspirin act directly against prostaglandins, doctors will often recommend these drugs for first-line symptom relief.)

No one knows for sure what causes endometriosis. Probably most women have some degree of what's called retrograde menstruation, where some of the sloughed-off tissue comes out through fallopian tubes and enters the abdominal cavity. Usually, a woman's immune cells destroy the tissue. "Endometriosis may be one of many manifestations of more fundamental immune or metabolic disease. Once the immune, metabolic, nutritional and hormonal problems are identified and corrected, the body heals as it is designed to do," observes Dr. Mabray.

"Current research suggests that women with endometriosis have a combination of immune and endocrine problems," says Wayne Konetzki, M.D., a doctor of internal medicine in Waukesha, Wisconsin, and member of the advisory board of the Endometriosis Association. "Some women actually seem to be allergic to their own hormones – especially luteinizing hormone, but also oestrogen and progesterone," Dr. Konetzki says. "Some also have problems with sensitivity to *Candida albicans*, an opportunistic yeast. They have antibodies to the yeast, and those antibodies seem to attack ovaries as well as the yeast organisms. The yeast also generates toxins that cause bodywide symptoms in the brain and nervous system, gastrointestinal tract and immune system."

## The Drug Route

Most doctors use surgery or a variety of hormone-suppressing drugs to relieve the pain of endometriosis, shrink implanted tissue and, hopefully, improve fertility in those women who hope to have children at some point. Which drug your doctor suggests depends on the severity of your symptoms, what you've tried previously and what side effects you can tolerate.

Unfortunately, many women experience a gradual return of pain within a year of ending drug treatment. And because all the drug treatments have side effects, "it's a constant trade-off between side effects and benefits," says Mary Ellen Ballweg, executive director of the Endometriosis Association, which is headquartered in Milwaukee. "Endometriosis is a chronic, long-term disease. Women who suffer from it will often search for and try a variety of treatments over time. At some point, many women opt for surgery to remove endometrial tissue."

Although the only way to accurately diagnose endometriosis is through laparoscopic surgery, your doctor may recommend medication before surgery. Some suggest starting with oral contraceptives, which may help shrink endometrial tissue. "Remember, a laparoscopy is needed to correctly diagnose endometriosis, so taking oral contraceptives may help, but since a diagnosis has not been made, this approach may not be a good idea," Ballweg notes.

**Birth control pills.** Today oral contraceptives are the most commonly prescribed treatment for endometriosis. Numerous reports show that in most women they relieve pain to a degree comparable with other treatments. "It's been a long-standing practice among gynaecologists to keep women with endometriosis on continuous birth control pills for about a year, so they have no periods at all," Dr. Wheeler says. The Pill's effect on reducing the size of implanted tissue has not been properly evaluated, however, and there is no evidence that it improves or preserves fertility.

**Progestin alone.** Progestins are a class of compounds that produce progesterone-like effects on endometrial tissue. A large number of progestins exist, ranging from those chemically derived from progesterone, such as medroxyprogesterone acetate (MPA, or Provera), to derivatives of male hormones such as norethindrone and norgestrel. All inhibit the action of oestrogen on endometrial tissue, so they make endometrial implants shrink.

MPA, or Provera, is the progestin most likely to be used for endometriosis. Its side effects include breakthrough bleeding, nausea, fluid retention, breast tenderness and depression. All these adverse effects disappear when the drug is discontinued.

**GnRH (gonadotropin-releasing hormone) agonists.** GnRH agonists include the injectible drug goserelin (Zoladex) and the nasal sprays nafarelin (Synarel) and buserelin (Suprefact). This class of drugs works by overloading and desensitizing the pituitary gland so it eventually shuts down and stops producing hormones that stimulate the ovaries to produce oestrogen and progesterone. The result: a medical, or reversible, menopause complete with hot flushes, headaches and insomnia. But endometriosis shrinks, and pain is reduced.

Because these drugs can undermine bone density and cardiovascular health, doctors won't prescribe them for more than 6 months or so without doing what they call "add-back therapy". They add back a bit of oestrogen and progesterone, similar to the hormone replacement therapy used for menopause.

**Danazol.** A synthetic testosterone derivation marketed as Danol, danazol was the first drug approved by the Committee on Safety of Medicines specifically for the treatment of endometriosis, but its masculinizing effects have caused it to be largely replaced by the newer drugs.

Danazol suppresses normal pituitary–ovary signalling, so it suppresses oestrogen production in the ovaries. It also inhibits oestrogen production in the adrenal glands, creating a low-oestrogen, high-androgen state. This drug also lowers autoantibodies and decreases the inflammatory response to endometrial cells. While danazol causes hot flushes and other symptoms of oestrogen insufficiency, it is unlike GnRH agonists because it does not cause bone loss. However, because danazol often caused weight gain and brought about acne and some masculinizing effects, it was an unpopular choice for many women.

# Alternatives for Endometriosis

Despite a host of medical options, when asked which work better for them – drugs or surgery – women report "neither", says Ballweg. "From what I've been hearing, alternative therapies, dietary changes and the newer immunotherapies – such as treating *Candida albicans* sensitivity – work best." (For more information on these alternatives, see "On the Web & Other Resources" on page 133.)

Doctors who provide alternative, or complementary, medicine approach endometriosis treatment differently, Dr. Mabray says. They may use the hard-hitting drugs, if need be. But they look at how the whole body functions and address hormone imbalances, allergies and fungal problems, and nutrition. They may try to help a woman rid her body of excess oestrogen through dietary changes and by avoiding exposure to xeno-oestrogens – hormone-mimicking chemicals (also called hormonally active chemicals). They also may recommend a liver detoxification programme since the liver breaks down hormones for excretion from the body. And these doctors tackle the immune dysfunction and inflammation that accompany endometriosis with anti-inflammatory herbs and dietary changes that dampen the body's production of inflammation-producing prostaglandins. Here are the details.

**Don't give yeast a chance.** Chronic yeast infections – in the gastrointestinal tract and the vagina – are common in women with endometriosis. The antibodies women develop to the yeast seem to cause a cross-reaction that spurs on endometriosis, and the toxins produced by the yeast suppress the immune system and cause other problems, Dr. Konetzki says.

"Although there may be actual infection, more often there's a covert yeast problem. Women with endometriosis tend to have increased yeast sensitivity. Because it is not usually an overt infection, some doctors may tend to overlook the possibility of the yeast factor," notes Dr. Mabray.

Treatment for yeast is complex: it involves yeast-killing drugs such as nystatin (Nystan). (Dr. Konetzki finds the powder form of nystatin most helpful.) It may involve desensitizing injections or oral drops. And to be effective, it must be accompanied by a strict diet that eliminates refined sugar, and strictly limits yeast and its products, Dr. Konetzki says.

**Do a fat exchange.** Cut back on saturated fats – those that harden at room temperature – and add more omega-3 and omega-6 fatty acids to your diet, says Allan Warshowsky, M.D., an holistic gynaecologist at Beth Israel Hospital's Continuum Center for Health and Healing in New York City. The easiest way to do this: switch to low-fat meat and dairy products or cut out meat and dairy foods altogether. "I advise women who have severe hormonal imbalances to avoid all animal and dairy products," notes Dr. Warshowsky. Eat cold-water deep-sea fish – such as salmon, cod, or halibut – three times a week. Tuna is another option, but it should be eaten in more limited amounts due to recent concerns that it may be high in mercury. Add flaxseed, olive oil and walnuts to your diet.

**Be a cabbage head.** Cabbage, broccoli, kale, Brussels sprouts – cruciferous vegetables – contain indole-3-carbonyl, a compound that helps your liver break down oestrogen, Dr. Warshowsky says. In fact, this compound is so powerful it is currently under development as an anticancer supplement. How much of these vegetables should you eat? More than you probably do now. "I would recommend at least one serving of these healthy vegetables daily," Dr. Warshowsky advises.

**Choose organically raised meat, poultry and dairy products.** Since xeno-oestrogens are fat soluble, they're concentrated in animal fat as it moves up the food chain. So the best way to avoid them is to avoid eating meat and poultry, Dr. Warshowsky says. If you must eat some meat, use hormone-free, antibiotic-free brands. "I believe antibiotic residues in meat also have adverse hormonal effects," Dr. Warshowsky says. (For information on finding hormone-free, antibiotic-free meat, see "Week 5: If You Eat Meat, Buy Organic" on page 270.)

**Give your liver some TLC.** The liver breaks down hormones so they can be eliminated from the body in bile. To help it do that, Dr. Warshowsky uses "lipotropic factors" that prevent fatty build-up in the liver. These include the B vitamins $B_6$ and $B_{12}$, related compounds such as choline and inositol, vitamin C, magnesium, herbs such as milk thistle and dandelion root, and amino acids such as methionine and cysteine, which supply sulphur to the liver. Sulphur supports healthy liver detoxification. To find dosages that are right for you, consult a practitioner who is well-versed in nutritional therapy.

Along with this goes a very high fibre diet. "Fibre sequesters bile so it is not reabsorbed into the body," Dr. Warshowsky says. Excess hormones are excreted with bile and then get flushed down the toilet. "Increased fibre also helps to keep the favourable intestinal bacteria healthy and happy, which helps with hormone excretion. The extra fibre also keeps you regular – having at least one bowel movement a day," Dr. Warshowsky explains.

**Use anti-inflammatory herbs.** Dr. Warshowsky's favourites: two Indian, or Ayurvedic, herbs: turmeric and boswellia. Both have strong anti-inflammatory properties. They inhibit leukotrienes and prostaglandins, biochemicals involved in generating inflammation in the body. They also have liver-protecting properties, Dr. Warshowsky says. The active ingredient in turmeric, curcumin, may also inhibit some effects of growth hormone, another hormone implicated in endometriosis.

For standardized turmeric extract, the dosage is one 450-milligram capsule three times a day. For boswellia, the dosage is three 400-milligram capsules of standardized extract two or three times a day. Dr. Warshowsky recommends use of both these herbs as part of an anti-inflammatory formula, available in health food shops. Some brands may also contain ginger.

## THE HORMONE CONNECTION
# NEW DRUG MAY MAKE HAVING PERIODS OPTIONAL

Ever since the Pill was introduced in 1960, gynaecologists have used it to control women's cycles. Instead of taking the seven blank pills at the end of the pack, which allow the uterine lining to shed, a woman can start a new pack, taking hormone-containing pills. That way she can delay her period for a week – say, while she's on holiday – or even skip it altogether that month, with no apparent ill effects, according to Freedolph Anderson, M.D., director of clinical research at the Technical Development Center at Eastern Virginia Medical College in Norfolk, Virginia.

So it's little surprise that two prescription pills have been developed that do exactly the same thing. Called Seasonale Low and Seasonale Ultra-Low in America, the new medications contain two different strengths of ethinyl oestradiol and levonorgoestrel. With either version, it's a packet of pills you take every day for 12 weeks, and then 1 week of blanks. Instead of having 13 periods a year, you have four. If the European Medicines Commission approval proceeds as expected, these pills could be on pharmacy shelves soon.

Seasonale pills may have real health advantages too. For women with endometriosis, PMS, or polycystic ovary syndrome, whose symptoms are exacerbated by cyclical hormone changes, the continuous pill could mean relief. Others should weigh the risk of exposure to 9 extra weeks of oestrogen a year – and a theoretical rise in risk of breast cancer – against the benefit of convenience.

# Fed Up with Fibroids?

Fibroid tumours are simply muscle cells gone wrong. They result from over-growth of uterine smooth-muscle cells, which mutate and then grow to form dense "balls" of fibrous tissue.

Essentially, fibroids can grow anywhere within the uterus. Sometimes they appear within the thick, muscular wall of the uterus, other times just below the endometrium, and from there they can then protrude into the uterine cavity. Sometimes they grow on the outer walls of the uterus. They can be as small as a pea or a big as a melon. They can be symptom-less, or they can cause menstrual bleeding, pressure or pain, constipation, urinary frequency, or uterine prolapse, which is a condition where the uterus becomes displaced downwards, protruding into, or even out of, the vagina.

Fibroids seem to "run in the family," says William Parker, M.D., profes-sor of obstetrics and gynaecology at UCLA–Santa Monica. A genetic muta-tion starts the uterine muscle cells off in the wrong direction, and once that happens, the cells may become more responsive to hormones, Dr. Parker says. Too much oestrogen, or an imbalance of oestrogen to proges-terone, can fuel their growth. But so, apparently, may too much progesterone, or high levels of glucose or insulin. This is controversial.

Among drug treatments, GnRH agonists, also used for endometriosis, are often first tried if fibroids grow large enough to cause pain, or to shrink them prior to surgery to remove them. These drugs – Zoladex, Synarel and Suprefact – shut down the ovaries, inducing reversible menopause, and can also cause hot flushes, headaches and insomnia. Other side effects can include irreversible osteoporosis and memory problems. They are generally used for no more than 6 months at a time.

Most fibroids can be removed surgically, in a procedure called myomectomy. There are three basic forms of this surgery, including surgery done via "keyholes", laparoscopic surgery, and endoscopic surgery, which is done with a fibre-optic tool called a hysteroscope that is inserted into the uterus. Another procedure, called uter-ine artery embolization, uses tiny plastic pellets to block the blood supply to the fibroids and cause them to die. There are pros and cons to each type of surgery, and many details you and your doctor will want to consider, before you make a final decision. In any case, do your homework. "Know your options early, before your fibroids become so large or bothersome that you'll do anything to be rid of them," urges Carla Dionne, director of the National Uterine Fibroids Foundation in Camarillo, California.

# The Alternative Route to Fibroid Relief

There are no easy, reliable alternatives to shrink fibroids with natural medicine, but a combination of dietary changes, herbs and lifestyle changes can help reduce their growth and relieve pain and abnormal bleeding, Dr. Warshowsky says. Some women may use fibroid-shrinking drugs initially, then rely on alternative therapies to control further fibroid growth. Here are the details.

**Perimenopausal? Add progesterone.** Fibroids tend to grow faster when oestrogen in the body is unopposed by progesterone, Dr. Warshowsky says. He prescribes progesterone and may recommend it be applied as a cream or gel. "The transdermal route is easy, but you can't always get enough progesterone in that way," he says. If this is the case, an injection (Gestone) is your only choice in the UK. Progesterone cream is sold over the counter at health food shops and over the Internet.

**Follow a hormone-balancing diet.** Eliminate animal protein, sugar and, in some cases, flour products, Dr. Warshowsky recommends. Add fish, such as salmon, tuna and sardines; flax and pumpkin seeds; green leafy vegetables such as kale and spring greens; and soya. (For more details, see "A Pain-Minimizing Menu for That Time of the Month" on page 120.)

**Consider calcium D-glucarate.** This is a nutritional supplement, available at health food shops or through a naturopathic doctor. "Calcium D-glucarate enhances the chemical processes that makes certain hormones, such as oestrogen and androgens, more water soluble," Dr. Shapiro says. "That way, it helps your liver to metabolize and excrete excess hormones and toxins found in tobacco smoke, pesticides and other chemicals." She suggests taking 500 milligrams twice a day.

**Use nutrients to your advantage.** The same nutrients that are helpful for so many other menstrual and hormone-related conditions can reduce the pain, cramps and excess bleeding of fibroids, Dr. Warshowsky says. B vitamins such as $B_6$ and $B_{12}$, magnesium and zinc help to ensure that all systems are functional, including the systems that break down and remove excess hormones from your body. Bioflavonoids and quercetin, plant nutrients that help stabilize and strengthen capillaries, are also helpful, he says. Take 500 milligrams of a bioflavonoid mix that contains quercetin (available at health food shops) twice a day for as long as needed to reduce the heavy bleeding that can occur with fibroids. "There do not seem to be any increased negative effects with prolonged use," Dr. Warshowsky notes.

**Try hydrotherapy.** An old-time remedy for lots of "female problems" is alternating hot and cold baths, Dr. Warshowsky says. The baths are supposed to increase bloodflow through the pelvic area, relieving congestion, and are still a big part of Chinese medicine, which holds that the baths restore "energy flow" through the body. You sit in as hot a bath as you can tolerate for 3 minutes, then sit for 30 seconds in another bath, which contains ice cubes. Do three rounds of both baths, several times a week. "If you don't have two tubs, purchase a galvanized metal tub to use," Dr. Warshowsky suggests. If you have heart or digestive problems or high blood pressure, don't take a cold bath without first seeking your physician's advice.

**Take a yarrow soak.** If the idea of ice cubes gives you chills, try another type of bath instead, Dr. Shapiro suggests. Make a strong infusion of yarrow. Steep about 100 grams (4 ounces) of the dried herb in a litre (1¾ pints) of freshly boiled water, covered, for about 20 minutes. Strain and add to your bathwater. Plan on parking yourself in the tub for about 20 minutes. "Yarrow acts as a pelvic decongestant, so it's a helpful addition to your treatment," she says.

**Slap on a castor oil pack.** In naturopathic medicine, castor oil is considered to have special properties, Dr. Warshowsky says. "It's thought to help draw the lymphatic system, so it's considered helpful to draw out infection and to move stagnant blood," he says. To test its healing properties for fibroids, use cold-pressed castor oil, a wool flannel cloth, a piece of plastic and a cloth-covered heating pad. Fold the cloth into four layers and saturate it with the oil. Lie down, place the cloth over your lower abdomen, cover it with the plastic, and then apply the heating pad, set to a moderate heat. Leave it on for at least 20 minutes, or as long as an hour. Try to do this for three consecutive days per week.

## ON THE WEB & Other Resources

If menstrual discomforts are making your life miserable, you have lots of company. Look for leaflets at your GP surgery, local gynaecology clinic or chemist.

For further information on endometriosis, contact:
**The National Endometriosis Society**
Suite 50, Westminster Palace Gardens,
1–7 Artillery Row, London SWIP IRL
Tel: 0207 222 2776

**Simply Holistic Endometriosis Trust**
Red Hall Lodge, Bracebridge Heath,
Lincs LN4 2JT
Tel: 01522 51992
*shetrust@shetrust.org.uk*

# CHAPTER 8

# Create More Love, Sex and Intimacy

Say the word "hormones" and lots of people will reply "sex". That's our strongest association. And it's true – hormones pretty much mould our sexual selves. In the womb, embryonic exposure to hormones determines sex (and perhaps even sexual orientation). At conception, every embryo starts out as a female and, unless hormonally altered, will remain so. Testosterone turns a foetus with a Y chromosome into a boy, converting into testes tissues that would otherwise become ovaries.

And it's not just the sex organs that are affected by foetal exposure to sex hormones. The brain, bones, muscles – every cell in the body is "primed" by this early exposure so that later, in adolescence, the same cells can respond when the body starts to crank up production of sex hormones.

The ability to reproduce depends on a whole orchestration of hormones, with the brain's hypothalamus and pituitary conducting. We need follicle-stimulating and luteinizing hormones to ripen and release an egg, and oestrogen and progesterone to prime the uterus for conception. (For more details, see chapter 9.)

And, whether sex leads to reproduction or not, there's evidence that sexual attraction, or drive, is hormone-based. Hormones circulating in our own bodies make us more or less receptive to the idea of sex, even if we decide the next morning it was a very bad idea. And as those hormones are metabolized, or broken down, in our bodies, we are also producing odourless airborne chemicals called pheromones that can have a subtle influence on those around us. We might like to think that humans have evolved beyond this point, but recent findings suggest just the opposite.

## WHAT'S GOING ON?

Among any group of couples, there are as many reasons for a flagging sex drive as there are men and women in the room. Some are hormonal. To help analyse your situation, do this quick quiz.

**1. Do you seldom think about sex these days and can't remember the last time you imagined the man in your life wearing nothing but a come-hither look?**
Testosterone levels in women drop by half between the ages of 20 and 40, and an additional 30 to 50 per cent with the onset of the menopause. Low testosterone does the same thing in women as in men – makes them think less about sex and have fewer fantasies about physical intimacy.

**2. Do you find that as much as you appreciate your main squeeze, you don't *crave* him? Do you initiate lovemaking less than you used to?**
Low testosterone levels may also inhibit your willingness to take the initiative.

**3. Does it take you a long time to become lubricated and aroused even with stimulation?**
Mention this to your doctor. You need adequate levels of both oestrogen and testosterone to get physically revved up for sex.

**4. Are you less likely than in the past to have an orgasm – even when you stimulate yourself? And when you do have one, is it only a tremor, and not an earthquake?**
Both the ability to reach orgasm and its level of intensity are influenced by hormone levels. Here again, it's mostly testosterone that's orchestrating the act. Added amounts may help.

**5. You're taking hormone replacement therapy (HRT), and when you first started it, you felt the spark rekindle. But now, 6 months later, are you wondering where that flame went?**
HRT and oral contraceptives may actually make less testosterone available for use in the body. A change in prescription may be in order.

Researchers at Rockefeller University in New York City and Yale University have isolated a human gene that they believe encodes for a pheromone receptor in the mucous lining of the nose. (A receptor is a patch on the surface of a cell that binds with specific molecules, like a lock that accepts only a specific key.)

Pheromones act on us at a primitive, subconscious level to influence behaviour and hormonal balance. For instance, the menstrual cycles of women exposed regularly to male pheromones are more likely to be regular. In one study, fresh male pheromones were dabbed on the upper lip of seven women with irregular menstrual cycles of 26 to 33 days. After 3 months, the average length of the cycles approached 29.5 days, the optimal length, associated with highest fertility. The researchers concluded that the male essence – derived from unwashed armpits – contained at least one pheromone that helps to promote reproductive health.

Women living together tend to synchronize menstrual cycles. Researchers at the University of Chicago found that armpit secretions from women in the late follicular phase of the menstrual cycle (shortly before ovulation) accelerated the preovulatory surge of luteinizing hormone of their roommates and shortened their menstrual cycles. Armpit compounds from the same "donors" that were collected later in the menstrual cycle (at ovulation) had the opposite effect: they *delayed* the luteinizing hormone surge of the roommates and lengthened their menstrual cycles.

The evolutionary advantage to this synchrony isn't clear, says Meredith F. Small, Ph.D., author of *What's Love Got to Do with It?* In the past, it might have promoted shared infant care or perhaps have increased male–male competition, she says. "But since we know little about the communal living conditions of our ancestors, it is still a mystery why some women are able to have such a driving effect on their close associates."

## What *Does* Love Have to Do with It?

Even what we call "love" – a mix of sex, kinship and defence behaviours called "bonding behaviour" in animals – has hormonal origins. Whether a species is monogamous or promiscuous, whether animals of the species nurture their young, protect their turf, bring home the bacon – or the worm or the wildebeest – all such behaviours have been associated with hormone levels. Bonding behaviour is particularly distinct in some animals. Birds tend to display it, and so do American prairie voles, creatures that have the distinction of being one of few monogamous species of rodents. But long-term bonding behaviour also seems to be operational in some primates, and, of course, as a species, humans form long-term pair bonds.

In both, the behaviour is related to oxytocin, the hormone that stimulates labour in pregnancy. Oxytocin has been thought of as an "affiliation" hormone because research on non-human mammals has demonstrated that it plays a key role in the initiation of maternal behaviour and the formation of adult pair bonds. A study published by researchers at the University of California, San Francisco, found that elevated oxytocin levels are associated with the ability to maintain good interpersonal relationships. Perhaps not so incidentally, oxytocin is also released during orgasm.

Males of our species may need oxytocin to stick around and do the right thing after birth because they probably aren't going to be "seeing any action" for a while. If a new mother is breastfeeding, high levels of prolactin, the milk-producing hormone, inhibit ovulation and possibly lessen sex drive for a while. Just knowing what's going on hormonally – and that it is a temporary situation – is enough to avert problems for many couples.

## The Main Player – Androgens

For both men and women, the main hormones behind sex drive are androgens, the stuff that predominates in males and makes men out of boys. These hormones are synthesized in the testes and the adrenal glands, but in women they are also made in small amounts in the ovaries. They include testosterone, dehydroepiandrosterone (DHEA) and androstenedione. (Only the last one is higher in women than in men.) Testosterone is the most potent of these hormones, and the most research has been done on it. Women produce about one-tenth (or less) of the amount of testosterone that men do, but they react to it exactly the same way. They gain sexual interest and energy and seem to experience a general elevation of mood and energy levels.

Anything that decreases androgen levels in either sex lowers sex drive. Women who have had their ovaries removed, for instance, often report an abrupt decline in sex drive, as do women who have had their adrenal glands removed. Stress, illness and heavy, chronic alcohol consumption also may decrease androgen levels and, so, make sex the last thing on your mind.

The flip side to this: increasing androgen levels boosts sexual interest or desire. Giving androgens (usually testosterone) to men and women complaining of low sexual interest has been found to result in an increase in the self-reported strength of sexual desire and frequency of sexual thoughts and desire for intercourse. Supplemental testosterone causes the spontaneous return of sexual feelings and desire in women with low androgen levels due to chemotherapy or ovary removal.

Orgasm, too, is influenced by this hormone of desire, testosterone. "Women who've had their ovaries removed often complain of 'deadness' of the clitoris, and many complain of being no longer able to have orgasm no matter what the stimulation," says Judith Reichman, M.D., assistant professor of medicine at the University of California, Los Angeles, and author of *I'm Not in the Mood*. "And even if they achieve it, orgasm is shorter, more localized and less powerful," she says. Doctors who give supplemental testosterone say women report that it is easier for them to achieve orgasm.

As wonderful as testosterone may sound, more is not better. Research indicates that only some "baseline" amount is needed for desire to occur. Once that baseline is reached, increasing levels further will have no effect on desire. In women, too high a dose, over time, can lead to irritability, increased downy facial hair, acne and lowered voice – all symptoms of hormone imbalance. These effects won't develop if testosterone is given properly. Some doctors also worry about possible long-term effects of testosterone on the heart and blood vessels.

"Evidence is accumulating that low amounts of testosterone are actually very helpful for older women and may prevent osteoporosis and frailty," says Susan Rako, M.D., author *of The Hormone of Desire: The Truth about Sexuality, Menopause, and Testosterone.*

## Where Oestrogen Fits In

Oestrogen, the "girlie" hormone, is important for sex, too, but for a different reason. "It may improve a woman's attitude towards sex indirectly by preventing and relieving vaginal dryness or lack of elasticity that often makes sex painful or uncomfortable," says Barbara Bartlik, M.D., clinical assistant professor of psychiatry at Weill Medical College of Cornell University in New York City. So oestrogen helps with the female version of physical arousal: lubrication. And because it also improves bloodflow to vaginal tissues, it may improve engorgement and orgasm. Both oral and vaginally applied oestrogen does a great job of preventing postmenopausal vaginal atrophy, and there are a variety of products on the market these days to choose from. (For details, see Vaginal Dryness and Irritation on page 305.)

Oestrogen doesn't appear to contribute to sex drive or desire – the

---

**ON THE WEB** & Other Resources

| | |
|---|---|
| If you want to learn more about the fascinating effects of testosterone and other hormones on sex and sexual health, visit these Internet sites. | *Testosterone,* check out: *www.susanrako.com* |
| | To keep abreast of worldwide research in the area of testosterone replacement for women, check out information from the Jean Hailes Foundation in Australia (use the search term "testosterone") at: *www.jeanhailes.org.au* |
| For enlightening information about testosterone from Susan Rako, M.D., author of *The Hormone of Desire: The Truth About Sexuality, Menopause, and* | |

---

initial "got to have it" impulse. In fact, supplemental oestrogen is given to male sex offenders in the US to reduce sex drive. The oestrogen in hormone replacement therapy (HRT) and, especially, the higher dosages in some oral contraceptives can increase blood levels of proteins that bind to androgens, making them unavailable for use. So the use of HRT or oral contraceptives, over time, can lead to diminished sex drive, Dr. Bartlik says. "A woman may start on oestrogen and have a wonderful feeling of sexuality and psychological well-being," she says. "But then, after she's been on it for 3 months, 6 months, or a year, she starts to lose her sexual feeling. I can't say how long it takes, exactly, but somewhere down the road, she finds herself unable suddenly to function sexually." So there's good argument for adding testosterone to HRT for women who complain of lack of sexual desire.

## Progesterone: Not a Major Player

Of the female hormones, researchers know the least about progesterone and how it affects sex drive. The most commonly used synthetic progesterone, medroxyprogesterone, is also used to reduce sex drive in male sex offenders, so it is a well-known anti-androgen.

But synthetic progesterone (called progestins) may act differently than natural progesterone, Dr. Bartlik says. "Synthetic progesterone seems to have a dampening effect on sex drive in women. A main ingredient in birth control pills, it can cause a reduction in sexual desire." But one study showed that some women who took supplemental progesterone after having their ovaries removed reported an increase in sex drive with supplemental progesterone, so there may be a wide range of individual variation with this hormone.

# A Troubleshooting Guide to Sex

If you're bothered by a noticeable drop in sexual desire or arousal, testosterone may or may not be the answer. Here's what to consider first.

**If you're taking birth control pills:** You may find switching from one contraceptive pill to another of different type helps improve your sex drive. Switching from a pill with one type of progestogen to another, or switching to a lower-dose pill, or to a pill such as Trisequens that has a "three phase cycle" in the month, may make a difference. Your doctor will explain the difference between the pills to you. However, some women find that their sex drive only returns when they stop the Pill altogether.

**If you're taking an antidepressant:** The chief culprits here seem to be selective serotonin reuptake inhibitors (SSRIs). About 58 per cent of SSRI users (men and women) report sexual dysfunction when asked about it. Most often, they're taking fluoxetine (Prozac), sertraline (Lustral), fluvoxamine (Faverin) and paroxetine (Seroxat).

**If you're taking drugs to lower blood pressure:** Some blood pressure medications impair the nerve impulses and bloodflow to the genitals that normally occur during arousal. Exercise, weight loss and a diet low in sodium and high in potassium may help you reduce your dosage or get off these drugs altogether. Or your doctor might be able to put you on a blood pressure lowering drug that has fewer sexual side effects.

# Is Testosterone Right for You?

If you've ruled out other options, your doctor may consider testosterone.

A blood test can measure total testosterone, free testosterone, DHEA and other androgens that circulate in both men's and women's blood. The most accurate and useful test – a blood test – measures free, or unbound, testosterone, says Dr. Rako. That test can be used to establish a "baseline" level against which later tests can be compared. That's useful in monitoring treatment if a woman takes supplemental testosterone, to see how her blood levels are changing. But using a blood test alone to determine if a woman needs testosterone in the first place isn't particularly useful, Dr. Rako says, "because the results can be normal even when a woman is having symptoms that clearly indicate a testosterone deficiency."

## Using Testosterone Wisely

Testosterone is not approved for use in women in the UK. The US form on the market for women, Estratest, contains both oestrogen and methyltestosterone, and its labelled use is for "menopausal symptoms not responsive to oestrogen alone."

"Some doctors won't even prescribe any testosterone for women with sexual problems, for fear of lawsuits," Dr. Bartlik says. Because its long-term use in women hasn't been studied, some doctors fear that if a woman taking testosterone develops a serious illness, such as heart disease or cancer, some might blame the doctor, whether or not the illness has anything to do with testosterone.

The pill form available for women in the US but not in the UK, Estratest (made by Solvay), combines 1.25 milligrams of esterified oestrogens (extracted from pregnant mares) with 2.5 milligrams of methyltestosterone. Estratest HS is 0.625 milligrams oestrogen and 1.25 milligrams methyltestosterone. The usual regime for either dosage is one tablet daily for 21 days per month. Some doctors think the 2.5-milligram dosage of synthetic testosterone is too high for most women. And they don't particularly like giving testosterone orally because that's how it is most likely to adversely affect HDL cholesterol.

Still, use of testosterone is becoming more common in women in the US, not just for sex drive but also because studies suggest it also helps rebuild bone, restores energy and may actually protect women's hearts, Dr. Rako says. For postmenopausal women or for women who've had their ovaries removed, "there is no question that testosterone can be helpful for some women," says Mark Elliott, Ph.D., a psychologist and sex therapist at the Institute for Psychological and Sexual Health in Columbus, Ohio. For women between the ages of 40 and 55, the perimenopausal and early menopausal crowd, women who might test within a normal or low normal range but still have symptoms of low testosterone, there's some controversy over prescribing. Some doctors will, some won't, and a lot just don't know much about it. Yet, says Dr. Bartlik, "These are the women who could benefit the most from testosterone. They are the ones feeling the effects of dropping levels."

Testosterone can be "made to order" in just about any form, from a compounding pharmacist. Some doctors in the UK will prescribe a testosterone cream, with methyltestosterone or micronized testosterone, that is applied first, directly to the vulva. Then, after a week or two when this tissue has been resensitized, the cream is applied to the inside of the thighs or the wrist 5 days a week, alternating with the vulva twice a week, at a concentration that provides 0.25 to 1 milligram a day. Some women prefer to switch either to taking a fraction of a methyltestosterone pill designed for men a few times a week, a specially compounded methyltestosterone pill in dosages suitable for women, 0.25 to 1 milligram per day, or a testosterone skin patch. (In the UK these are licensed only for androgen deficiency in men.) Both patch and gel forms of testosterone for women are currently being tested in the United States.

If you're interested in finding out whether testosterone might be helpful for you, look for a reproductive endocrinologist or a gynaecologist who specializes in menopause and knows about testosterone treatments for women. You may need to look within a larger region than you normally would for a doctor. (For tips on achieving hormonal balance, see The Hormone-Balancing Programme, starting on page 258.) For more nonhormone options, try these.

**Try a herbal helper or two.** Various herbs are promoted for improving sexual drive and performance, mostly in men but some in women, too. But the herbs most likely to help women are black cohosh and chasteberry (vitex).

"In both cases, it's because they tend to normalize women's cycles, especially during perimenopause, when women are beginning to feel the effects of dwindling hormone levels," says Sarah Brewer, Bachelor of Surgery, a doctor specializing in women's medicine in Norfolk, and author of *Increase Your Sex Drive*. (For details on the use of these herbs during perimenopause, see chapter 10.)

Another herb, damiana, works very differently. It rapidly stimulates circulation and increases sensitivity of nerve endings in the clitoris and, so, may produce throbbing, tingling sensations. "It can be used for decreased genital sensitivity, loss of sex drive associated with anxiety, or difficulty achieving arousal," Dr. Brewer says. It should only be taken once or twice a week, when needed, because long-term use might affect iron absorption. Usual dosage is one 200- to 400-milligram capsule once or twice a day.

**Let your nose lead the way.** Those odourless attractants we all exude, pheromones, accumulate mostly in our armpits and groin area. You can make the most of these natural sex stimulants by not washing squeaky-clean and by not using antiperspirants and deodorants, Dr. Brewer says. Women who want to increase their own sex drive can use the male pheromone, which is available commercially, in their perfume.

**Take the aromatherapy route.** Smells have a profound effect on behaviour because they affect parts of the brain that are not "screened" first by the thinking brain. For thousands of years, humans have used smells to fan the flames of sexual desire. Cleopatra doused the sails of her ship with rose oil to let Marc Antony know she was on the way. "You can use aromatherapy to boost your own sex drive or that of your mate," Dr. Brewer says. Dilute a few drops of an essential oil with a carrier such as almond oil and rub it into your skin. Masculine oils (to be rubbed on him) include sandalwood, ginger and lemon. Feminine oils (for your use) include lavender, ylang-ylang and vanilla.

## Let's Get Physical

Hormones, pheromones and herbs may help, but they are not the answer to everyone's problems. "There are no easy answers to long-term relationship problems, chronic stress, age-related health issues," Dr. Elliott says. And for some women, as they get older, sex just isn't a priority, he says. "It might be the last thing on their mind."

If sex – sexual energy – *is* something you want to keep in your life, you may have to work at it, says Patricia Love, Ed.D., a marriage and family therapist in Austin, Texas, and co-author of *Hot Monogamy*. Here are ways to keep sexual energy alive.

**Accept responsibility for your own arousal.** Don't expect your partner to do all the work. Accept that you may need extra stimulation to become fully aroused, in the form of sexual fantasies, erotic videos, or a vibrator. "The more graciously you and your partner can accept this reality, the more harmonious and satisfying your sexual relationship will be," Dr. Love says.

**Pay attention to subtle sexual cues.** When you feel even the slightest pulse of desire, follow through on it. "If you wait for a tidal wave of passion to wash over you, you may wait a long, long time," Dr. Love says. See if you can detect any cycles of desire. Are you more receptive at a certain time of day or in a particular place? Note these times and take advantage of them, Dr. Love says.

**If it helps, set some conditions for sex, but be clear and reasonable.** Would you be more in the mood if you got a relaxing massage first? A long soak in the tub? If your husband pitched in with the housework or brushed his teeth more often? Make such requests, but be aware that a long list of "preconditions" for sex indicates unresolved issues, Dr. Love says.

**Make time for sex.** If sexual desire doesn't come to you spontaneously, you might still enjoy sex once you're aroused. But if you aren't highly motivated, you may have to deliberately schedule time for lovemaking. Make "dates" and keep them.

**Clear away anger.** Studies have shown that women react to anger with greater loss of libido than men. You may be angry because of sexual demands on you – you may begin to see your husband's attempts at "romance" as sexual pressure and possibly coercion, Dr. Elliott says. That can be especially true after you've had a baby, he says. "A woman's husband may become very insensitive to her needs for sleep, downtime,

THE HORMONE CONNECTION

## WOMEN'S HORMONES REVEAL THE STATE OF THEIR MARRIAGES

Is your marriage going to last? Only time – or perhaps an astute mother – knows for sure. But researchers at Ohio State University in Columbus have found they can gauge a couple's chances of a happy marriage by measuring hormonal changes in a woman's body.

Women whose stress hormone levels rose when they were asked to discuss the history of their relationship – how they met their spouse, what attracted them to each other, how they decided to marry – were twice as likely to be divorced a decade later as women whose stress hormone levels dropped during the discussion, says researcher Janice Kiecolt-Glaser, Ph.D. No similar relationship between stress hormones and future divorce was found among men. "Women appear to function as the barometer of distressed marriages and are in part more sensitive to negative marital interactions than men," Dr. Kiecolt-Glaser says.

She has also found that women's stress hormone levels rise during marital arguments and tend to stay high longer than those of their husbands, as women think about and relive the argument throughout the day. Evidently, men tend to "tune out" their wives during an argument, seeking to escape from the conflict. Wives, on the other hand, are more likely to criticize or demand change in the relationship. "The husband's withdrawal is acutely frustrating to these women, so they tend to stew over things," Dr. Kiecolt-Glaser says. "There is strong evidence that marital discord impacts women's health. High levels of stress hormones have been associated with weakened immune response, slow wound healing and depression." All the more reason to take steps to resolve any discord in your relationship.

etc., and completely turn her off," he says. "That's a hard hurt to heal." Your husband may have had an affair. In any case, you need to talk openly, outside of the bedroom. And if that doesn't work, see a marriage counsellor.

# CHAPTER 9

# Making Babies:

## Fertility, Conception and Birth Control

Fertility – being able to conceive and bear a child – depends on a host of hormones. The ripening and release of an egg from the ovary requires follicle-stimulating hormone (FSH) and luteinizing hormone (LH), both secreted from the brain's pituitary gland on signal from the hypothalamus. The wavelike fallopian tube movements that waft an egg along to its "date" with some lucky sperm are enhanced by oxytocin, a hormone released during orgasm. The thick, blood-rich uterine lining that can nurture a fertilized egg is prepared by oestrogen and progesterone. And the thinning of cervical mucus that allows several million sperm (including the lucky one) to enter the uterus is influenced by a peak in oestrogen just prior to ovulation.

A lot can go wrong in the process, but the two most common hormone-related fertility problems in women in their late thirties or older are failure to ovulate and failure to implant an embryo (fertilized egg). In women in their twenties and early thirties, another common problem is polycystic ovary syndrome (PCOS).

### Your Ageing Ovaries

Failure to ovulate becomes more common as a woman ages, says G. David Adamson, M.D., director of Fertility Physicians of Northern California in Palo Alto. "The ageing ovary simply doesn't respond to FSH and LH way it used to," he says. "It becomes resistant, and levels of these two hormones go up." Older eggs are harder to fertilize and less likely to properly implant in the uterus. They can contain genetic abnormalities, such as Down's syndrome. In women no longer ovulating regularly, the process is often induced

## WHAT'S GOING ON?

**While female reproductive health is only half of the fertility quotient, this short quiz can help you identify hidden hormonal factors that may influence your fertility.**

**1. Have you and your partner been having sex without using contraception for more than a year, yet you still haven't become pregnant?**
For some women, the first clue to infertility is being "careless and lucky". You don't take precautions, yet you don't get pregnant.

**2. Have you had irregular periods for the past few years and wonder if it means that you'll have trouble conceiving when you're ready to start a family?**
Irregular periods can be a sign of hormonal imbalances. So, yes, your risk for infertility is higher than normal. So have your hormonal status checked now.

**3. Have you or your husband been treated several times in the past for sexually transmitted diseases (STDs)?**
A history of STDs puts both of you at risk for infertility. (Male problems account for 30 to 40 per cent of infertility cases.) Sometimes the STD has been inadequately treated, but antibiotics, taken properly, can help prevent an infertility problem.

**4. Have you had two early miscarriages in the past year and worry about your ability to carry a baby to term?**
This is sometimes correctable. See a doctor before you try again.

**5. Do you seem to have male-pattern hair growth on your face, or excessive body hair? Does your skin still break out in spots even though you're way past puberty? Are you kind of chunky? Have you had abnormal periods since your mid-twenties?**
You should be checked for polycystic ovary syndrome, a common yet treatable cause of infertility in young women.

through the use of drugs. The eggs are retrieved via a needle passed through the vagina to the ovary, examined for quality, and, often, fertilized outside the body before being implanted in the uterus.

Some women simply can't use their own eggs. "Old eggs can really make things tough," Dr. Adamson says. Using a donor egg from a younger female often greatly improves an older woman's chances for a successful pregnancy.

Most doctors think there's not much that can be done to improve the quality of an old egg. Others, however, think the woman herself can improve its odds by providing the egg with a good "nesting site" and by getting optimal nutrition during the time an egg is maturing in the ovary.

"Fertility doctors may be able to get an older woman to ovulate, but they don't look at the total environment and they don't improve a woman's nutritional status, so they often have a high failure rate," says Serafina Corsello, M.D., director of the Corsello Centers for Integrative Medicine in New York City and Melville, New York, and author of *The Ageless Woman*.

"You can improve the quality of an older egg, but more important, you can improve the environment into which it is received, by making sure a woman has optimal levels of nutrients that are needed by the egg as its cells rapidly divide in the womb," she adds. Here's what Dr. Corsello recommends for optimal fertility.

**Try chasteberry.** This herb, also known as vitex, acts indirectly to modify the body's balance of hormones, Dr. Corsello says. "It stimulates the pituitary to increase the production of luteinizing hormone, resulting in higher levels of progesterone during the second phase of a woman's menstrual cycle, called the luteal phase," she says.

Progesterone is important for fertility because it helps to develop the thick, blood-rich uterine lining into which a fertilized egg can implant. Studies have shown an increase in progesterone levels during chasteberry therapy. Many women between the ages of 30 and 45 have a drop-off in progesterone, Dr. Corsello says. This can lead to shortened cycles and the inability to implant an egg.

Chasteberry also lowers levels of prolactin, the hormone that stimulates breast tissue to produce milk and that, in excess, can inhibit ovulation. Prolactin levels are increased during stress of any kind. In one study on breast pain, chasteberry worked as well as bromocriptine, a drug used to lower prolactin levels.

"Low progesterone and high prolactin levels may play more of a role in infertility than many realize," Dr. Corsello says. In one study, low progesterone levels and high prolactin levels were diagnosed as the cause of infertility in 62 per cent of 753 women.

Studies show that chasteberry is reasonably safe, even when taken for long periods of time, although it may reduce the effectiveness of birth control pills. While chasteberry is not generally recommended during pregnancy, it has been used to prevent miscarriage in the first trimester for women with progesterone insufficiency. "I use it in women trying to become pregnant, and then I prefer to use adequate amounts of progesterone, the natural micronized (powdered) form, to maintain the pregnancy," Dr. Corsello says. You should use chasteberry for several months before attempting to become pregnant. A standard dose is 40 drops of standardized extract once a day or one 650-milligram capsule up to three times a day.

**Add in progesterone.** "This is actually the 'pro-gestational' hormone and is very important at maintaining early pregnancy because it promotes a healthy uterine lining," Dr. Corsello says. If you're low on progesterone, you may become "pregnant" and never know it, because your fertilized egg never properly implants. Your period may come a few days late, accompanied by more painful cramps than you normally have, and be a little heavier than usual, but it was actually an early miscarriage.

Using progesterone during the second half of your menstrual cycle, as oral micronized progesterone, such as Duphaston, a prescription product, can help prevent this. You can also use a progesterone cream. If you suspect you have just become pregnant and you have miscarried before, talk to your doctor about using progesterone suppositories to elevate progesterone to a level that can maintain the pregnancy initially, Dr. Corsello says. (For fertility problems, progesterone is best used with medical supervision because it's tricky to know how much to use. Dr. Corsello relies on blood tests.)

**Get super nutrition.** Experts know more about what you should eat once you get pregnant than what you should eat while you're trying to conceive. But one thing they know for sure: a folic acid deficiency during the time of conception and shortly afterwards can cause birth defects. (There's also some evidence that folic acid deficiency can cause early miscarriage.) Doctors advise that women start taking 400 micrograms daily of folic acid 3 months before they stop using contraception and then while they are trying to conceive. The same daily dose should be continued for at least 3 months into pregnancy.

But other nutrients play important roles in fertility and conception, Dr. Corsello says. Vitamin E, for instance, was first noted to be essential because pregnant female animals with vitamin E deficiency reabsorbed their foetuses back into the uterus, preventing the animals from bearing young. Giving the animals even a single drop of vitamin E-rich wheat germ oil restored fertility. In fact, vitamin E got its scientific name, tocopherol, from Greek words that mean "to bring forth offspring".

It's best to take an all-around approach with nutrition to get all the nutrients you may need. That means eating a healthy diet that offers at least five servings of fruits and vegetables, along with whole grains and some good-quality protein, such as meats, fish, eggs and milk. If you need to, you should lose weight before you try to get pregnant. Most doctors recommend women take a prenatal vitamin supplement that meets their folic acid and vitamin E needs, along with all the other vitamins and minerals. Check the supplement's label for the percentage of the RDA of each vitamin supplied. Remember, every one is essential for life. That's the definition of a vitamin. And they are essential for creating new life.

## Polycystic Ovary Syndrome on the Rise

In young women, the leading cause of infertility is polycystic ovary syndrome (PCOS). PCOS affects about one in every 10 women of reproductive age. More often than not, a woman doesn't realize she has the condition until she seeks treatment for infertility.

PCOS gets its name from the look of the ovaries, which are covered with cysts, fluid-filled structures somewhat like blisters, that form on the ovaries' surface. Normally an ovarian follicle grows throughout the menstrual cycle, eventually releases an egg and then dissolves. When this process does not take place normally, the follicles may continue to enlarge and eventually form cysts. That's what happens with PCOS.

In addition to infertility, women with PCOS often have irregular periods, acne, oily skin and masculine-type hair growth – facial or abdominal hair. (Caucasians of northern European descent and Asian women are less likely to have unusual hair growth.) Some are overweight, and most are insulin resistant – that is, their cells won't let insulin work normally, so in many of them, both their insulin and blood sugar levels are increased, especially after eating a food or meal containing a lot of glucose.

Nobody really knows what causes PCOS, but a genetic tendency probably starts things off in the wrong direction, says Walter Futterweit, M.D., clinical professor of medicine in the division of endocrinology at Mount Sinai School of Medicine in New York City. One thing is conclusive, however, he says.

"Weight gain and insulin resistance play a key role in the perpetuation of the disease."

The woman's increased weight reduces her cells' sensitivity to insulin and causes high insulin levels. High levels of insulin, in turn, increase androgen production in the ovaries. High levels of insulin also enhance the androgens' effects, causing the masculine symptoms and, perhaps, increasing appetite and the tendency to gain weight. "Women with PCOS often say it's hard to lose weight, and in fact their body chemistry may be working against them," Dr. Futterweit says. "They get into a vicious cycle that's hard to break."

Here is what experts recommend.

**Slim down if you're overweight.** Some 50 to 60 per cent of women with PCOS are obese, and for these women, losing between 4½ and 7 kg (10 to 16 pounds) may be enough to reduce insulin resistance, normalize menstrual cycles, reduce symptoms of excess androgens, and reduce the risk of heart disease and diabetes. Plus, "even a minimal reduction in weight results in women's conceiving much more easily and having a better chance of carrying their baby to full term," Dr. Futterweit says.

Typical low-fat diets don't seem to work well for women with PCOS, says Martha McKittrick, R.D., a certified diabetes educator and dietitian with New York Presbyterian Hospital–Cornell Medical Center in New York City, who specializes in working with women with polycystic ovary syndrome. "I find many do better on a low glycaemic index diet, which means limiting the amount of carbohydrates to 45 per cent or less; sticking with high-fibre, wholegrain carbohydrates, vegetables, beans, whole fruit; and limiting juice and sugar." Many women also do better on a diet that has more protein and less refined carbohydrates than normal and that keeps blood sugar levels stable. (For more details on using diet to control diabetes, see "Eating for Insulin Control" on page 245.)

Even with these dietary changes, women with PCOS need to limit calories and take care not to eat excessive amounts of fat, especially saturated fat, McKittrick says.

**Include exercise in your programme.** Exercise goes hand-in-hand with weight loss and is the number-one tool for weight maintenance. Both aerobic exercise and weight training (to build muscle) reduce insulin resistance, which can improve other symptoms of PCOS, McKittrick says. And in fact, exercise is part of the Hormone-Balancing Programme.

**Find someone who's well-versed in PCOS.** Ask any prospective doctor, reproductive endocrinologist, gynaecologist, or nurse practitioner how much work she's done with PCOS.

**If a blood test shows you're insulin resistant, ask your doctor about insulin-sensitizing drugs.** The one used most often is metformin (Glucophage), which reduces insulin resistance and blood levels of insulin and testosterone and, so, helps limit signs of masculinity. Clinical experience also suggests that this drug can help women with PCOS become pregnant. "It's definitely worth trying for a few months before a woman turns to ovulation-inducing drugs," Dr. Futterweit says. (Doctors who treat PCOS are also awaiting approval of a new insulin-sensitizing drug, d-chiro inositol.)

**Use birth control pills.** Oral contraceptives have long been a mainstay of PCOS therapy and are still used to regulate periods, suppress excess male hormones and keep ovaries from developing more cysts, Dr. Futterweit says. Women with PCOS should avoid forms of the Pill that contain a progestin called levonorgestrel, which mimics male hormones. The best one to take contains the progestin called norgestimate (found in Cilest). Stop the pills a month or two before attempting to become pregnant.

Using birth control pills for a month or two before a round of ovulation-stimulating drugs may even increase a woman's chance of achieving pregnancy, Japanese researchers have found. They think the Pill lets the ovary "rest" and therefore provides conditions for the development of a healthier egg, with an increased pregnancy potential up to two menstrual cycles later. Using the Pill beforehand increased both fertilization rates and the number of fertilized eggs that continued to develop to the pre-embryo stage, increasing a woman's odds for pregnancy from 9 to 23 per cent.

## When Pregnancy Triggers Diabetes

Some women develop diabetes during pregnancy, or gestational diabetes. This condition is pretty much the same as type 2 (non-insulin-dependent) diabetes mellitus, and runs in families with type 2, but it usually disappears once the baby is born. (Women who develop gestational diabetes are more likely to get type 2 later in life, however.)

Testing for diabetes is scheduled 16 to 20 weeks into pregnancy because insulin resistance has increased considerably by that time, and making the diagnosis early still allows time for treatment.

"It's not just one hormone that causes problems but several, including oestrogen, human chorionic gonadotropin and cortisol," says Donald Coustan, M.D., professor and chairman of obstetrics and gynaecology at

Brown University School of Medicine in Providence, Rhode Island. The hormones make some women's cells resistant to the action of insulin, so you have elevated insulin and blood sugar levels. This action might have been helpful during humankind's early evolution; that's because during times of plentiful food, extra glucose would go to a developing foetus, rather than to Mum. But these days gestational diabetes produces extra-large babies, posing problems at delivery. (Babies aren't likely these days to die as a result of gestational diabetes, but in the old days they used to.)

Gestational diabetes is treated pretty much the same way as type 2 diabetes, except that it usually doesn't include weight loss, simply a slowing of weight gain, says Jil F. Shangraw, R.D., a clinical dietitian at Dartmouth-Hitchcock Medical Center in Lebanon, New Hampshire. "We teach women to read labels and do carbohydrate counting, and they cut back on carbohydrates and get more protein," she says. They eat three snacks and three meals a day. Each meal has protein and 45 to 70 grams of carbohydrate. Each snack has a mix of protein and 15 to 30 grams of carbohydrates (a piece of bread or fruit, two small biscuits, or 100 millilitres of ice cream contains 15 grams of carbohydrates).

The women Shangraw sees often are "juice junkies". "They know enough not to load up on soda, but they think they can drink as much juice as they want, even though it has as much sugar as soda," she says. While eating lots of sugar doesn't *cause* diabetes, it can trigger trouble in someone with a tendency toward the disease, she says.

Oral diabetes medications are generally off-limits to pregnant women because of the potential risk of foetal death or birth defects. So they have to use insulin injections to control their blood sugar if diet and exercise don't work. But, Shangraw says, "we catch it early, and dietary changes work very well for most women. Most women with gestational diabetes never have to take insulin."

## Beyond the Baby Blues: Postnatal Depression

The soaring hormones that can make a pregnant woman glow drop sharply after delivery and can take time to return to normal, says Deborah Sichel, M.D., an instructor of psychiatry at Harvard Medical School and co-author of *Women's Moods: What Every Woman Must Know about Hormones, the Brain, and Emotional Health*. The abrupt drop-off can trigger a period of anxiety, irritability and melancholy in most women 1 to 2 weeks after delivery. But some who are more sensitive to hormonal changes may over time spin off into true depression after the birth of a child. Marie Osmond of the singing Osmond family, the celebrity "poster girl" for postnatal depression, has spoken in magazines and on television of her excruciating experience with it after the birth of her seventh child, Matthew, in 1999.

The usual treatment for postnatal depression is the same as for regular depression: antidepressants. Replacement hormone therapy – oestrogen or progesterone – has been used in the past and is sometimes still used these

## ON THE WEB & Other Resources

For depression after delivery contact:
**The Association for Postnatal Illness**
145 Dawes Road
London SW6 7EB
0207 386 0868
*www.apni.org.uk*

For information about postnatal
depression, call the following number,
leave your name and address, and an
information pack will be mailed to you. Or
you can purchase a brochure, by
contacting the address below.

**Depression After Delivery (D.A.D.)**
Depression After Delivery Inc. –
 Brochure
PO Box 278
Belle Mead, NJ 08502
(800) 944-4773
*www.depressionafterdelivery.com*

For information on infertility, there are
several important addresses. They
include:

**CHILD, The National Infertility Support
Network**
Charter House
St. Leonard's Road,
Bexhill on Sea
East Sussex TN40 1JA
Tel: 01424 732361
E-mail: *office@child.org.uk*

**The British Infertility Counselling
Association (BICA)**
69 Division Street
Sheffield S1 4GE
Tel: 01342 843880
E-mail: *info@bica.net*

**The Human Fertilisation and
Embryology Authority (HEFA)**
Paxton House
30 Artillery Lane
London E1 7LS
*www.hfea.gov.uk*

**The National Fertility Association
(ISSUE)**
*www.issue.co.uk*

A private medical organization dealing
with fertility problems:
**The Bristol Centre for Reproductive
Medicine**
4 Priory Road
Clifton
Bristol BS8 1TY
Tel: 0117 902 1100
*www.ReproMED.co.uk*

As with other aspects of women's
illnesses, the BMA produce excellent
Family Doctor booklets on infertility from
all causes:
*www.bmj.com*

A useful self-help organization for PCOS
sufferers is:
**Verity**
52–54 Featherstone Street
London ECIY 8RT
*www.verity-pcos.org.uk*

days. But, Dr. Sichel says, "antidepressants work best in the long run. They help restore brain chemistry in a way that hormones can't – they treat the whole picture, not just one symptom of it. The hormones usually straighten themselves out once the antidepressant kicks in."

Here's when you may need the additional help of hormones.

**If you've had postnatal depression before and want to prevent it with your next pregnancy:** Some doctors will start a woman on an oestrogen patch shortly after delivery to help prevent the development of postnatal depression.

**If you've been taking an antidepressant and haven't improved much:** Using an oestrogen patch for a while may help the antidepressant work better, Dr. Sichel says.

**If you started taking oral contraceptives soon after delivery:** You may need to stop them. "They may not be such a good idea for a woman with post-natal depression," Dr. Sichel says. "If we then try to treat the women on the Pill with antidepressants, we find that birth control pills may actually worsen the situation." She believes it's the progestins (synthetic proges-terone) in the formula that cause the problem.

**If you're breastfeeding:** Be aware that doing so can contribute to postnatal depression, Dr. Sichel says. Women continue to have high levels of pro-lactin as long as they breastfeed, and prolactin depresses oestrogen levels. "We never tell a woman to stop breastfeeding since it's so beneficial to the baby, but we can put her on an antidepressant that is compatible for breastfeed-ing," she says. These compatible antidepressants include sertraline (Lustral), fluoxetine (Prozac) and paroxetine (Seroxat). Dr. Sichel advises that women also discard milk from the breast about 8 hours after taking an antidepres-sant since that milk tends to have the highest levels of the drug.

**If you're not just depressed but totally exhausted:** Get your thyroid hor-mone levels checked. "A fair number of women develop an underactive thy-roid after pregnancy, and low thyroid activity can cause depression or masquerade as depression," says Ricardo Fernandez, M.D., medical director of Princeton Family Care Associates in New Jersey and member of the board of Depression After Delivery (D.A.D.), a self-help group for mums. (See Web site in "On the Web & Other Resources" on page 155.) Correcting a thyroid problem also helps antidepressants work better. (See "On the Web & Other Resources" on page 77.)

# CHAPTER 10

# Perimenopause:
## The Change before The Change

**M**ost women don't just suddenly reach the menopause one day, when their menstrual periods stop permanently with no warning. Instead, they go through years when their hormone levels peak and plummet unpredictably, when their periods become erratic, shorter, or lighter, sometimes very heavy, or sometimes missed altogether. Most women have hot flushes and mood swings in varying degrees of intensity. Some develop PMS.

Now officially defined as the 2 to 8 years preceding the menopause until 1 year after the final menses, perimenopause typically begins in a woman's forties, although it may start in her thirties, with subtle hormonal changes that slowly become more exaggerated. Fluctuations of oestrogen can become extreme, with occasional elevations to levels similar to those seen during early pregnancy, followed by prolonged low levels. Some hormone-influenced health conditions – such as migraine headaches, endometriosis and fibroid tumours – get worse during this time but then often improve once a woman is in postmenopause.

Just how bad these symptoms become, or how well a woman copes with them, varies enormously from woman to woman. Some take the situation in their stride with no extraordinary measures, knowing things will eventually settle down. "Doing nothing" is always an option. But, with menopause out of the closet and more options than ever available, including safe and effective alternatives to drugs, "fewer women than ever are toughing it out," says Nanette Santoro, M.D., professor of obstetrics and gynaecology at Albert Einstein Medical School in the Bronx. "For some women, it may be a very good idea to take some hormones during this time to make it a smoother ride

(continued on page 160)

## WHAT'S GOING ON?

Changes associated with perimenopause may be subtle, dramatic, or somewhere in between. Or you may be experiencing something else entirely. Conditions not related to perimenopause – such as obesity, diabetes, thyroid disorders, or high blood pressure – often develop at midlife. Do this quick quiz to help sort out where you stand.

**1. Do you find that while your periods used to be fairly regular – now there's no telling when one will show up, or how long it'll last, or how heavy it will be?**
You're not ovulating regularly, so progesterone, the hormone that regulates the second half of your menstrual cycle (the luteal phase) is often low. That makes for all sorts of irregularities. Your menstrual cycle may shorten by as much as 3 to 7 days, perhaps as a result of ovulation occurring earlier than day 14 of your cycle. Some women may skip several cycles and then, to their amazement, return to regular cycles. Still others may have irregular spotting or regular menstrual cycles until the onset of the menopause.

That said, if your periods occur more often than every 3 weeks or if you have spotting between periods, see your doctor. The same goes if you have heavier uterine bleeding than usual, prolonged uterine bleeding (1½ to 2 times a long as your periods used to be), or bleeding after sexual intercourse.

**2. Are you feeling that as far as sex goes, you could just as soon leave it? And are quickies are pretty much out of the question because you need more time than ever to warm up?**
Levels of the female sex hormone oestrogen are falling, but so is testosterone, present in small quantities in women. Called the hormone of desire, testosterone drops by about 50 per cent in women between their twenties and their forties.

**3. Are you finding that while you've never really had a problem with PMS, now you're starting to wonder if you're making up for all those menstrual cycles when you were nice?**
Women experiencing PMS for the first time in their mid-thirties or later may actually be showing signs of perimenopause.

**4. Do you sometimes wake up in the middle of the night hot, sweaty and uncomfortable – but you're the only one in the midst of the heat wave?**

Many women have their first hot flushes at night and wake up wondering what's happening to them.

**5. Have you had prolonged bouts of tiredness and lost interest in normal activities? Are you sad and irritable?**

You may need a prescription for progesterone (identical to that made in our bodies naturally), not Prozac. Dropping hormone levels can play a role in depression, in which case hormone therapy may help. But you should see your doctor to be checked out for signs of clinical depression, a thyroid imbalance, or other possible (and treatable) causes.

**6. Do you find that lately your brain is foggy or your thinking is fuzzy and that you're just not as clearheaded as you used to be?**

Don't resign yourself to feeling out of sorts just because you may be entering perimenopause. Get your thyroid gland checked, especially if you are also feeling tired. Hypothyroidism can cause mental symptoms and amplify symptoms of perimenopause.

**7. Do you wake up most mornings thinking, "I hate my body. I can't stand what's happening to me, I'm losing my looks. This is just awful"?**

You're catastrophizing perimenopause and could probably benefit from techniques in acceptance or attitude adjustment, discussed on page 167. If you find yourself putting on weight or losing your figure, hormonal changes may indeed play a role. Turn to chapter 6 for an eating programme designed to counteract those changes.

**8. Are you and your husband at odds with each other more often lately and seem to get on each other's nerves a lot? Do you worry that he's going to head for the hills now that you're headed towards the menopause?**

Don't blame perimenopause for relationship problems. This time of transition might put things in clearer focus, thereby bringing up problems in your relationship that might have lain latent. But it will create nothing new. For relationships that are better off over, this could be the beginning of the end. For strong relationships, it will be a time to re-evaluate where you are and what you want from each other. (For details on how to talk to your husband about perimenopause, see page 169.)

than it is going to be otherwise. For short-term relief especially, hormones are a very reasonable thing to consider, and do not pose the long-term issues (such as breast cancer) that longer-term, postmenopausal hormone replacement therapy has."

There's even a potential sunny side to the situation, says Ann Webster, Ph.D., director of the Menopause/Perimenopause Program at the Mind/Body Center for Women's Health at Beth Israel Deaconess Medical Center in Boston. "This is a time of transition anyway, and with a little encouragement, women can make a lot of big changes and create a more satisfying life," she says. Getting out of a bad relationship or going back to school to finish a degree works as well as any pill at providing a psychological lift, she says. "Some women just blossom."

Women who seek out alternatives – dietary, lifestyle and the like – are likely to find that a combination of things works best for them. And since this is a time of transition, what works to make you feel better may change as your body changes, from your early forties to late forties to early fifties, says Connie Catellani, M.D., director of the Miro Center for Integrative Medicine in Evanston, Illinois. "At first, dietary and lifestyle changes may be all you need.

## THE HORMONE CONNECTION
# HIGH IQ MAY SIGNAL LATE MENOPAUSE

The cleverer you were as a kid, the later you may reach menopause, according to researchers with the Medical Research Council's National Survey of Health and Development in Britain. They've been studying about 1600 women since their birth, in 1946. Based on IQ tests taken at 8, menopause occurred by 50 in 26 per cent of the women with the lowest mental ability, 21 per cent of women with medium ability, and 16 per cent of women with the highest mental ability.

Even after the researchers took into account factors such as smoking, social class and education, the association remained.

"We know that oestrogen and other steroid hormones help programme brain development early in life," says Marcus Richards, Ph.D., of the Medical Research Council and Honorary Senior Lecturer at University College London. "So we think that measurements of mental ability early in life may provide clues to the brain's role in reproductive ageing."

But later, you might want to add in some natural hormones or herbs." But you'll reap long-term benefits as well.

"Dietary changes can help keep bones strong and prevent cancer and heart disease," says Hope Ricciotti, M.D., an obstetrician gynaecologist at Beth Israel Deaconess Medical Center in Boston and co-author of *The Menopause Cookbook: How to Eat Now and for the Rest of Your Life.* Foods like soya and flaxseed have the highest levels of phyto-oestrogens – substances in plants that are chemically similar to the hormone oestrogen in humans.

Here are experts' top recommendations for this time of life.

**Enjoy soya.** Soya contains isoflavones, a form of phyto-oestrogens. "Even though isoflavones have been isolated from soya and used to make nutritional supplements that can alleviate hot flushes, some experts still recommend getting your isoflavones from whole foods," Dr. Ricciotti says. Some data does support supplement use, especially for hot flushes, but soya foods are proven safe and may actually be more effective in the long run for cardiovascular and bone health. Research suggests that to reduce hot flushes by 40 per cent, you need to eat 85 to 110 grams (3 to 4 ounces) of soya a day. Try silken tofu or firm tofu, soya milk, or soya powder, which can be mixed into juice or water. Look for other soya products in your local health food shop.

**Help yourself to flax.** Compounds in flaxseed called lignans are also phyto-oestrogens and can do some of the same things as isoflavones, helping to smooth out hormones, Dr. Catellani says. Plus, flaxseed is a rich source of alpha linolenic acid, essential for healthy skin. (It's even fed to elephants and rhinoceroses in zoos to maintain healthy skin.) Add a tablespoon a day of flaxseeds, ground in a blender, to hot cereal or a "smoothie". Because flaxseeds can become rancid quickly, buy them in small quantities and store them in tightly covered jars in the refrigerator. Grind only as needed.

**Shore up bones with calcium and vitamin D.** You still have a bit of time to get some bone in the bank to head off low bone density or outright osteoporosis so often associated with menopause. But unless you're a big milk drinker or eat a vast amount of leafy green vegetables, you may need supplements to do so. Make sure you get the RDA – 1000 milligrams of calcium a day (more if you take steroid drugs for asthma) and 400 to 800 micrograms of vitamin D. If you're over 50, experts recommend 1200 milligrams of calcium daily.

## Get a Herbal Edge

Before you consider taking hormones for perimenopausal changes, you may want to give herbs a chance, Dr. Catellani says. The following are two favourites for perimenopause.

**Black cohosh.** Research focusing on standardized black cohosh extract has found it performs as well as synthetic oestrogen (Premarin) in reducing the physical symptoms of the menopause and is comparable with both oestrogen and diazepam (Valium) in improving psychological complaints. It is also useful for PMS, Dr. Catellani says. "It helps lessen symptoms of oestrogen

---

*Escape from* **HORMONE HELL**
## HER PERIODS ARE AWOL

**Q:** When I was in my twenties and thirties, my periods were so regular, I could virtually set my watch by them. Now that I'm 47, I never know when I'm going to menstruate. My period might come in 21 days, 45 days, or somewhere in between. Worse, I have no idea whether the flow will be light or heavy. Some months I have no period at all, sometimes it's just a spot, and other times it's heavier than ever. An unexpected spot or two, I can handle. It's gushing blood at highly inopportune times that has had me at my wit's end! There I am, standing in the queue at the grocery store, bread and milk in hand, praying that my tampon doesn't leak and leave embarrassing stains on my white shorts.

I'm tired of lugging a hodgepodge of tampons, pads and panty liners with me on every holiday, never sure what I'll need or when. I hate being on "period alert" week in and week out!

I'm grateful that I'm not experiencing hot flushes or any other perimenopausal symptoms. And my doctor has ruled out fibroids. But these "surprise menstrual periods" are not acceptable. What can I do?

Marcey Shapiro, M.D., an holistic physician and herbalist in Albany, California, replies: you're not alone! Many women your age have the same complaint. Luckily, there are several ways to smooth the hormonal fluctuations responsible for irregular periods before menopause.

Start with chasteberry. Also known as vitex, this herb normalizes the luteal phase of your cycle responsible for on-time menstruation. Try taking either a 500-milligram capsule one to two times a day or ¼ to ½ teaspoon of tincture twice a day. Give yourself a break during each period, then resume

excess and improves oestrogen deficiency symptoms. So it's very good for PMS and cramping, hot flushes, mood swings – anything that feels like something is amiss with your hormones," Dr. Catellani says. "Black cohosh would be my first choice, along with diet and lifestyle changes, for perimenopause symptoms before I tried other things."

A frequently used dosage for standardized extract of black cohosh is ½ to 1 teaspoon (60 to 120 drops) twice a day. (The standardized element in black cohosh is deoxyacteine.) In Germany, where the herb is used regularly, a drug regulatory agency considers black cohosh safe for use in women with

once it's gone.

Be patient; with chasteberry it can take up to 3 months before your periods are regular and your flow normal. Continue taking the herb until your periods seem to wind down at menopause (usually around the age of 51, on average).

Cautions and side effects are few. However, chasteberry may counteract the effectiveness of birth control pills. Some women experience nausea and headaches, especially women who tend to feel cold. If you get headaches from chasteberry, take a "warming" herb such as ginger (one or two 500-milligram capsules a day).

If you've been constantly stressed, you may suffer from adrenal burnout, which can cause an overproduction of cortisol and a drop in sex hormones. Adrenal problems can be a major cause of irregular menstrual cycles. Relaxation methods such as yoga or deep breathing can help. In addition, take the following for 3 to 6 months,

to nourish the adrenals:

**Pantothenic acid** Known to restore proper adrenal function. Take 100 milligrams two to three times a day.

**Stinging nettle tea** Used by traditional herbalists to soothe the adrenals. Use 1 tablespoon of the dried herb for every cup of water; let the herb steep for 10 minutes in hot water. Drink twice a day. You can drink this tea anytime during the day since it isn't a stimulant. If you have allergies, your symptoms may worsen, so take only one dose a day for the first few days.

**Licorice root** Thought to prolong the action of cortisol so it spares the adrenals from becoming overtaxed. Take 100 milligrams two to three times a day in tincture or capsule form. Discontinue use after 4 to 6 weeks as this herb may lead to water retention, high blood pressure caused by potassium loss, or impaired heart and kidney function.

## ON THE WEB & Other Resources

To find out about an integrated approach to perimenopause, contact:
**The British Holistic Medical Association**
59 Lansdowne Place
Hove
East Sussex BN3 1FL
E-mail: *bhma@bhma.org*

The British Wheel of Yoga exists to encourage greater knowledge and understanding of yoga. Contact the association at:
**The British Wheel of Yoga**
25 Jermyn Street
Sleaford
Lincs NG34 7RU
Tel: 01529 306851
*www.bwy.org.uk*

Loretta LaRoche, a stress management and humour consultant, is the founder of the Humor Potential. She also contributes her skills to the Perimenopause/Menopause Program at the Mind/Body Medical Institute in Boston. If you need to laugh about menopause, growing older, growing wider, or just about anything else, contact her at:
**LaRoche, Inc.**
50 Court Street
Plymouth, MA 02360
(800) 99-TADAH (998-2324)
*www.lorettalaroche.com*

The Perimenopause/Menopause Program at the Mind/Body Medical Institute at Beth Israel Deaconess Medical Center, Boston, is designed to help women cope with menopause and its symptoms. The programme focuses on healthy behaviours that can help prevent heart disease and osteoporosis.
**Mind/Body Medical Institute**
Division of Behavioral Medicine
Deaconess Hospital
1 Deaconess Road
Boston, MA 02215
*www.mbmi.org*
Click on "Medical Programs",
then scroll down and click on
"Perimenopause/Menopause Program".

OTHER SOURCES
The Yoga Site provides an extensive teacher directory covering all 50 US states and 17 foreign countries. Individual teacher listings include mailing addresses, phone numbers and e-mail addresses.
*www.yogasite.com*

Belief Net is a spiritually oriented Web site that includes information about meditation, and provides numerous links to yoga sites that specialize in online lessons. You can find it at:
*www.beliefnet.com*

Need a hot flush or PMS cartoon? Check out the selection of "Minnie Pauz" humour at cartoonist Dee Adams's Web site:
*www.minniepauz.com*

oestrogen-sensitive cancers as well as with uterine bleeding, liver or gallbladder disease, endometriosis, uterine fibroids and fibrocystic breast disease, all conditions that rule out synthetic hormone use. Since black cohosh dosages are highly individualized, talk to your health care provider about what's right for you, Dr. Catellani says.

**Chasteberry, or vitex.** This herb is likely to be used during perimenopause for irregular bleeding, whether flow is frequent or infrequent, heavy or light, long or short. "It acts on the hypothalamus and pituitary gland to stimulate the release of luteinizing hormone, resulting in higher levels of progesterone during the second phase of a woman's menstrual cycle," says Serafina Corsello, M.D., director of the Corsello Centers for Integrative Medicine in New York City and Melville, New York, and author of *The Ageless Woman.* "When there is progesterone deficiency, oestrogen continues to dominate the luteal phase of the cycle, contributing to problems such as heavy periods and PMS," she says. Studies have shown an increase in progesterone levels during chasteberry therapy. In clinical trials, chasteberry also lowered levels of a third hormone, prolactin. In excess, prolactin can cause breast tenderness, imbalances in the menstrual cycle and even infertility.

Chasteberry can be taken as a tincture, capsule, tablet, or tea. In clinical trials, the dosage used was 40 drops of standardized chasteberry extract taken once or twice a day for anywhere from 1 month to 19 months. For capsules or tablets, Dr. Corsello recommends taking one 650-milligram capsule up to three times a day or, in tincture form, 40 drops up to three times a day. When the problem is severe, Dr. Corsello recommends starting the full dosage at once. For premenstrual syndrome, she has seen results within one to two cycles. For tea, drink 1 cup 2 to 3 times a day, she says.

Use chasteberry under medical supervision, Dr. Corsello says. If you're trying to regulate menstrual cycles, you may need to have an endometrial biopsy first to rule out the possibility of endometrial cancer. It's best not to mix chasteberry with hormone replacement therapy (HRT), Dr. Corsello says. "Too little is known about how these two may interact." Be aware also that chasteberry may counteract the effectiveness of birth control pills.

## Restore Hormone Balance

Oestrogen levels during perimenopause are erratic, so measuring them is somewhat unreliable. But doctors who practise alternative medicine tend to view perimenopause as a time of relative oestrogen dominance, compared to progesterone, which tends to drop quickly and erratically during cycles when a woman does not ovulate, Dr. Catellani says. "During cycles when a woman does not ovulate, there will be relatively more oestrogen to progesterone during the second phase of the cycle. So even though both hormones are dropping, progesterone drops more, earlier."

**Try natural progesterone.** For women in their forties, who may not yet need oestrogen, natural progesterone (identical to that made in our bodies) alone may relieve hot flushes, help normalize periods and alleviate PMS-like symptoms, Dr. Catellani says.

You can use a progesterone cream that you simply rub on your arms or chest. Your doctor may be able to recommend a reliable brand. (See "Which Natural Hormone Is Right for You?" on page 209 for buying tips; not all over-the-counter brands deliver the goods. Buy only brands that say "progesterone BP".) The typical dosage is ¼ to ½ teaspoon twice a day. You can also use a pill form of progesterone, such as Duphaston, or forms available in compounding pharmacies, if you prefer, Dr. Catellani says. (Duphaston, which is micronized natural progesterone, is available by prescription only.)

If you're still having periods, you should use progesterone in a cyclic fashion, starting 10 to 12 days before your period, then stopping during the time you have your period. If PMS symptoms seem to start the minute your period ends, though, and you're "flushing" all month long, you may need to start the progesterone as soon as your period ends. If you continue to have problems with that schedule, then you can try taking a smaller dose of progesterone during the time you have your period, and a larger dose the rest of the month, Dr. Catellani says. Consult your health care provider for a personalized programme, she says.

After a few months of progesterone use, you might feel stable enough to cut back to the 12-days-a-month regimen, starting at the middle of your normal cycle.

Using progesterone during this time could also reduce your risk for endometrial hyperplasia (overgrowth of the lining of the uterus) and endometrial cancer (cancer of the uterus) by continuing to keep the oestrogen balanced, says Margery Gass, M.D., director of the University Hospital Menopause and Osteoporosis Center in Cincinnati. "We know that if a woman has a predominance of oestrogen over a long period of her life, she is going to be more prone to endometrial cancer," Dr. Gass says. "Overweight women in particular are more at risk for endometrial cancer, which may prompt a doctor to do an endometrial biopsy sooner rather than later. But if a woman is simply having a recent onset of irregular menstruation, I think it's worth trying to regulate the cycle first with a progestin (synthetic progesterone) or progesterone."

**If nothing else does the trick, add oestrogen.** Consult your doctor if you think you need oestrogen to smooth things out. Some doctors will prescribe an oestrogen patch for symptoms during this time. A recent study showed that 80 per cent of women with perimenopause-related depression who used an oestrogen skin patch had full or partial alleviation of their symptoms. If you have your uterus and use the patch, you will also need to use progesterone, and you may also need to use contraception.

**Consider oral contraceptives.** If you see a traditional doctor about perimenopausal symptoms, and you don't smoke or have problems with blood clots, you will most likely be offered a prescription for oral contraceptives, Dr. Santoro says. "A lot of doctors who treat women in perimenopause will enthusiastically prescribe oral contraceptives," she says. On the other hand, she says, "a lot of general obstetrician gynaecologists are more suspicious about their use in older women, thinking the dose is too high and that women may develop blood clots that could lead to a stroke or heart attack."

It's true that oral contraceptives used to be considered somewhat dangerous to use after the age of 35, especially in smokers, Dr. Santoro says. "But new, low-dose formulas, some with as little as 20 micrograms of oestrogen, have made oral contraceptives safer to use." The Committe on Safety of Medicines has approved them for use in nonsmokers up to the time of menopause. (The cutoff for smokers is still 35. Of course, there are plenty of other good reasons to quit smoking, regardless of what form of hormone therapy you're considering. See the smoking cessation programme in "Week 1: If You Smoke, Quit" on page 259.)

Oral contraceptives do a great job of regulating menstrual cycles during perimenopause, but they also come with their own potential side effects, which can include headaches, loss of sexual desire, breast tenderness and fluid retention. (To decide whether oral contraceptives are a good bet for you, and to figure out which one to take, see chapter 9.)

## Change What You Can – And Accept the Rest

Remember the Serenity Prayer? It says: "God, grant me the serenity to accept the things I cannot change, the courage to change the things I can, and the wisdom to know the difference." You can use it to approach everything in life, including perimenopause, Dr. Webster says. You will have to accept the fact that you're getting older, but there are lots of things you can do to make that process easier. Here's what she suggests.

**Find ways to relax.** Feeling like the stress just never ends is a sure way to make the ups and downs of perimenopause feel even worse, Dr. Webster says. The flip side: reducing your response to stress helps to reduce side effects such as hot flushes, anxiety and memory problems. "Learning ways to relax and cope with perimenopausal problems is really at the heart of our programme," Dr. Webster says, referring to the Menopause/Perimenopause Program at the Mind/Body Center for Women's Health at Beth Israel Deaconess Medical Center in Boston. There women learn a variety of ways to chill out, including something called the "relaxation response". (For instructions on how to practise the relaxation response and more ideas on how to relax, see Phase 2 of the Hormone-Balancing Programme on page 275.) They also learn breathing techniques that can cool hot flushes. (For instructions, see "Other Personal Cooling Tactics" on page 302.)

**Exercise regularly.** Schedule 30 minutes of moderate-intensity exercise a day (such as walking, jogging and biking) at least 5 days a week. Experts also recommend strength training for 20 to 30 minutes 2 to 3 days a week. It's bone in the bank, a great way to relax, sleep better, improve your mood and make you feel better about your middle-aged body, Dr. Webster says. (For specific bone-building exercises, see "Stop Osteoporosis with These Moves" on page 222. For details on how to start an exercise programme, see "Week 8: Move That Body" on page 295.)

"In particular, I recommend yoga, not only for strength but for healthy bones, joints, posture and self-esteem," Dr. Webster says. "Yoga reorganizes your energy and quiets the mind, so it's great during this time of physical change." To locate a yoga instructor in your area, see "On the Web & Other Resources" on page 164.

**Rethink your thinking.** We all have a running monologue in our heads about life, and sometimes we need to change the script, Dr. Webster says. It's a form of psychotherapy called cognitive restructuring, and it involves learning to pay attention to negative automatic thoughts, "being able to see that we make ourselves upset with some of our ways of thinking," she says. "If you walk around all day saying 'I hate my body, I can't stand what's happening to me, I don't like the way I look, this is just awful', you are not going to feel too terrific. We learn to challenge that mode of thinking. 'Is this really true? Is this thinking helping me? Is there another way I might be able to think?'" One woman in the programme, for instance, came up with this substitute "positive affirmation" to her negative thoughts: "I may not be perfect, but parts of me are excellent."

**Use that midlife crisis to your advantage.** Many women in the Menopause/Perimenopause Program no longer have children as their main focus, and wonder what's next for them, Dr. Webster says. "We have a goal-setting project where we ask them to look at eight areas of their lives and figure out what they really want," she says. The areas include career, relationships, health, creativity and spirituality. Women have decided to do things like go back to school, get divorced, buy a sports car, join an ashram, move to the country, or dye their hair red. "Seriously, the old stuff might not be relevant anymore, and if they get going in the right direction, women make a lot of big changes during this time," Dr. Webster says.

**Try "humour replacement therapy".** Finding humorous things to chuckle about isn't silly. "Studies show that laughter actually reduces blood levels of stress hormones and enhances immunity," Dr. Webster says. "It helps people to look at things from a fresh perspective, to lighten up and not take everything so seriously."

One of the best humour resources that people in the Menopause/Perimenopause Program tap into is comedian Loretta LaRoche, whose "speciality" is middle-age angst. (Imagine needing the Jaws of Life rescue apparatus to be extricated from the sexy lingerie you squeezed into, and you'll get the picture.) "The women all get fake diamond tiaras and sit around and watch one of her videotapes," Dr. Webster says.

And that diamond tiara comes in handy later when you decide to make yourself "queen" for a day, an hour, or however long it takes to make yourself feel special again and let people around you know it. (For more details on how to make better use of humour in your life, see "Week 2: Laugh It Up" on page 279.)

## How to Talk to Your Man about Perimenopause

Men and women agree: men are pretty much clueless about menopause. They may know some of the basics, but they know surprisingly little about the details. That's because in general they would rather avoid the topic.

"Most men don't want to know about menopause because it means we're getting older, too," says Dick Roth, author *of "No, It's Not Hot in Here": A Husband's Guide to Understanding Menopause.* "Even a caring husband will go into denial and try to ignore it. This can be a very emotional topic, and that makes it doubly hard for men to have a rational discussion about it."

Like many women, you may find that your husband is more comfortable joking about perimenopause (or menopause) than discussing it with you seriously.

It's okay to laugh, as long as the joke's not on you. "Laughing about 'Who turned up the heat?' can be a great opening to have a serious talk, instead of waiting for an emotional blowup," Roth says. If you want your mate to understand what you're going through, which is what many women say they want most, you're the one who'll have to bring the topic up and share your personal experience. Here's how you can get started.

**Tell him your concerns and what you are doing about them.** Your concerns might include fatigue, irritability, anxiety, sleeping problems, lack of interest in sex, irregular cycles, having to make complicated decisions about treatment, and needing to focus on taking care of yourself right now. "Your husband is not going to be able to fix this. Your body is going to do what it will," Roth says. "But your husband can listen to you, and perhaps you'll need to tell him that just listening is all you want from him right now." The payoff for you in sharing your experience, Roth says, is that "once he understands what's going on, he'll become more supportive. The sooner you can enlist his support, the better it will be for the entire menopausal transition."

**Be specific about your needs and expectations.** Most men are willing to help out, given the opportunity, Roth says. Give your mate that opportunity by telling him what you need right now, he suggests. "What you need right now may be different from what you needed an hour ago, or the same time yesterday."

If you feel overwhelmed or irritated because you do most of the housework, set a time to sit down and have a conversation about who is going to do what. "The sharing of chores can be appreciated as much as empathy and understanding, if not more. It's an important way to show love, caring and respect," Roth says. "A woman going through menopause may need more help than she used to, and that discussion needs to happen."

**Give him fair warning about your moods.** A common concern among men is that their wives are going to become terminally crabby as they approach menopause. So tell your husband what kind of mood you are in before he inadvertently sets you off, says Roth. After all, men have feelings, too.

"It really helped me when my wife could say, 'I'm really on edge right now. I'm tired. I'm in the middle of a hot flush. Will you please just not say anything right now?' Or 'I need half an hour alone. Could you make dinner?' If I knew what kind of mood she was in and what was going on inside of her, my natural desire to be helpful saved the day. When I thought she was mad at me or something, I was not the nicest person in the world."

**Be kind – and pick the right time – when talking about sex.** A big concern of men is that, with the menopause, their sex life will go south. "Reassure him that your changing feelings have to do with the menopause, not with him, if that's the case," Roth says. Are there simple things that would make sex more comfortable for you? Would you prefer more communication? More cuddling? More foreplay? Let him know, honestly and directly, preferably outside bed. At the same time, "try to stay warm and open. Try not to lose the closeness," says Mary Cerreto, Ph.D., a psychologist specializing in family relationships at Boston University Medical Center. If sex doesn't interest you, try for hugs and conversation or just spending quiet time together. "It may take conscious work to keep the closeness, to keep from drifting apart," she says.

# CHAPTER 11

# A Step-by-Step Guide to the Menopause

Over the past few generations, the average age at which girls in the United Kingdom start menstruation dropped from 14.5 to 12.10 years old, thanks mostly to better nutrition and better health. Fertility is wisely dictated by body fat – we don't become fertile until we accumulate enough body fat to incubate a growing foetus for 9 months. Well-nourished bodies reach that point earlier.

But the end of women's reproductive years has stayed relatively constant at about 51. (The normal range is 46 to 54.) Women who are in poor health, or who smoke, or who are underweight may reach that point a few years earlier. But females whose reproductive years extend much beyond the half-century point are rare.

In fact, there may be some evolutionary advantage to having older, experienced nonfertile females in the family, tribe, or community, says Meredith Small, Ph.D., a Cornell University professor of anthropology and author of *What's Love Got to Do with It?: The Evolution of Human Mating*. "It's called the Grandmother Hypothesis, and it seems that the survival rate is higher among infants whose mothers get help from *their* mothers than among mothers who don't get help," she says. This occurs in some tribal communities, but it's also the case in Western cultures too, where lots of grandmas are bringing up their kids' kids.

## The Shelf Life of Eggs

Survival of the species aside, why does the female body have a "biological clock" that runs out of time, while men remain fertile virtually their entire lives?

The answer is simple: sperm is a renewable resource; eggs are not.

Men produce sperm – millions of them every day – from the time they reach puberty until the day they die. Cells in their testes are virtual nonstop sperm factories. A woman, on the other hand, has her total supply of eggs determined by the time she is born. She's born with approximately 400,000 eggs – more than enough to produce a family before menopause.

As each menstrual cycle approaches, several eggs are in different stages of development. Usually, only one egg becomes dominant. The others degenerate. So for the first 25 years of a woman's reproductive life, about five or six eggs are lost during each cycle. Somewhere between the ages of 35 and 40, however, "there appears to be an accelerated depletion of eggs from the ovary," says David Archer, M.D., professor of obstetrics and gynaecology at Eastern Virginia Medical School in Norfolk. Your ovaries begin to spit and sputter. You have fewer cycles in which you ovulate, and sometimes you ovulate more than one egg – one reason why twins are more common in women who give birth in their thirties than women who give birth at a younger age.

With each cycle, more eggs degenerate. Even though the pituitary gland sends out more and more follicle-stimulating hormone (FSH) and luteinizing hormone (LH) – the hormones that stimulate egg maturation and release – the ovary becomes less responsive to these signals. Its cells show signs of ageing. Older eggs become harder to fertilize and are less likely to successfully implant in the uterus. Instead of developing normally, the eggs are more likely to undergo a process called apoptosis, genetically programmed cell death.

Finally, there are no more eggs available to be released, so there is no egg follicle to secrete oestrogen or, after an egg is released, to switch over and secrete progesterone. There is no more getting ready for egg implantation if you become pregnant, or shedding of the uterine lining if implantation does not occur. Progesterone drops to a very low level, but the ovary continues to make declining amounts of oestrogen for a few years after the menopause (officially defined as 1 year with no menstrual cycles). Finally, ovaries become nonfunctional as endocrine organs. The adrenal glands, however, continue to make small amounts of sex hormone precursors, such as DHEA (dehydroepiandrosterone), found in normal urine and synthesized from cholesterol; its level increases with age. These can be converted to oestrogen (or testosterone) in the fat tissues of the body. That's why normal or moderately overweight women often have an easier time at menopause than very thin women, Dr. Archer says. (Very obese women tend to have their own unique hormonal abnormalities that make menopause difficult.)

## WHAT'S GOING ON?

Like so many other health experiences, the menopause is a process more than an event. It's not as though you wake up one morning and say, "Well, I am now menopausal." Rather, changes occur gradually and go beyond absence of menstruation. This quiz can help you assess your hormonal status.

**1. Have your periods stopped completely? No more missed periods, light periods, shortened cycles, or flooding?**
Your ovaries have probably stopped functioning, so there is no more oestrogen/progesterone cycle to stimulate monthly growth and shedding of uterine lining.

**2. Are you still having hot flushes? In fact, are they worse now rather than better?**
Low or fluctuating hormone levels are still playing tricks with the part of your brain that regulates body temperature. For relief, see page 298.

**3. Are you less moody than you were during perimenopause but still feeling down and forgetful?**
Doctors aren't exactly sure how low hormone levels affect your brain, but they suspect links with mood and memory. For details, see chapters 3 and 5.

**4. Are you wondering where your sex drive went?**
In addition to oestrogen, your blood levels of testosterone, the "hormone of desire", drop off by about 50 per cent between 20 and 40 and then more slowly trail oestrogen after menopause. That's why some women benefit from getting both oestrogen and testosterone. For details, see chapter 8.

**5. Are you having more vaginal irritation than ever, and urinary tract problems on top of it?**
The cells of these tissues rely on oestrogen for growth and proliferation. The vaginal wall actually thins after menopause, and the cells produce less mucus. That makes you more vulnerable to infection and irritation during sex. Protective mucus-producing cells of the urinary tract also count on oestrogen. For solutions, turn to pages 305 and 309.

# Why Not Just Let Menopause Happen?

The Menopause is a natural process, not a disease. For aeons, women have been doing nothing about the menopause, although some cultures appear to make things easier. The traditional Japanese diet, for instance – loaded with soya products and fish – seems to ease hot flushes. And in traditional Chinese medicine, formulas that include ginseng, licorice root, and other herbs have been used for centuries (and still are) to treat symptoms that could be related to menopause, such as "false heat" (hot flushes) and "heart cold" (lack of libido).

If you do decide to let nature take its course, you may sail through the 5 or 6 years around menopause with no problems, or at least none severe enough to warrant a visit to the doctor. The majority of women have bothersome but tolerable symptoms. Women who have had their ovaries removed as part of a hysterectomy have a particularly tough time. They experience immediate onset of menopause and more severe symptoms.

But denial will get you only so far. Even if you have no immediate obvious symptoms that affect your quality of life, you "absolutely" will eventually have some symptoms, a result of diminishing hormone levels and ageing, Dr. Archer says. These include thinning and drying of the mucous membranes of the vagina and urethra, gradual thinning of the skin, slowly rising total cholesterol levels and a drop in "good" HDL (high-density lipoprotein) cholesterol, and loss of bone mass. These far-reaching effects may not show up for decades, but they are reasons some women decide, sooner or later, that they're not ready to let nature take its course.

"Many women live one-third of their lives after menopause, and although they have no choice about getting older, they *can* and often do decide to do whatever they can to stay healthy, which is why hormone replacement therapy (HRT) and its alternatives draw such interest," says Ricki Pollycove, M.D., director of patient education at the California Pacific Medical Center in San Francisco. "Until we reach menopause, many of us are on automatic pilot and take things for granted. Then we start to notice that a lot of things don't not quite work the way they used to, and we start paying more attention to pretty much everything. Women realize this is no longer a dress rehearsal, that this really is the second half of their lives, and they often begin exercising and eating better, and if they've been meaning to stop smoking, they get serious about it now. They realize if they don't, they'll soon pay the consequences."

So consider the physical changes around the time of the menopause as a wake-up call that leads to an overall healthier lifestyle. Then follow this 12-step strategy to decide what's best for *you*.

# Step 1: Find Out Where You Stand

You might know perfectly well from your symptoms and your age that you are approaching menopause. You don't need a doctor to tell you. But how far off are you from that final period? Months? Weeks? Years? Menstrual cycles tend to be erratic during this time. You may skip a few months and then have a period. You might skip 6 months and then have a period. Surprise! So it's only in retrospect that any woman knows for sure she has reached menopause, after a full year of not menstruating.

Some tests can be done to help confirm that you have indeed reached menopause. But still-fluctuating hormone levels make any of the available tests too inaccurate to be the sole means of diagnosis. So most doctors also "diagnose" menopause the same way you do – by your symptoms and age.

You don't necessarily have to do anything at this point – with one important exception. If you don't want to get pregnant, you still need to think about contraception. "Doctors are likely to prescribe low-dose birth control pills during your perimenopause years, and then switch you over to HRT once you reach menopause," says Dr. Pollycove. "HRT is available in several different dosages, but even the highest dosage is lower than even the lowest-dose birth control pills – and it doesn't offer any kind of contraceptive protection." In fact, HRT can jump-start your fertility for a while.

With that in mind, here are tests your doctor might order to check your menopausal status.

## Follicle-Stimulating Hormone (FSH)

This is the pituitary gland hormone that stimulates your ovaries to produce oestrogen. As oestrogen production in your ovaries drops, FSH levels rise to induce the ovaries to produce oestrogen. It is generally accepted that you have reached menopause when your FSH blood level rises above 30 mIU/ml (milli international units per millilitre).

This test might be done to diagnose a problem in a younger woman who's having symptoms of menopause or in an older woman who hasn't had a period for a few months and wants to know for sure that she has reached menopause, says Dr. Pollycove.

## Oestradiol

Women with high FSH levels are often still producing oestrogen and, so, are not fully menopausal. To avoid a premature diagnosis, your doctor should also test your blood levels of oestradiol, the major oestrogen produced by your ovaries. If your oestradiol levels are low (under 50 picograms per millilitre) and your FSH levels are high, chances are you've reached menopause.

To get accurate results, women taking oral contraceptives or any other type of hormone will need to stop the drug for a week before FSH and oestradiol tests. For more reliable results, stop for 1 week before your period, then get tested on day 2 or 3 of your period, says Dr. Pollycove. If your periods have stopped, it doesn't matter when during the month you are tested.

If tests say you're not in menopause, but you're still having bothersome symptoms, your doctor might recommend temporary measures – taking birth control pills, for example, or using cyclic progesterones or taking micronized progesterone (progesterone that's been broken down into fine particles that are more easily absorbed) during the second half of your menstrual cycle, says Dr. Pollycove. Then you might want to be tested again 6 months or so down the road to see if the levels have dropped. When the levels have reached the "menopause range", your doctor will switch you over to HRT.

## Other Helpful Tests

Most doctors do not monitor levels of hormones once a woman starts HRT. Instead, they monitor dosages of oestrogen and progesterone via symptoms and side effects: start with a standard dose, then raise or lower the dose if necessary, according to symptoms. However, if circumstances warrant, still other tests may be helpful.

## Saliva Testing

Some doctors use saliva testing to monitor a woman's individual response to treatment. "I might use saliva testing after a woman's been taking HRT for a few months, to see if the dose is adequate or, if she's using a patch, to see if she's absorbing the hormone," Dr. Pollycove says.

Saliva testing can be used to test for the three forms of oestrogen (oestradiol, oestriol, and oestrone), progesterone, testosterone and DHEA (which is sometimes used as a form of hormone replacement therapy). Some doctors and researchers think saliva testing for hormones may be better than blood tests because it measures only "free" levels of hormones, not those bound up by proteins in the blood (and, so, unavailable for use). But others point out that, as with blood tests, saliva tests can vary in reliability from woman to woman and can be misleading unless the sample is carefully handled and interpreted by an expert.

## Testosterone

Some doctors will check a woman's testosterone levels, especially if she

---

# Making the HRT Decision

Deciding whether or not to use hormone replacement therapy, natural alternatives, or a combination of therapies can be a complex, highly individualized process. To help work through the risks, benefits and quality-of-life issues, use this handy worksheet. As you read through each step of the menopause guide in this chapter, put ticks next to criteria that apply to you.

When you've worked through all 12 steps of the decision-making process, review this chart, looking for patterns that steer you towards certain options and away from others. Do you have more ticks next to oestrogen and progestin than for progesterone and herbs, for example? Or is it the reverse? Reread the chapter to focus on treatments that seem most applicable to you. Then review your options, along with appropriate test results, with your doctor or alternative health care practitioner.

AGE AND MENOPAUSAL STATUS
❒ Perimenopausal
❒ Menopausal due to surgery (hysterectomy) or chemotherapy
❒ Ovaries removed
❒ Ovaries not removed
❒ Uterine or endometrial cancer
❒ Menopausal not due to surgery or chemotherapy
❒ Over age 65
❒ Under age 65

PERSONAL OR FAMILY HISTORY
❒ Existing heart disease
❒ Risk factors for heart disease
❒ Breast cancer
❒ Uterine or endometrial cancer
❒ Abnormal uterine bleeding
❒ Risk factors for osteoporosis (see page 191)
❒ Normal bone density
❒ Low bone density (osteopenia)
❒ History of fractures
❒ Blood-clotting disorder
❒ Endometriosis or fibroids
❒ Gallbladder disease

complains of a lack of interest in sex, says Dr. Pollycove. This can be a blood test, requesting a reading for "free" testosterone, or a saliva test (see above), which tests only for free testosterone. The normal range depends on the laboratory doing the test, but if levels are low or low-normal, your doctor may suggest supplemental testosterone (sometimes called androgens). "There is new appreciation for role androgens (such as androsterone and testosterone)

MOST TROUBLESOME SYMPTOM OR
SYMPTOMS
❐ Hot flushes/night sweats
❐ Irregular menstrual cycles
❐ Vaginal dryness or irritation
❐ Low sex drive
❐ Breast tenderness
❐ Depression

HRT OPTIONS
❐ Oestrogen (estinyl oestradiol,
    conjugated equine oestrogen,
    esterified oestrogens, tri-est, etc.)
❐ Progestin (medroxyprogesterone,
    norethindrone, norgestimate)
❐ Oestrogen and progestin
    combination (such as Prempro)
❐ Synthetic testosterone
❐ Micronized testosterone
❐ Progesterone
❐ Pill
❐ Patch
❐ Cream
❐ Gel
❐ Ring
❐ Cyclical

SOYA DERIVATIVES
❐ Ipriflavone

DIET AND NUTRITION
❐ Soya foods
❐ Calcium (food and supplements)
❐ Vitamin D supplements
❐ Multivitamin/mineral
❐ Vitamin E
❐ Vitamin C with bioflavonoids

HERBS
❐ Red clover
❐ Black cohosh
❐ Milk thistle
❐ St. John's wort
❐ Coenzyme $Q_{10}$
❐ Hawthorn

EXERCISE
❐ Aerobic exercise (average 30
    minutes per day)
❐ Weight training

play in a woman's general wellness, not just sexuality," Dr. Pollycove says. Women low in testosterone who take supplemental amounts of the hormone often report better mood, energy and sex drive. Testosterone also benefits lean body mass and bone strength.

## Other "Menopause Ready" Tests

As you decide whether or not to take HRT, certain other, non-hormonal tests can supply information equally critical to your decision. They include a Pap smear; a mammogram; and a complete lipid profile, to measure total cholesterol, HDL (high-density lipoprotein), LDL (low-density lipoprotein), and triglycerides (blood fats that can contribute to heart disease in some women). Total cholesterol tends to rise after menopause, and "good" HDL tends to drop. The oral oestrogens tend to raise HDL, but they can also raise triglycerides – not so good – so some doctors won't start a woman on HRT if her triglyceride level is higher than 3.3 mmol/l. If you get a baseline measurement before you start any kind of HRT, it's easier to see later what kind of an impact the hormones are having on your risk for heart disease (discussed later, starting on page 183).

Some doctors feel strongly that as you approach menopause, you should get a baseline reading of your bone density, a predictor for developing osteoporosis. (To find out which test is best, see "The Right Way to Test Your Bones" on page 193.)

And the American Association of Clinical Endocrinologists recommends that all women of 40 or older get a thyroid-stimulating hormone (TSH) test to screen for an underactive thyroid. That's because low-thyroid problems tend to start about this time and are more prevalent than previously realized, says Connie Catellani, M.D., medical director of the Miro Center for Integrative Medicine in Evanston, Illinois. "When your thyroid gland is out of balance, that magnifies all menopausal symptoms, including weight gain and mood swings. So part of a good evaluation at menopause will include looking at the thyroid gland, making sure it isn't contributing to symptoms."

# Step 2: Weigh Your Risks versus Benefits

Once the test results are in, the next step is to prioritize your personal hormonal needs, based on quality-of-life issues and far-reaching ramifications.

Potential risks and side effects are as disparate as vaginal dryness and breast cancer, osteoporosis and blood clots, gallstones and low sex drive.

"It's like comparing apples and oranges," says Mary Jane Minkin, M.D., clinical professor of obstetrics and gynaecology at Yale University School of Medicine. "There are lots of pieces you need to integrate into the whole when making decisions about HRT."

**Start by simplifying.** Write down your top three current concerns about menopause, whatever they are, she says. Vaginal dryness? Lack of sex drive? Terminal crabbiness? Then consult the section of this book that offers solutions. Depending on your problems, there may be one solution for all of them. If HRT isn't the answer for you, non-hormonal remedies or medications might help.

**Review your medical history.** If HRT offers relief for whatever bothers you, your doctor will explore your "contraindications" – any reasons HRT might *not* be advisable for you. These include a recent history of breast or endometrial cancer; abnormal uterine bleeding of unknown cause (in which case your doctor will want to do an endometrial biopsy before giving you the go-ahead); a history of blood-clotting disorders; liver disease; a history of endometriosis or fibroids; a history of gallbladder disease; seizure disorders; migraine headaches; and high triglycerides (more than 3.3 mmol/l).

"These contraindications don't all necessarily mean you can't use HRT," Dr. Pollycove says. "Some women with breast cancer may not have an increased risk of recurrence, for instance. But it does mean that if you decide to take HRT, you will need to be closely monitored for adverse effects."

**Weigh the pros and cons.** Finally, you and your doctor will need to wade through the pros and cons of long-term treatment, based on what is currently known about the topic. You might not do this at an initial visit if you're interested in simply treating your hot flushes. But sooner or later, you will want to work out if HRT is something you want to take long-term, for its reported benefits on bone and its possible benefits on the heart and cardiovascular system, brain, skin, and whatever else research uncovers in the postmenopausal years ahead.

**Stay informed.** For ongoing updates on the risks versus benefits of hormone replacement therapy and other menopausal strategies, see "On the Web & Other Resources" on page 220.

One study doctors are eagerly awaiting that may help them to offer clearer choices to women is the US National Institutes of Health (NIH) Women's Health Initiative. One component of this large, randomized clinical trial is a hormone replacement therapy (HRT) intervention that looks specifically at the effects of long-term HRT on coronary heart disease and osteoporosis-related fractures as well as other diseases that might be affected by oestrogens. The study was started in 1991. Final results won't be available until the study ends. To find the latest on HRT and heart disease, check the excellent BMA Web site at www.bma.org.

Between authoritative updates you locate on the Internet and information here, you should be able to have a productive conversation with your doctor about your own risks and benefits. "Ultimately, it is a decision you shouldn't make alone – you make it with your doctor's guidance – and you should pick a doctor who's willing to spend the time with you helping you to make a decision and following through on it," Dr. Minkin says.

### Escape from **HORMONE HELL**
## HER HEART THROBS COULD BE HORMONES

**Q:** I've started to have heart palpitations – out of the blue, my heart starts to beat very rapidly for no reason at all. Sometimes it feels like it is beating erratically; sometimes it feels like skipped heartbeats or a powerful beat. I don't really have any other symptoms, like chest pain or breathing trouble. But it makes me anxious, and then I start breathing rapidly, too. At the age of 50, I'm close to menopause, and I am wondering if this is related to the menopause – or could it be a sign of a heart condition?

Mary Jane Minkin, M.D., clinical professor of obstetrics and gynaecology at Yale University School of Medicine, replies: it's not uncommon to get palpitations – a sensation of the heart's beating erratically or fast – around the time of the menopause. And there may well

be an association between hormones and heart rhythm, although the association is probably not a simple or direct one. Oestrogen receptor sites are found on every cell in your body, including the cells of your heart. Endothelial cells, for instance, which line the inside of blood vessels and the heart, respond to oestrogen by producing nitrous oxide, a potent vasodilator. So it's possible that fluctuations in oestrogen levels are causing vasospasms (ischaemia) that affect bloodflow to your heart, causing palpitations, or to your brain, triggering a migraine headache.

Around the time of the menopause, the risk of serious heart disease starts to increase, so first you need to rule out heart rhythm abnormalities or more serious heart problems, especially if the palpitations

# Step 3: Consider Your Heart Health History – And Future

For years, doctors were saying oestrogen replacement therapy was good for your heart. They based their case on what seemed like pretty solid evidence: oestrogen lowers LDL and raises HDL, and it improves the function of the endothelium, the cells lining the blood vessels, improving the ability of blood vessels to dilate. Women who go through surgical menopause –

(continued on page 186)

are associated with light-headedness or shortness of breath. Your doctor may fit you with a portable device called a Holter monitor, which you'll wear for 24 hours, or an event monitor, which you use intermittently for up to 1 month. These recorders help determine whether you have an abnormal heartbeat.

A new imaging technique especially accurate at diagnosing heart disease in women is the stress echocardiogram. It combines a treadmill stress test with cardiac ultrasound to detect bloodflow through the heart. Beta-blockers are used to treat heart arrhythmias, angina pectoris and high blood pressure.

If you're over 50, you should be screened for thyroid disease. Too much or too little thyroid hormone can have a profound effect on your heart and is an often-overlooked signal to thyroid malfunction.

If your palpitations are in fact related to menopause, oestrogen replacement therapy is usually quite effective in relieving them, and it should work fast. In a study where oestrogen was injected intravenously while women underwent angiography, the oestrogen had an immediate relaxing effect on blood vessels. Synthetic progesterone – while it's helpful in most regards – *causes* vasospasms. So it's one hormone you don't want to get more of than you need.

I'd also suggest cutting out caffeine – it's a surefire palpitation producer in some people – and getting more sleep. Too little sleep raises levels of stress hormones, which can make your heart race.

# An At-a-Glance Guide to Hormone Terms and Options

**Amenorrhoea** – going without a menstrual period for longer than a year (excluding pregnancy and breastfeeding).

**Androsterone** and **testosterone** – androgens.

**Atypical cells** – cells in which details appear coarsened or abnormally active.

**Bisphosphonates** – family of drugs that works by blocking the normal breakdown of old bone (bone remodelling). These drugs inhibit osteoclasts, the cells that break down bone.

**BMD** – bone mineral density. The single best predictor of the risk for fractures.

**Cardiotonic agent** – enhancing the function or well-being of the heart.

**Compact bone** – very dense bone.

**Complete lipid profile** – measures total cholesterol, HDL (high-density lipoprotein), LDL (low-density lipoprotein) and triglycerides.

**Cortisol** – stress hormone associated with bone loss.

**DHEA (dehydroepiandrosterone)** – an androgen found in normal urine and synthesized from cholesterol; its level increases with age. Sometimes used as a form of hormone replacement therapy.

**Double-blind, randomized clinical trials** – neither the participants nor the investigators are aware of the specific treatments assigned.

**Dual energy x-ray absorptiometry (DEXA) test** – measures density of the bones in the hip, spine and wrist and compares this with the bone of a young woman at peak bone mass (about age 25).

**Endometrial biopsy** – uterine lining tissue sample.

**Endometrial hyperplasia** – buildup of the uterine lining.

**Endothelium** – the cells lining the blood vessels.

**Esterified oestrogen** – oestrogens produced from natural sources or synthesized.

**Flavonoids** – compounds found in citrus fruits similar to the isoflavones found in soya.

**FSH (follicle-stimulating hormone)** – the pituitary gland hormone that stimulates the ovaries to produce oestrogen.

**Gastric reflux** – heartburn.

**HDL (high-density lipoprotein)** – the "good" cholesterol.

**HERS** – the Heart and Estrogen/Progestin Replacement Study (an American trial).

**HRT** – hormone replacement therapy.

**"Hyperproliferative"** – overactive gland growth.

**"Inflammatory marker"** – also called CRP, or C-reactive protein. It increases in response to oestrogen.

**Ipriflavone** – a synthetic cousin of natural soya isoflavones.

**Isoflavones** – ocstrogen-like compounds found in foods such as soya and red clover.

**LH (luteinizing hormone)** – this hormone stimulates egg maturation and release.

**Metabolites** – breakdown products that linger in the body for a long time.

**Micronized progesterone** – progesterone that's been broken down into fine particles that are more easily absorbed.

**Mineralization** – the addition of mineral matter to the body.

**"Natural" hormone** – has the exact same chemical structure as that made in your body – that is, biochemically identical.

**Neuropeptides** – several types of molecules found in brain tissue.

**Oestradiol** – the major oestrogen produced by your ovaries.

**Oestring** – an oestrogen-impregnated ring inserted into the vagina.

**Osteoblasts** – bone-building cells.

**Osteoclasts** – cells in the bone responsible for bone breakdown.

**Osteoid tissue** – the "scaffolding" that gives bone its flexibility and great tensile strength.

**Osteopenia** – low bone density.

**Palpitations** – fast or erratic heartbeat, especially common around the time of the menopause.

**Phyto-oestrogens** – plant versions of oestrogen.

**Premarin** – conjugated equine oestrogen.

**Progestin** – synthetic progesterone.

**RUTH Trial** – "Raloxifene Use for the Heart" Trial.

**SERM** – US term for oestrogen receptor blockers or antagonists.

**"Statin" drugs** – lipid-lowering drugs used for the treatment of excessive cholesterol in the blood; also known as HMG CoA reductase inhibitors.

**Sublingual pill** – pill that's dissolved under the tongue.

**Surgical menopause** – having both ovaries removed.

**Synthetic hormone** – not chemically identical to that made in your body.

**Systemic hormones** – hormones that circulate throughout your body.

**Trabecular bone** – a spongy, high-turnover bone found in the spine.

**Transdermal oestrogen** – applied to the skin.

**Triglycerides** – blood fats that can contribute to heart disease.

**T-score** – the number of standard deviations above or below the mean bone density for young normal adults.

**Venous thromboembolism** – dangerous blood clots deep in your veins.

having both of their ovaries removed – are less likely to develop heart disease if they take oestrogen than if they don't. And in "observational" studies, including the large, ongoing Nurses' Health Study from Harvard, women taking HRT had a 35 per cent to 50 per cent lower rate of heart disease.

True, there were some doubts and negatives. In the Nurses' Health Study, for instance, there was no way to know if HRT was offering heart protection or if the women taking HRT were simply healthier and had access to better health care than those not taking oestrogen. All oral forms of oestrogen can raise triglycerides. In other women, oestrogen increases the risk of developing dangerous blood clots deep in your veins – venous thromboembolism. And taking synthetic progesterone along with oestrogen appears to negate some of oestrogen's HDL-raising effects.

In general, though, the benefits of oestrogen seemed plausible enough for doctors to think it might help to prevent heart disease or provide benefits to women with heart disease.

Some of that thinking has been questioned, though, by the findings of a new US study that suggests a slight initial increase in risk for heart disease in women who use HRT. Called the HERS study (the Heart and Estrogen/Progestin Replacement Study), it found a 52 per cent increased risk for coronary heart disease "events" (heart attack or death due to heart disease) during the first year of treatment in women with established heart disease who took HRT. Some 4 per cent of women using HRT in the study developed heart problems (or died from them), compared with 2 per cent of non–HRT users. By the fourth year of the study, however, the risk for heart disease in the women in the study still taking HRT was lower than the risk for women who were not taking HRT.

Bear in mind that HERS study findings may apply only to women with heart disease. But preliminary data from another large, ongoing US study (the Women's Health Initiative mentioned earlier) has also found a slight increase in stroke and heart attacks in the first 2 years of HRT use, compared with women using a placebo. "In the WHI study, the increase was small, only about 1 per cent, but it was still there. And it was found in mostly healthy women," says David Herrington, M.D., associate professor of internal medicine–cardiology at Wake Forest University Baptist Medical Center in Winston-Salem, North Carolina, and one of HERS's main researchers. (This WHI finding was not published, but the study participants were informed of it.) And when researchers involved in other large, epidemiological studies have gone back and looked over their preliminary data, some have also found the evidence of the same pattern, of increased risk for heart disease in normal, healthy women who were new users of HRT, Dr. Herrington says. "There is an accumulating body of evidence that this is not a fluke and that we need to be cautious about it," he says.

Just what women and their doctors should do about it, though, depends on whom you talk to. Some doctors are very cautious about recommending HRT to women these days. Others still feel that HRT is, overall, a good thing, and that there is lots of research to back up their position. All acknowledge that many questions still need to be answered about HRT and heart disease.

For now, deciding on the role of HRT in your "menopause portfolio" is a lot like researching an investment portfolio. While no one can predict the consequences with certainty, you need to make the best decision based on what *is* known – and your own comfort level and instincts. Here's what you need to know about oestrogen and progesterone – the "stocks and bonds" of the HRT issue. No one mix of hormones is perfect.

## Not All Progesterone Is Created Equal

Some doctors contend that the drug regime used in the HERS study was part of the problem. The drug used was a continuous oestrogen/progestin combination, Prempro (which is not available in the UK), at a daily dosage of 0.625 milligrams of conjugated equine oestrogen and 2.5 milligrams of medroxyprogesterone. "A lot of the big players in my business think that daily progestins are not a good thing, that women would do much better taking a cyclical progestin, taking it for 12 days every 2 or 3 months, meaning you would have a period once every 2 or 3 months," says Dr. Minkin. She and some other leading women's doctors also believe you're better off if you use a "natural" (biochemically identical) form of progesterone, such as Prometrium (not available in the UK), and avoid taking Provera, a synthetic progestin, which increases LDL and can cause vascular spasms. "The addition of Provera undoes a lot of the good of Premarin," Dr. Minkin says.

But blaming the regime used in the HERS study doesn't fully explain the risk, Dr. Herrington says. In the WHI study, which also found a slight increase in risk, some of the women were taking oestrogen alone.

Some doctors also say that once you're past this apparent initial period of risk, you might benefit from taking HRT. "But you can't say to women, 'If you don't die in the first year, you are going to do better'. That's not the way we practise medicine," says Nanette Wenger, M.D., chief of cardiology at Grady

Memorial Hospital and professor of cardiology at Emory University School of Medicine in Atlanta. The truth is that no one, not even Dr. Wenger and other researchers involved in the studies, knows what the heart attacks are due to, or how to identify the women at early risk for heart attacks. That's what they are working on right now.

"We do know that oestrogen causes an increased risk of blood clots in the veins, so it's not unreasonable to wonder whether there is a chance it might increase the risk for blood clots in the arteries, such as arteries in the heart, where clots could cause a heart attack," Dr. Herrington says. No one knows if blood clots, rather than fatty plaque, caused the heart attacks. And so far, none of the possible associated risk factors they've looked at have shown a strong correlation. These include smoking, diabetes, high blood pressure, high cholesterol, and a prior history of heart attacks.

Researchers will be testing the blood of the women in the HERS and WHI studies to see if they can come up with any new correlations, Dr. Wenger says. They are particularly interested in blood substances associated with clotting and inflammation. One of these proteins – an "inflammatory marker" called CRP, or C-reactive protein – increases in response to oestrogen. "That is a fairly new finding, and it may be a problem in being associated with a higher risk," Dr. Wenger says. CRP has recently been shown to be an independent risk factor for coronary events in both men and women. It is possible to have your blood measured for this protein, and more doctors in the US are recommending it, Dr. Wenger says. But do tell your doc-

## A Heart Drug That Also Protects Your Bones

If you're taking a "statin" drug (HMG CoA reductase inhibitor) to reduce cholesterol, you'll be happy to hear that these drugs also seem to help prevent bone loss. In two recent observational studies, researchers found that older people taking a statin drug had about a 50 per cent reduction in the risk of fractures. Statins appear to increase bone mineral density at the spine and hip in postmenopausal women.

These drugs aren't strong enough to be prescribed for osteoporosis alone – other drugs do a better job of that. But if you're equally concerned about heart disease and osteoporosis, statins may be a good choice although unfortunately they are also linked to an increased rise of neuropathy.

tor if you've had phlebitis or a blood clot in your vein or lung, or if blood clots run in your family. Blood clots at an early age are a good tip-off of a family predisposition.

Right now, there is no good way to tell which healthy women are at higher risk for a heart attack once they start HRT. There's no good way to "screen" yourself to determine your risk. Even if you have the tests most doctors recommend at menopause – cholesterol, HDL, LDL, triglycerides, blood pressure, blood sugar – and they're all normal, "it doesn't mean we can guarantee it's safe for you to take HRT," Dr. Herrington says. "We just don't know."

## What to Do Now

Some doctors still think there could be long-term heart benefits from HRT – and they point to the fact that the women on HRT who remained in the HERS study at 4 years did have a reduction in heart disease risk. That benefit has yet to be confirmed in double-blind, randomized clinical trials (where neither the participants nor the investigators are aware of the specific treatments assigned).

**If you already have heart disease and have never taken HRT:** The message seems pretty clear, Dr. Herrington says. "Don't take HRT with the expectation that it will benefit your heart." Any increased risk seems to occur during the first year or two of use.

Instead, use tactics proven to help your heart, says Dr. Herrington. Stop smoking. Treat high blood pressure. Use "statin" drugs (lipid-lowering drugs used for the treatment of excessive cholesterol in the blood) or a low-fat diet to get your total cholesterol to 200 mg/dl or lower. (For non-hormonal strategies and treatments for heart disease, see "The Menopause Menu" on page 218, "When Your Heart Needs Help" on page 226, and "Diet and Exercise" on page 227.)

**If you've been taking HRT for less than a year:** Talk to your doctor and consider switching to an HRT regime that includes daily oestrogen, with only 10 to 14 days every 2 or 3 months of natural progesterone, Dr. Minkin says. You may also want to take transdermal (applied to the skin) oestrogen rather than oral oestrogen. Oestrogen affects blood clotting through its action in the liver, and that action is stronger when you take drugs orally.

**If you have heart disease and have been taking HRT for more than a year or two with no problems:** You may not need to stop, but you still may want to talk to your doctor about switching to a cyclical regime if you're not already on one, Dr. Minkin says.

**If you haven't been diagnosed with heart disease but have some of the**

**risk factors:** If you smoke, have diabetes, or have high cholesterol, for instance, your first health concern should be reducing your risk for heart disease by proven means, such as statin drugs or keeping your diabetes under tight control or using aspirin, says Dr. Minkin. HRT might still be appropriate for you – to treat osteoporosis, for instance – but here again, natural progesterone and a cyclical regime using transdermal oestrogen might be your best bet.

**If you don't have heart disease and have no risk factors for it:** Other than that you're a postmenopausal female, don't let the HERS finding scare you away from HRT, Dr. Minkin says. But keep alert for results from the US Women's Health Initiative Study. "That's the study that should give some definitive statement about the prospective prevention of heart disease with HRT use," Dr. Minkin says.

# Step 4: Assess Your Fear, Risk, or History of Breast Cancer

Risk factors for breast cancer include a family predisposition in first-degree relatives (sisters, daughters, or mothers), history of endometrial or ovarian cancer, history of breast cancer, the "hyperproliferative" (overactive gland growth) form of fibrocystic disease (benign tumours in the breast) with atypical cells (details of individual cells appear coarsened or abnormally active), early onset of menstruation (before 13), late menopause (after 52), and first pregnancy and breastfeeding after 30.

One of the big reasons women say they won't use HRT is a fear of getting breast cancer. Those fears aren't entirely unfounded. Population studies on HRT and cancer show a moderate but significantly increased risk of breast cancer if you use HRT for more than 5 years. (There appears to be no increased risk if you use it for a shorter period of time.)

Scary as that sounds, consider what it really means: in a randomly selected group of 1,000 women who have never taken conventionally prescribed hormones, 77 will get breast cancer by the age of 75. Compare that population to women who've had five years of HRT; that figure nudges up to 79 women. After 10 years of HRT, the figure remains 79; and after 15 years, the figure jumps somewhat to 89. In other words, the large majority of women using HRT long term will not get breast cancer as a result.

To put the risk into perspective, compare it to the risk of lung cancer in women who smoke. "Depending on which study you look at, the relative risk for breast cancer is 1.2 or 1.6, which is not very high," Dr. Minkin says. "If you're a smoker, on the other hand, your relative risk of lung cancer is 25 or 26 – much, much higher. So when it comes to deciding for or against HRT, it becomes a matter of weighing other health benefits and quality-of-life issues against this slight increase in risk."

Within the small but potential increased risk of breast cancer associated with HRT, some evidence indicates that the highest risk comes from combined oestrogen and progestin. So here again, some doctors believe it could be wise to reduce your exposure to synthetic progestins, Dr. Minkin says. Some doctors prescribe continuous oestrogen (in oral or patch form), and progestins at infrequent intervals, such as every 2 or 3 months. Or you might try a combination of continuous oestrogen and a progesterone vaginal gel (Crinone).

There are fewer side effects associated with micronized progesterone. However, because this regime has not been studied in large groups of women, there is no concrete evidence that its use is less likely to increase breast cancer risk than synthetic oral progestins. (For more on Crinone, see page 209, "Which Natural Hormone Is Right for You?")

# Step 5: Take Stock of Your Bones

If you're planning to live another 20 or 30 years past menopause – and we assume you are – you need to think about osteoporosis, which literally means "porous bones". As you age, all your bones will become less dense and easier to break. Unless you start taking protective measures early in adulthood and at menopause, your spine will become prone to tiny fractures that can crumble your vertebrae, bending your spine forward and causing chronic pain. The effects nibble away at your quality of life. You're also more likely to fracture your hip. And if that happens when you're 75 or older, you have only a one-in-three chance of getting back to normal.

"If you intend to make the third of your life after menopause active, quality time, you need to be concerned about osteoporosis before it happens," says Ethel Siris, M.D., director of the Toni Stabile Center for the Prevention and Treatment of Osteoporosis at Columbia-Presbyterian Medical Center in New York City.

Your doctor can determine whether you have osteoporosis, or are at high risk for developing osteoporosis, by assessing your risk factors and by measuring your bone density. There are lots of risk factors for osteoporosis. In addition to being female, the US National Osteoporosis Foundation's "top four" are:

- *Smoking currently*
- *Weighing less than 57 kg (9 stone)*
- *Having had a bone fracture as an adult*
- *Having a mother, father, sister, or brother who has had a fracture due to osteoporosis*

Other risk factors include:

- *Being white (Caucasian) or Asian*
- *Poor eating habits, especially low dietary calcium*
- *Vitamin D deficiency*
- *Getting little or no physical activity*
- *Alcoholism*
- *Going without a menstrual period (amenorrhoea) for longer than a year (excluding pregnancy and breastfeeding) during your reproductive (premenopausal) years*
- *Early menopause, especially if earlier than the age of 45 or due to surgery*

Researchers are discovering new risk factors for osteoporosis all the time – some even your doctor may not know about:

**If you've taken prescription steroid drugs, such as prednisone, for asthma, emphysema, rheumatoid arthritis, or other chronic conditions:** These drugs rapidly accelerate bone loss. In one study, for example, a group of patients (aged 18 to 55) treated with 7.5 milligrams of prednisone daily for 12 weeks experienced an 8 per cent loss of bone in the spine. Some experts suggest that anyone who has received orally administered steroid drugs (such as prednisone in a dose of 5 milligrams or more for longer than 2 months) is at high risk for excessive bone loss. Other research indicates that people who use inhaled steroids for asthma run a higher risk for osteoporosis. (Fortunately, there are drugs that can help prevent this bone loss.) For more about minimizing the effects on bone from steroids, see "Corticosteroids: Breath Savers, Bone Breakers" on page 358.

**If you've been treated for thyroid disease:** You might have taken an excess amount of thyroid replacement hormone, thyroxine, which can promote bone loss. Your doctor should check for bone loss, using bone mineral density, and periodically check your dosage of thyroxine by doing a blood test called TSH (thyroid-stimulating hormone), the most sensitive test available, says Felicia Cosman, M.D., clinical director of the US National Osteoporosis Foundation and a bone specialist at Helen Hayes Hospital in West Haverstraw, New York.

**If you have a history of chronic depression:** Older women who are depressed may be more susceptible to osteoporosis because they secrete more cortisol, a stress hormone associated with bone loss.

**If you have prematurely grey hair:** No one knows why, but a study found that women who were mostly grey by 40 tended to have lower overall bone density than those who went grey later in life.

**If you have lost more than two permanent teeth in adulthood:** Because tooth loss may reflect poor bone health in postmenopausal women, some researchers believe that it may become the earliest warning sign of osteoporosis. Bone loss in the jaw may also signal bone loss in the skeleton, says Dr. Cosman.

## The Right Way to Test Your Bones

Risk factors only hint at your bone health. To actually determine how strong your bones are, doctors use special X-rays to measure your bone mineral density (BMD) – the single best predictor of the risk for fractures. Then they compare your BMD to an optimal density measure – the average density of a young adult woman at the time of peak bone mass (about the age of 25). Depending on how your bone compares with young, dense bone, your doctor determines if your bones are normal, if you have low bone density (medically referred to as osteopenia), or if your bone density is so low that you have outright osteoporosis.

If you've had a regular X-ray recently and your doctor said your bones look just fine, don't assume you don't have osteoporosis. Standard X-rays are not sensitive enough to reveal osteoporosis until 30 per cent of bone has already been lost. By then the damage is done, and the way back to health is more difficult.

### The DEXA Test Is Best

There are several ways to measure BMD, but the current gold standard is the dual energy X-ray absorptiometry (DEXA) test. DEXA measures the density of the bones in your hip, spine and wrist and compares this with the bone density of a young woman at peak bone mass. A normal DEXA result would tell you that your bones are within one standard deviation of peak bone mass. A standard deviation score of −2.5 yields a diagnosis of osteoporosis. For every standard deviation below 0, fracture risk is increased about twofold. This SD, or distance from the norm, is translated into something called a T-score (the number of standard deviations above or below the mean for young normal adults).

The World Health Organization has established these definitions based on bone mass measurements at any skeletal site in white women. Your doctor can – and should – explain your score to you.

**Normal:** BMD is within 1 SD of a "young normal" adult (T-score above −1).

**Low bone mass (osteopenia):** BMD is between 1 and 2.5 SD below that of a "young normal" adult (T-score between −1 and −2.5).

**Osteoporosis:** BMD is 2.5 SD or more below that of a "young normal" adult (T-score at or below −2.5). Women in this group who have already experienced one or more fractures are deemed to have severe or "established" osteoporosis.

"Waiting until you have a fracture to do something about osteoporosis is like waiting to have a stroke before you get treated for high blood pressure," says Dr. Siris. According to doctors' guidelines issued by the US National Osteoporosis Foundation, BMD testing should be performed on:
  • *Postmenopausal women under 65 who have one or more additional risk factors for osteoporosis (besides menopause)*
  • *All women aged 65 and older regardless of additional risk factors*
  • *Postmenopausal women who have bone fractures (to confirm the diagnosis of osteoporosis and to determine its severity)*

## Urine Tests Have Potential

Bone mineral density testing can catch osteoporosis before a hip or spinal fracture knocks you for six and when treatments to save your bones can be very effective. It's sometimes also used to determine if a particular treatment is having an impact on bone density. But because bone density builds up so slowly, it may take 2 or 3 years of a treatment before a BMD test such as DEXA can detect an improvement, Dr. Cosman says. The improvement may also be so small that DEXA can't really detect it accurately, she says. Urine tests and some blood tests that measure the amount of bone turnover may also be useful for treatment monitoring.

So doctors are interested in biochemical tests of urine that can measure levels of bone breakdown products. "Ideally, these tests should be able to tell you in a matter of weeks if a treatment is working," says Douglas Bauer, M.D., associate professor of medicine, epidemiology, and biostatistics at the University of California, San Francisco. Unfortunately, these tests "aren't really ready for prime time," as Dr. Bauer puts it. "The way they're usually done now, there's just too much normal day-to-day variation in the results to make much sense of them," he says. You might be able to do the test every day for a week or so, and average the results and get some accuracy that way, but that would be very expensive, he says. "Lots of doctors just don't use them because they believe they are not yet reliable enough to base a treatment decision on," Dr. Bauer says.

But stay tuned. In a few years, you may be able to closely monitor your osteoporosis treatment – whether it be exercise or HRT or other drugs – with a reliable urine or blood test.

## Non-hormonal Strategies Are Essential

Diet and exercise – with or without HRT – can help protect your bones.

**Make a lifelong commitment to calcium.** No matter what else you do, make sure you get 1200 milligrams of calcium a day – including calcium supplements, if necessary. (The typical Western diet provides less than 600 milligrams a day.) And keep taking it. In one study, women taking 500 milligrams a day of supplemental calcium had a 9 per cent reduction in the rate of bone remodelling, which means they had that much less bone breakdown. But if they stopped taking the calcium, within 2 years their bone density had returned to pretherapy levels.

**Go easy on the antacids.** If you're getting your calcium from an antacid, choose tablets that are aluminium-free. Aluminium can prevent adequate mineralization (the addition of mineral matter to the body) of bones.

**Include vitamin D.** Your body requires vitamin D to be able to use calcium. True, you can make some from the sun. But the older you get, the less efficient your body is at converting sunlight to vitamin D. Women older than 50 need 400 IU a day and often need a separate vitamin D supplement to reach that amount. Because lots of older people don't get enough vitamin D to keep their bones strong, many women older than 65 will benefit from taking up to 800 IU daily, Dr. Cosman says.

**Take a well-rounded multivitamin and mineral.** To weave together the tissues that form the scaffolding for strong, flexible bones, your body needs several other nutrients besides calcium and vitamin D – namely, boron, magnesium, vitamin K, vitamin C, manganese, copper, and zinc. If you eat lots of fruits and vegetables, whole grains, and beans, then you're getting these nutrients. If you don't eat properly, then do your bones a favour and take a good multivitamin with minerals – one that supplies 100 per cent of all nutrients, Dr. Cosman says. And take your multi separate from large amounts of calcium since calcium can interfere with the absorption of certain minerals, such as iron.

**Walk, work out, or weight lift.** Research shows that high-impact weight-bearing exercise (like running) and weight training are the best bone builders, says Jennifer Layne, C.S.C.S., a certified strength and conditioning specialist and a senior research associate in the Nutrition, Exercise Physiology, and Sarcopenia Laboratory at the Jean Mayer USDA Human Nutrition Research Center on Aging at Tufts University in Boston. The stress that weight-bearing activities, such as running, put on your bones activates bone cells to produce new bone. Same goes for exercise such as lifting weights or other forms of resistance training (like working with machines). Weight training stresses muscle tissue to cause new growth.

Postmenopausal women can increase their bone density by regularly doing such exercise, although exactly how much bone they'll gain is highly variable, Layne says. Nevertheless, the more inactive you've been, the more benefit you'll get from low-impact weight-bearing activities, such as walking, stairclimbing, dancing, even gardening, Dr. Siris says. "Even if it does not build bone a whole lot, walking can improve your balance and muscle strength, making falls less likely," she says. (For Layne's top six suggestions to maintain spine and hip bone strength, see "Stop Osteoporosis with These Moves" on page 222.)

**If you already have low bone mass or osteoporosis:** Ask your doctor to be very specific about what you can and can't do, Layne says. Your doctor can refer you to a physiotherapist to get you started. Make sure you see someone who specializes in osteoporosis.

## Osteoporosis Drugs: For Bones at Risk

The lack of firm evidence showing a clear reduction in fracture rates with long-term use of HRT in women with osteoporosis – plus the risks of long-term use, such as breast cancer – have made other osteoporosis drugs very attractive, especially for women aged 65 or older, Dr. Cosman says. "Some of these drugs, particularly the bisphosphonates, have been clearly shown to reduce osteoporotic fractures, without all of the associated effects on other organs, such as the breasts and uterus, that HRT has," she says.

**If you have normal bone density:** You're not likely to be prescribed an osteoporosis drug to prevent bone loss, although you might take HRT for other reasons during menopause and get the advantage of protection from bone loss, Dr. Cosman says. For osteoporosis prevention, HRT remains a good choice.

**If you already have osteopenia (low bone density) or osteoporosis:** Medication can slow or stop the loss of bone and in some cases even restore some bone mass. A compilation of mostly small studies indicated that, in women relatively close to the menopause, HRT could reduce osteoporosis-related fractures. This ability to decrease fractures is not so clear in older women further from the menopause.

These are the current choices among osteoporosis drugs: oestrogen (the most common brand names approved for prevention include Prempak-C, Adgyn Combi, Climageot, Climesse, Cyclo-Progynova and Elleste); three bisphosphonates, alendronate (Fosamax), etidronate (Didronel) and risedronate (Actonel); raloxifene (Evista), an oestrogen receptor antagonist); and calcitonin (Miacalcin).

Researchers measure the success of a new drug by finding out how much new bone is formed, usually over a 3-year period, and by calculating how many broken bones are prevented. They look at two areas where fractures are common – the vertebrae and the upper femur, the long bone in your thigh whose "ball" fits into the "socket" of the pelvis to form the hip. The spine has more of a spongy, high-turnover bone called trabecular bone, and the benefits of a drug are seen faster here. The femur, on the other hand, is mostly very dense bone, called compact bone. "These distinctions between types of bone are important because some drugs work better on the spine than the hip, and some don't work at all on the compact bone of the hip," Dr. Cosman says.

Each drug has its own benefits and limitations, so no one osteoporosis drug is the best, or is right for everyone, Dr. Siris says. For example, alendronate (Fosamax) has been compared with an oestrogen/progestin combination in a prevention study to see which treatment better delayed osteoporosis. But other than that, many treatments have not been directly compared with others, making it difficult to evaluate which treatment is "best".

Also, don't substitute drugs for diet and exercise. When researchers test a new osteoporosis drug, they make sure all the people in the study are getting adequate calcium and vitamin D, using supplements if necessary.

"Even these powerful new drugs don't work as well if you don't have on hand the nutrients needed to build bone," Dr. Cosman says. Drugs, exercise, and nutrients all benefit bone in different ways, and one doesn't substitute for another. "Everyone should be eating right and exercising," Dr. Cosman says. "Then, if they're still at high risk, drugs might be the way to go."

That said, the more familiar your doctor is with these drugs – and with you – the better able you are to decide the treatment that's ideal for you. Here are your choices.

## Hormone Replacement Therapy

Until the 1980s, HRT was the sole treatment available for osteoporosis. And hormone therapy does seem to do the job when it comes to preventing this debilitating condition, at least in women close to the menopause.

Oestrogen helps the bone directly, by reducing the rate of remodelling from elevated postmenopausal levels to normal premenopausal levels. It also stimulates production of vitamin D, which helps the intestines absorb calcium. It makes your kidneys hoard calcium, so less is excreted. If you start taking oestrogen at the time of the menopause, it prevents the rapid loss of 3 per cent to 5 per cent of bone mass that occurs per year in the 5 to 10 years following menopause.

The problem is that if you stop taking HRT, as many women eventually do, you lose bone quickly – in a few years, it's as though you never took it. And if you start taking it later in life – say, aged 60 or older – its benefits aren't quite so clear-cut.

"We used to say that starting oestrogen anytime would be helpful to bones," says Dr. Cosman. "And we definitely do see a positive effect on both bone mass and bone turnover, the process by which bone breaks down and rebuilds."

Unfortunately, very few definitive studies look at the relationship between HRT and fractures, an even more important gauge of bone strength. The largest clinical trial, the HERS study, did not show a reduction in risk for hip or other fractures with HRT. Several small clinical trials indicate that oestrogen can reduce the risk of spine and some non-spinal fractures.

As for the bone-building process, it's the oestrogen in HRT that protects bones, not progesterone or progestins, which appear to have little impact – positive or negative, Dr. Cosman says. All chemical forms of oestrogen work, and both pills and patches work well at protecting bones. (Do note that vaginal creams, rings, and suppositories have not been adequately tested, nor have topical oestrogen creams. In the UK creams, rings and suppositories are only used to produce oestrogen effects – on, for example, a dry vagina – and not to prevent osteoporosis.)

The form of oestrogen most studied regarding bone health is conjugated equine oestrogen (Prempak), at a standard dose of 0.625 milligrams. "But even doses as low as 0.3 milligrams have proven bone protection in some women, if they are also taking supplemental calcium and vitamin D," Dr. Siris says.

**If you're aged 60 or younger:** Oestrogen may be selected as the first choice for the prevention or treatment of osteoporosis around the time of menopause, and for 5 to 10 years postmenopause although recent findings about an increase in risk in heart disease for the first year of use and an increase in risk of breast cancer with long-term use mean that it is no longer the top choice. When women are older, Dr. Cosman says, "Because of that, and because we have alternative drugs that are very good for bone at that stage in life, I don't think many doctors will start women on HRT for osteoporosis treatment much after the age of 60."

**If you're taking testosterone therapy for low sex drive:** You might derive bone-building benefits, Dr. Cosman says. Testosterone replacement therapy might improve bone mass in both men and women, but it hasn't been tested or approved for use for osteoporosis in women. There also may be side effects, such as acne, facial hair growth, and deepening of the voice, says Dr. Cosman.

## Bisphosphonates

This family of drugs works by blocking the normal breakdown of old bone (bone remodelling). Bisphosphonates inhibit osteoclasts, the cells that break down bone. The bisphosphonates include etidronate (Didronel), alendronate (Fosamax), and risedronate (Actonel); Fosamax is the most commonly prescribed drug for osteoporosis in the UK.

Studies show that bisphosphonates consistently reduce the risk of spinal fractures by 40 to 50 per cent over 3 years. And they are the only sure bet among currently available drugs for reducing hip fracture. Several other bisphosphonates are currently being considered for osteoporosis treatment by the European Medicines Commission.

"Alendronate and risedronate reduce the risk not only of spine fractures but of fractures throughout the body. They are the only drugs definitely proven to reduce the risk of hip fracture – by about 50 per cent in patients with osteoporosis – so they're great if you're really concerned about the hip," Dr. Siris says. Researchers followed women taking alendronate for up to 7 years and found that it continued to build bone in the spine, maintained bone at the hip, and was generally well-tolerated.

**Follow the instructions carefully.** These drugs can be hard on your stomach, especially if you have any oesophagus or stomach problems to begin with, such as ulcers, heartburn (gastric reflux), or chronic indigestion. Swallow the drug with a full 200 ml (7 fl oz) of water first thing in the morning, before eating anything. Then, for at least 30 minutes, don't lie down. (A long-lasting 70-milligram tablet of Fosamax, taken once a week, seems to be as effective as daily dosage and may be associated with fewer side effects.)

## Oestrogen Receptor Antagonists

Oestrogen receptor antagonists are designed to fit into oestrogen receptors on a cell's surface. And so, like oestrogen, they are "keys" that fit into the "locks" that allow a hormone to "turn on" a cell. But since they are not a perfect fit, they work on only some tissues and not others, and this can be a big advantage when it comes to treatment. They are designed to maximize the effects of oestrogen on bone and to minimize or even counter oestrogen's effects on the breast and uterine lining.

Raloxifene (Evista), the only oestrogen receptor antagonist on the market approved in Europe for osteoporosis, has been shown in large clinical trials to reduce the risk of spinal fracture by 30 to 55 per cent. It has not been shown to reduce hip fractures, so "it's attractive if the bone density of the hip isn't too bad," Dr. Siris says. "It's for someone who doesn't have severe osteoporosis (other than in the spine) and who is concerned about breast cancer since it appears to reduce the risk for that disease."

**If you're between the ages of 55 and 65 and have low bone density (osteopenia):** Your doctor may suggest raloxifene, which can maintain bone mass in women past menopause and reduce spine fracture occurrences. At this age, the risk of spinal fractures is greater than the risk for hip fracture, which doesn't start to climb until close to the age of 70. Raloxifene also seems to offer some protection against breast cancer. "So it's a good choice for women who are concerned about breast cancer," Dr. Cosman says. Whether it also reduces fractures other than of the spine isn't clear.

**If you're postmenopausal and have heart disease:** Because raloxifene offers a number of apparent cardiovascular benefits, it is being studied to see whether it reduces the risk of heart attack and heart disease-related deaths in postmenopausal women. That study, called the RUTH Trial (for "Raloxifene Use for the Heart") will be finished in 2005. Scientists hope that the results will provide a wider range of treatment and prevention options for postmenopausal women in the future.

**If you have had blood clots in your veins:** You shouldn't use raloxifene. It's about as likely as oestrogen to cause blood clots. It increases your risk about threefold, although your absolute risk is still low, about 1 in 1000. The greatest risk occurs during the first 4 months of use.

**If you're taking raloxifene and experiencing breast tenderness or vaginal bleeding:** See your doctor to find out the cause. It's not likely to be due to raloxifene, says Dr. Cosman. Even though it has oestrogen-like effects on bones, raloxifene does not produce oestrogen-like effects in the uterus or breasts. There are no studies that tell how oestrogens and raloxifene act together, so the combination can't be recommended at this time.

**If you experience other side effects:** Raloxifene causes hot flushes in about 10 per cent of women and can start hot flushes in women who weren't bothered by them before. That tends to happen during the first 6 months of use and then decline. Seven per cent of women also get leg cramps, and 5 to 6 per cent get swelling of the hands or feet. Usually these side effects are minor, and you can continue taking the medication. If side effects are severe, talk to your doctor.

## Calcitonin

You can get a nasal spray or injection version of calcitonin, a hormone produced in the body by special cells in the thyroid gland. This hormone reduces the bone-dissolving activity of osteoclasts, cells in the bone responsible for bone breakdown. As a drug, it's very safe and has few side effects, but it may not be quite as effective as the other agents. Studies show it can reduce fractures of spinal vertebrae and may relieve pain in women who have already had recent spinal fractures. The usual dose is about 200 IU a day, Dr. Siris says.

"I typically prescribe calcitonin to elderly women (aged 80 or older) with spine fractures who can't use any of the other drugs," says Dr. Siris. "It may reduce the risk of spine fracture, and it is a very benign drug with few side effects." Calcitonin is used in injectable form (Calsynar, Forcaltonin and Miacalcic); Miacalcic is also used as a spray.

## Soya Substances: A Nondrug Alternative?

No doubt you've heard of isoflavones, oestrogen-like compounds found in foods like soya and red clover that some experts claim may help relieve hot flushes. Ipriflavone is a synthetic cousin of natural soya isoflavones, and in

## THE HORMONE CONNECTION

# PARATHYROID HORMONE – A NEAR-FUTURE CURE FOR OSTEOPOROSIS?

Doctors say that there's no cure for osteoporosis – yet. The best that any drug currently on the market can do is to stop bone loss and allow bones to play catch-up.

But a few call one new drug a "cure". Now in the final stages of FDA review (though it has not yet come before the European Medicines Commission), daily injections of parathyroid hormone (which, like insulin, you learn to give yourself) may actually grow new, stronger bone.

We all make parathyroid hormone in our bodies, from four peppercorn-size glands located in the region of the thyroid gland. Parathyroid hormone regulates the metabolism of calcium and phosphorus in the body, the two minerals in highest concentration in bone.

What's more, the hormone actually stimulates the growth of new bone. Given in one brief, high dose a day, parathyroid hormone increases the number of bone-building cells, called osteoblasts. And it stimulates those cells to churn out osteoid tissue, the "scaffolding" that gives bone its flexibility and great tensile strength.

"Drugs currently on the market simply prevent bone breakdown, or resorption," says Claude Arnaud, M.D., professor emeritus at the University of California, San Francisco, and a leading researcher in this field. "This one actually forms new bone tissue. It makes your body build bones the way you did when you were younger."

In a study of postmenopausal women with osteoporosis, those who got both parathyroid hormone and HRT for 2 years had a 26 per cent increase in bone density in the spine and 8 per cent at the hip. Women who got parathyroid hormone but were not taking HRT had about a 15 per cent increase in spine and a 4 per cent increase in hip bone density. The hormone increases bone mass in women with corticosteroid-induced osteoporosis and has been used to prevent bone loss in women with endometriosis who have had to take oestrogen-suppressing drugs such as danazol (Danol).

When parathyroid hormone becomes available for use, women with osteoporosis will probably use it for a short time to rebuild their bone. Once the bone is back to normal, they'll switch to a drug, such as raloxifene (Evista) or alendronate (Fosamax), that can maintain that bone density.

your body it converts to daidzein, which is also the major isoflavone found in soya beans. Overall, more than 150 animal and human studies show that ipriflavone may help prevent bone loss and build bone tissue. Ipriflavone is found in some nutritional formulas sold as bone builders.

About a dozen of those studies were done on postmenopausal women between the ages of 50 and 65. Most were small, short-term studies in which the women were given 600 to 1000 milligrams of ipriflavone a day combined with 1000 milligrams of calcium. Those taking ipriflavone plus calcium generally had either no bone loss or a slight *increase* in bone density, compared with the groups taking only a calcium supplement.

How does ipriflavone compare with osteoporosis drugs? "It's probably providing only partial protection from bone loss, about the equivalent of a very small dose of oestrogen," says Bruce Ettinger, M.D., senior investigator in the division of research at Kaiser Permanente Medical Care Program in Oakland, California, an authority on alternative treatments for osteoporosis.

Conventional doctors tend to prefer the tried-and-true over soya derivatives. "We simply have inadequate information to know if the isoflavones and ipriflavone are useful or not," Dr. Siris says. Some alternative doctors, on the other hand, say these treatments are useful for women with osteoporosis who can't or won't take HRT or an osteoporosis drug such as Fosamax.

**If you want to try ipriflavone:** Ipriflavone is available over the counter in the UK as OsteoPro. Experts suggest you buy a product that contains only ipriflavone and take a separate calcium supplement so that you are getting a total daily calcium intake of about 1000 milligrams. You may also need to take 400 to 800 IU a day of a vitamin D supplement.

# Step 6: Oestrogen, Progesterone, or Both?

If you've worked through Steps 1 to 5 and have decided you don't need to – or can't – take HRT, skip to Step 12, on page 217, for alternative treatments to consider. If you conclude that, all things considered, it's in your best interest to try HRT, read on. (Same goes if you're taking HRT for one of the individual health conditions, starting on page 298.)

Not so long ago, if you opted for hormone replacement therapy, your choices were pretty limited – it was kind of one-size-fits-all. If you hadn't had a hysterectomy, you'd be given a combination of oestrogen and progestin (synthetic progesterone). And usually, the products were Premarin (conjugated equine oestrogen, made from the urine of pregnant mares) and Provera (medroxyprogesterone, made from soya beans but still chemically distinct from the hormone made in your own body). You had one or two dosages to choose from. If you'd had a hysterectomy, you'd get oestrogen alone – usually Premarin. If you didn't want to go that whole route, you could use an oestrogen-containing cream, at least, for vaginal dryness. It, too, was made from Premarin.

Now there are dozens of types of oestrogens and progesterones on the market, and more on the way, including those most popular in other countries.

"There is no magic formula to pick the right drug for each woman, but there is an orderly procedure a doctor can follow," Dr. Minkin says. That includes ordering some of the tests we mentioned earlier, such as a total lipid profile, reviewing test results, and getting answers to questions to guide the doctor in the general direction of which drugs would be best. Here are things you need to consider.

# Step 7: Natural or Synthetic?

Once you've determined which hormones you need – oestrogen, progesterone, or both – you and your doctor will need to select a chemical "type" of each. Some doctors stick pretty much with "synthetics", others stick pretty much with "the naturals", and some combine the two. If you lean towards one or the other, it makes sense to find a doctor who will support your preference. Most general practices have one doctor who is particularly interested in the management of the menopause who will be pleased to discuss aspcts of it that affect you. And most hospitals have a specialist menopause clinic, run by the gynaecology department. You will be sure to find a sympathetic ear. Still, to be sure that you're selecting the type of HRT that fits you the best, it's best to keep an open mind, Dr. Minkin says. "Everyone is unique, and for some women, synthetic hormones actually have fewer side effects than the 'naturals'," she says.

When it comes to hormones, even experts don't always agree on how to define "synthetic" and "natural". For purposes of this discussion, a "natural" hormone has the exact same chemical structure as that made in your body – that is, biochemically identical. A "synthetic" hormone is not chemically identical to that made in your body. The source of the components used to synthesize the hormone – be it plant, animal, or laboratory – doesn't matter. It's the chemical structure that counts.

## Synthetic Oestrogen: Side Effects

Synthetic oestrogens available in the UK are ethinyloestradiol and mestianol. The side effects and potential dangers of the synthetics are well-known, but the real differences between synthetics and natural oestrogen have not been studied much, so it's hard to say what those differences are.

Some transdermal patch forms of oestrogen contain 17-beta oestradiol, the chemically identical form of the strongest oestrogen made in the body. Patches that contain this form include Estracombi, Estrapak, Evoriel, Femapak, and Nuvelle. Estring, an oestrogen-impregnated ring inserted into the vagina, also contains 17-beta oestradiol.

Premarin, the oestrogen made from pregnant mares' urine, is not the same as that found in humans. Made from soya or yams, pharmaceutical oestradiol, whose composition is not the same as that of human oestrogens, is sometimes considered natural.

## Synthetic Progestin: Not Free of Side Effects

Synthetic progestins – which include medroxyprogesterone, norethindrone, norgestimate, and levonorgesterol – are used in a variety of HRT agents. Synthetic hormones have been widely studied, and they have their place – some women do very well on them.

But some doctors believe synthetics sometimes cause problems. They are stronger than the hormones your body normally makes, and because they are foreign to your body, your liver has a harder time breaking them down. Some of the breakdown products, called metabolites, linger in your body for a long time.

"Some experts think that's a virtue of synthetic hormones," Dr. Catellani says. "They are harder to break down, the breakdown products still have some activity, and they are guaranteed to have an effect because the body can't dismantle them. The influence persists for a long period of time." While there currently is no consistent evidence to support the claim, some researchers speculate that, more than natural hormones, synthetic oestrogens and progestins may contribute to the development of cancer.

Synthetic progestins can cause such an array of unpleasant side effects – including bloating, mood swings, breast tenderness and irritability – that they're often the reason women abandon HRT entirely.

**If you have not had a hysterectomy and want to take HRT:** It's important that you take both oestrogen and progesterone or a progestin. Oestrogen causes the uterine lining − the endometrium − to proliferate and grow. Progesterone changes the structure of the endometrium, making it more organized and causing blood vessels to grow into the tissue. The natural drop in both hormones at the end of the menstrual cycle causes the endometrial tissue to slough off, but the tissue does not shed if progesterone is missing during the second half of the cycle. Instead, the uterine lining continues to build up, a condition called endometrial hyperplasia, which has the potential to progress to cancer.

Women and their doctors learned this the hard way when oestrogen replacement therapy − first approved in the 1940s − became widely used, in the 1960s. During the 1970s, use declined as the risk for endometrial cancer was recognized. Women who take synthetic oestrogen without also taking progesterone have up to 24 times the risk of developing endometrial cancer. Nobody knows what the risk for endometrial cancer is if you take natural (biochemically identical) oestrogen, but there is assumed to be some risk.

**If you take a standard HRT oestrogen/progestin combination:** You're pretty much assured of getting adequate amounts of both hormones to prevent endometrial cancer. "There doesn't seem to be an increased risk. If anything, there seems to be a decreased risk," Dr. Catellani says.

**If you're switching from oral contraceptives to HRT:** There are two different routes you can take. You can simply keep taking a low-dose oral contraceptive (OC) until about the age of 51, the average age for menopause, and then switch to HRT. Some doctors keep their patients on OCs even into their mid-fifties.

Or, at any time between the ages of 48 and 51, you can stop the Pill for 4 weeks, then have your FSH levels measured. Since FSH levels fluctuate during perimenopause, however, a more accurate way to do this is to stop the Pill for several months and have your FSH levels measured several times. Of course, you'll want to use some other form of birth control during this time.

The switch from OCs to HRT should be made when FSH has risen to at least 30 mIU/ml (milli international units per millilitre) or higher.

**Whether you are taking synthetic or natural hormones, if you have abnormal bleeding, and especially if you have it a few times within a few months:** Your doctor may want to do an endometrial biopsy. This is a common procedure, done in the doctor's surgery. A thin suction tube is inserted into the uterus to remove a small amount of tissue. A microscopic examination of the tissue sample can provide answers as to what exactly is going on and, more important, determine if you have endometrial cancer. A uterine ultrasound instead can determine if you have endometrial overgrowth, but if overgrowth is discovered, you'll still need a biopsy to get a definite answer about cancer.

**If you're postmenopausal because you had your ovaries removed along with your uterus, especially if this was done before 50:** You may be likely to benefit from getting testosterone along with oestrogen and progesterone. Testosterone levels are lower in women who have had their ovaries removed. Symptoms of low testosterone levels are lack of sex drive, fatigue and depression.

**If you're taking phyto-oestrogens from soya foods or herbs, instead of oestrogen:** You won't need to take progesterone to avoid endometrial cancer. "These act as very weak oestrogens, and have oestrogen-blocking qualities as well. The soya foods in particular have a long history of safe use," says Dr. Catellani. (For more details, see "Step 12: Alternative Remedies to Try" on page 217.) However, because researchers haven't definitively resolved safety issues for phyto-oestrogens, it's best to take phyto-oestrogenic herbs such as black cohosh, or soya isoflavones, under medical supervision. And as with oestrogen/progesterone combination therapy, if you have unexplained bleeding, always check with your doctor about it. You may be overstimulating your uterine lining. "All of us physicians have had patients taking enough herbal combinations without progesterone that they have had vaginal bleeding," Dr. Minkin says. "This suggests that there is action on the endometrium with these 'benign' herbal remedies."

**If you've had a hysterectomy:** The conventional consensus is that you can take oestrogen alone – no progesterone needed. However, some "alternative" doctors are recommending an oestrogen/progesterone combination even to women who have had a hysterectomy, Dr. Catellani says. "It's a misconception that if you don't have a uterus, you don't need progesterone. Progesterone is the balancing partner to oestrogen, and it does many things that are beneficial besides preventing endometrial cancer," she says. Natural progesterone (not synthetic, discussed below) can improve sleep, has a natural calming effect during the day, helps maintain fluid balance in the body, may actually help to protect against breast cancer, helps to normalize libido, aids in the body's ability to use and eliminate fats, and builds bone mass.

Those who don't advocate progesterone use in women who have had a hysterectomy – Dr. Minkin included – point out that two recent studies suggest that the progestin (synthetic progesterone) component of HRT is what puts women at increased risk for breast cancer. "Besides that, progestin is the culprit in the HRT balance that frequently causes bloating and other side effects," she says. "Most women have more trouble adjusting to the progestin component than the oestrogen component of HRT."

**If you decide to stop HRT:** You'll have fewer symptoms if you reduce your dose gradually. Try this, Dr. Catellani suggests: reduce your dosage of oestrogen by half and stay at that dose for 1 to 2 months, giving your body a chance to adjust to the lower dose. If you're still having lots of symptoms after that time, stay on that dose until your symptoms begin to abate. Then drop the dosage by one-half again, bringing the amount of oestrogen to one-quarter of your original dosage. You can stop altogether after that, once your symptoms have disappeared.

## What Natural Hormones Have to Offer

As for the natural hormones, the biochemically identical form of progesterone is simply called progesterone or sometimes micronized progesterone. "More doctors are coming to realize there are definite advantages to using natural progesterone," Dr. Minkin says. One of the clearest advantages: unlike the most widely used synthetic progestin, medroxyprogesterone (MPA), natural progesterone does not undo oestrogen's beneficial effects on HDL cholesterol. "Oestrogen has a very positive effect on lipid levels," Dr. Minkin says. "It raises HDL and lowers LDL. When you add medroxyprogesterone, just the opposite happens. So a lot of the lipid benefits you get from oestrogen go away when you also take medroxyprogesterone. The micronized progesterone doesn't have that effect."

One study, on the other hand, found that women who switched from synthetic to natural progesterone reported significantly fewer problems with quality-of-life symptoms. They also reported fewer problems with sleep disorders, menstrual problems, hot flushes, anxiety, symptoms of depression and sexual function.

Natural progesterone's main side effect with high doses – drowsiness – can even be a boon to menopausal women suffering from insomnia if it's taken at bedtime. "But I've not had any patients complain of drowsiness on the doses that I use routinely for HRT," Dr. Minkin says.

## Natural Testosterone

It's also possible to get a "natural" form of testosterone, simply called micronized testosterone in the US. In the UK testesterone is not recommended for women as a rule.

## Which Natural Hormone Is Right for You?

The following advice can help you and your doctor arrive at your best option among natural hormones for menopause.

**If you've been taking a synthetic progestin and have experienced side effects:** Dr. Minkin recommends switching to an equivalent dose of micronized progesterone. For women on a daily continuous cycle (2.5 milligrams of Provera) the equivalent of Prometrium is 100 milligrams a day. For women on a cycled dose – taking 2.5, 5, or 10 milligrams of Provera during 12 days of the cycle – the equivalent dose of Prometrium is 200 milligrams. (But note that Prometrium is very rarely prescribed in the UK.)

**If Prometrium causes side effects:** Ask for micronized natural progesterone in a vaginal gel (Crinone). Available by prescription only, this product delivers a protective amount of progesterone to the uterus, with fewer side effects than pills. "I use it for women for whom Prometrium causes side effects," Dr. Minkin says. Studies have demonstrated that it can prevent endometrial hyperplasia (overgrowth of the uterine lining) in postmenopausal women taking oestrogen. Crinone is guaranteed not to leak out, but it is strange to use. It's an expanding foam you insert into your vagina just before bedtime and leave in. "It looks like plastic foam, and it's messy but it really sticks in there," Dr. Minkin says.

**If the pills cause side effects and gel is too messy to use:** Talk to your doctor to see if you should consider a progesterone cream, available over the counter. But be careful: some don't contain much in the way of absorbable progesterone. Use a cream that contains pharmaceutical-grade progesterone – it should say "progesterone BP" on the label. Look for a minimum of 400 milligrams per ounce, the amount proponents say is needed to alleviate menopausal symptoms. And be especially wary of "wild yam" creams that say they contain diosgenin, "a precursor to progesterone". Though it implies that your body can turn constituents in the yam into progesterone, it can't.

**If you are also taking oestrogen:** Don't count on a nonprescription progesterone cream to counterbalance the oestrogen, even though it may relieve your hot flushes. "It may not contain enough progesterone to do that," says Dr. Catellani. "See your doctor to get a proper dosage of progesterone."

# Step 8: Determine the Right Dose

In addition to a trend towards use of natural hormones, doctors now tend to use lower doses of all hormones, especially for women well past menopause (aged 60 and above). "Oral oestrogen started out with 2.5 milligrams, then 1.25, 0.625, and now may go as low as 0.3 milligrams," Dr. Minkin says. The lower dosages have led to fewer side effects such as bloating, blood clots, gallbladder disease and, probably, endometrial cancer. Some doctors hope these lower doses will lead to a reduction in other risks, including cancer, in the long run. Research shows that even low-dose oestrogen increases bone mineral density by as much as 5.2 per cent, provided it's combined with adequate calcium and vitamin D.

Same goes for progestin and progesterone. Dosages have dropped over the years, and there are more "standardized" dosages than ever to choose from. For both hormones, your doctor should select a dosage that relieves your symptoms adequately and protects you from endometrial overgrowth, without causing undue side effects.

# Step 9: Do You Prefer Periods or No Periods?

Taking hormones in a cyclical pattern that mimics the natural rise and fall of hormone levels in the body maintains the menstrual cycle. Taking hormones in a continuous combined dosage (such as Climesse or Estracombi, which is a combination of oestradiol and norethisterone, a progestin) eliminates monthly periods. Natural hormones can be used in a cyclical or continuous pattern; which way often depends on a woman's age. Older women may use low-dose continuous natural hormones. Women who have had their uterus or ovaries removed will use oestrogen daily, but not progestin.

Is there any advantage to combined continuous HRT over cyclical? "The definitive answer isn't in on that yet," Dr. Catellani says. The combined continuous dosage is convenient, certainly. One big reason older women stop HRT, or won't start it, is that they feel uncomfortable having periods at, say, the age of 65. Another advantage of continuous HRT for women in their fifties is that with monthly cycling, some get hot flushes during the week they are not taking hormones.

"A lot of women tell me if I put them on a cyclical regime, they feel so much better when they're taking it, but those 5 days when they have to stop taking anything, they feel miserable and have hot flushes and then have to start HRT all over again," Dr. Catellani says. "So sometimes I prescribe a lesser dose of progesterone for 5 days, instead of no dose. But some are miserable even then, so I keep them on continuous progesterone and their periods stop altogether, and they are usually very happy."

And whether you take cyclical or continuous hormones, as you get older, you're less and less likely to have periods anyway. That's especially true in the case of low-dose biochemically identical hormones, Dr. Catellani says.

"Some women just stop menstruating no matter what they're taking, and that's just fine," she says. It's also possible to cycle every 2 or 3 months, Dr. Minkin says. She prefers every 2 months, to help prevent the possibility of endometrial overgrowth.

# Step 10: Pill, Patch, Vaginal Cream, or Ring?

If you decide to go the pill, patch, or transdermal cream route, you'll be getting "systemic" hormones – they circulate throughout your body. There is a big difference between taking a pill and using a patch or transdermal cream, though, with regard to the way they interact with your liver.

With pills, after the hormones pass through your intestines and into your bloodstream, they travel directly to your liver (the "first pass") before entering general circulation and into tissues throughout the body. So your liver experiences more of the impact from the hormones. This can be good or bad, depending on the desired effect. For instance, oestrogen raises "good", HDL levels most during its first pass through the liver, so if your HDL levels are low, your doctor might recommend oral oestrogen. But oestrogen also raises triglycerides and blood glucose levels, both also in the liver. So if you already have high triglycerides or have diabetes, you're better off avoiding oral HRT and sticking with a transdermal patch, says Dr. Minkin.

Alternatively, you could also use a vaginal or skin cream or take a sublingual pill (dissolved under the tongue). These forms bypass the liver.

Synthetic progestins tend to negate oestrogen's HDL-raising effects and, again, work in the liver. To avoid that effect, you might use a transdermal patch or a skin cream, a vaginal cream, a sublingual pill, or natural micronized progesterone, which doesn't seem to have that effect.

Blood-clotting factors are also made in the liver, and some doctors believe that the tendency for synthetic oestrogens to make blood likelier to clot comes in part from that first pass through the liver. Because of that, some doctors believe that the transdermal patch is less likely to cause clotting problems than oral oestrogen, Dr. Minkin says. "But the transdermal hasn't been around long enough, and there aren't yet enough women in studies to know for sure if it really is safer than oral oestrogen when it comes to blood clots," she says.

Testosterone also has an impact on your liver, although the impact tends to be slight in the small dosages women use. It tends to lower HDL and raise total cholesterol. This is less likely to happen when testosterone is applied to the skin or used as a gel used around the clitoris and labia, as it sometimes is.

The mucous membranes of your vagina are a good route for absorbing hormones, but their main impact tends to be on the vagina and urethra, so vaginal creams, rings, or gels are most likely to be recommended if a woman's main complaint is vaginal dryness or urinary tract problems associated with low oestrogen levels and she needs to reduce her systemic exposure to hormones, Dr. Minkin says. The vaginal route might be used in some women who can't take oral or transdermal hormones since blood levels remain lower.

Creams and gels tend to be messy and must be applied daily. A more convenient choice is a vaginal ring, such as Estring, similar to the outer rim of a diaphragm and inserted into the upper third of the vagina. The ring releases a controlled dose of oestrogen for 90 days. A woman can both insert and remove the ring herself. The most recent choice is Vagifem, a tablet that's inserted into the vagina. (For information on hormonal and non-hormonal treatments for vaginal dryness and irritation, see page 305.)

The possible combinations of hormone delivery routes are numerous. You can use an oestrogen patch and take progesterone orally, or use an oestrogen patch and progesterone cream, either cyclically or continuously. You can use oral oestrogen and a progesterone cream, vaginal oestrogen and progesterone cream. It's also possible to use an oestrogen cream. Instead of having an adhesive patch you stick on every couple of days, you rub a cream into your skin once or twice a day. You and your doctor will need to figure out what's best for you.

# Step 11: Individualize Your Prescription

More than ever, it is possible to individualize HRT. But you have to work with your doctor. "It can take some trial and error to find the HRT regime that works best for you," Dr. Minkin says. "Whatever we try, I emphasize to women I treat that this is just the first trial with HRT. I say, 'If you don't like it, that's all right. Call me.'"

**Give it 3 months.** Dr. Minkin asks women to try the first type and form of therapy she suggests for at least 3 months before deciding if it's not for them because initial side effects sometimes subside during that time. "But I also tell them that if they just can't get through the first month, then call me and we'll work something out," she says. "If they're uncomfortable enough to want to stop the medication, I want them to call me immediately." (See "Solutions for a Side Effect-Free HRT" below.)

Only about 45 per cent of women ever try HRT, and of those who do, two out of three stop taking it within a year because of side effects or fears, and often without discussing it with their doctors. "It's amazing how many women are walking around with unused prescriptions in their handbags," Dr. Minkin says. "Their doctors haven't answered all their questions, and until those questions are answered, they're not taking it."

Many of these women don't realize that they have more than one type, form, or dosage of hormone therapy from which to choose, Dr. Minkin says. "Their doctors just never tell them."

**Re-evaluate your therapy every few years.** What works for a woman initially usually doesn't suit her later in life. "A woman may take a particular type and dosage of HRT at menopause to relieve a particular symptom, such as hot flushes, and then reconsider her prescription later in regard to long-term use," Dr. Minkin says. She sees a fair number of women who didn't fare well initially on HRT and just stopped taking it. Now, later in life, they are willing to reconsider it, perhaps because they've been diagnosed with low bone density or osteoporosis. In fact, very low dose oestrogens are now being marketed specifically at women who are considering reinitiating oestrogen replacement therapy later in life to prevent osteoporosis.

**Don't be afraid that you're "bothering" your doctor.** Doctors who specialize in HRT expect adjustments. They're the norm, not a sign of failure. They're important in terms of maximizing benefits and minimizing side effects and dangers over the course of a woman's postmenopausal years.

## Solutions for a Side Effect-Free HRT

Hormone replacement therapy shouldn't have to be a trade-off. You should not have to trade hot flushes for breast tenderness, or osteoporosis protection for irregular bleeding. That's the whole point of tailoring a formula to meet your needs: to minimize the side effects that, at least in the past, have convinced many women that HRT isn't worth the trouble or risk.

True, some of the benefits, such as osteoporosis protection, seem pretty far down the road. "That's one reason periodically monitoring your bone density can be an incentive," Dr. Cosman says. "To get a woman who is basically healthy to take a medication and keep taking it when she has absolutely no symptoms at all, for protection 5 years later from fracture, you want to have something objective that says, 'Yes, this is working.'"

But HRT should also help you feel good right now, says Dr. Pollycove. And the trend has certainly been in the right direction: lower dosages of oestrogen and progestin or progesterone, the availability of natural (biochemically identical) forms of both oestrogen and progesterone, and the realization that some women do better when they also get a pinch of androgens have all made HRT a lot more user-friendly, Dr. Pollycove says.

Here's how to sidestep side effects.

**If you experience irregular or unwanted bleeding:** Tell your doctor, so she or he can rule out cancer or overgrowth of the uterine lining. An endometrial biopsy (uterine lining tissue sample) will help determine if you need more oestrogen, more progesterone, or both, Dr. Pollycove says. If you're younger than 55, switching from continuous combined to a cyclical regime may restore normal cycles and let your body do what it wants to do a while longer, Dr. Catellani says. If you're 55 or older, switching from a cyclical regime to combined continuous may help you stop having periods altogether sooner, she says. Always consult a health care professional about irregular bleeding or bleeding between cycles.

**If you experience breast tenderness:** More than one-third of women who take HRT report breast tenderness, and in clinical practice, older women taking HRT seem more likely to experience trouble with breast pain than younger women. "Oestrogen stimulates breast tissue proliferation and can cause swelling and fluid retention that is just plain uncomfortable," says Serafina Corsello, M.D., director of the Corsello Centers for Integrative Medicine in New York City and Melville, New York, and author of *The Ageless Woman*.

To reduce breast tenderness: take natural forms of hormones, and make sure you take progesterone along with oestrogen, even if you've had a hysterectomy, Dr. Corsello says. "Progesterone counteracts oestrogen's effects on breast tissue," she says. Lower the oestrogen dose, cut back on salt intake, cut back on caffeine and take 400 to 800 IU of vitamin E a day.

Dr. Corsello also uses iodine to treat breast tenderness, but only after she has determined that a woman has no problems with her thyroid gland.

"This is one of the most important things you can do," she says. "Iodine modulates the effects of oestrogen on breast tissue." Breast tissue lacks an enzyme that is needed to convert the most common form of iodine found in the diet, iodide, to iodine, the form that is used in the body. She uses elemental iodine (4 to 8 drops a day, depending on body size) or an organic source of iodine, such as kelp, to provide a dosage of no more than 500 micrograms a day.

For other, non-hormonal strategies for breast lumps or tenderness, see page 408 Breast Lumps and Tenderness.

**If you experience headaches:** Switch from synthetic progestins to natural micronized progesterone. If taking oestrogen alone, add natural micronized progesterone; reduce your dosage of oral oestrogen; switch from oral oestrogen to a transdermal patch, which causes less variability in blood levels of oestrogen throughout the day; change to an everyday, continuous dosage schedule; restrict salt intake to reduce fluid retention.

**If you experience bloating or weight gain:** Studies show that women who take HRT are no more likely to gain weight than women who don't take it. But "while that might be true on average, there are some women who definitely gain weight with HRT," Dr. Catellani says. Some postmenopausal women experience water retention with hormone therapy, especially synthetic hormones, just as some women retain water in response to oral contraceptives or during the later phase of their menstrual cycle.

These women may need to lower their dosage, switch to natural forms of hormones, or add natural progesterone to an oestrogen-only regime, even if they have had a hysterectomy, Dr. Catellani says.

Restricting salt intake and taking a herbal diuretic, such as uva-ursi, or a mild prescription diuretic can also help. Dr. Catellani recommends one to two capsules of uva-ursi three times a day.

**If you've gone from muscle to fat or if you've had no luck building muscle even though you exercise:** You might be low in testosterone, Dr. Corsello says. Get your blood levels of free testosterone measured, and start on low-dose testosterone if indicated, she recommends. In studies, testosterone has increased the ratio of muscle to fat, and improved muscle strength in frail, elderly women.

**If you experience depression, emotionality, or tearfulness:** Switch from synthetic progestins to natural micronized progesterone. Compared with women who took synthetic progestins, women who took micronized progesterone report significantly fewer symptoms of this sort. Take progesterone, even if you've had a hysterectomy. Talk to your doctor about cutting your oestrogen dosage or switching to a natural form. Stop the HRT for a few months to see if hormones are the cause. Check testosterone levels and add testosterone if needed. Do this especially if fatigue and a lagging interest in sex are accompanying problems.

**If you experience anxiety:** Try a natural product called Stabilium, Dr. Corsello suggests. Also called Garum Armoricum, this product is made from the fermented intestines of the great blue fish. Rich in neuropeptides (several types of molecules found in brain tissue), it's popular in Spain, France and Japan as an alternative to Valium. It is available in the UK by mail order from, among others, www.positivenation.co.uk.

**If you have no sexual desire:** The usual thinking is that HRT will not cause a lack of sexual desire. If anything, HRT should improve sexual desire by eliminating vaginal dryness and improving general well-being, says Barbara Bartlik, M.D., clinical assistant professor of psychiatry at Weill Medical College of Cornell University in New York City. In fact, oestrogen does do this. But it has another, unwanted effect. It makes your body produce more of the proteins that bind to testosterone, the male hormone that drives sexual desire and arousal. So the more oestrogen you get, the less testosterone you end up with, ultimately.

"A woman may start on oestrogen, and have a wonderful feeling of sexuality and psychological well-being," Dr. Bartlik says. "But then, after she's been on it for 3 months, 6 months, or a year, she starts to lose her sexual feeling. I can't say how long it takes exactly, but somewhere down the road, she finds herself unable to function sexually."

The solution: supplemental testosterone, in very small doses. In the US one pill form available for women, Estratest, combines oestrogen with 1.25 milligrams of methyltestosterone, a synthetic form of testosterone. But it's also possible to take testosterone in much smaller dosages than this by using a gel (which you may be able to get prescribed in the UK). The gel is usually applied to the clitoris and labia. This lower dose avoids some of the possible side effects.

A gynaecologist is most likely to know about testosterone treatment for women, but if you have no luck with your doctor, try calling around to find a psychologist or psychiatrist who specializes in sex therapy. That doctor can steer you towards a gynaecologist who is familiar with the use of supplemental testosterone for menopause. (For more information on this topic, see chapter 8.)

**If you feel nauseated:** Take oestrogen tablets at bedtime or with meals; switch to a transdermal patch.

**If you're a diabetic, and your blood sugar level rises:** Switch to transdermal oestrogen or esterified oestrogen (oestrogens produced from natural sources or synthesized).

# Step 12: Alternative Remedies to Try

If you've decided that hormone replacement isn't for you, or you haven't been able to settle on a type, form, or combination that you can tolerate to your satisfaction, or you've found that natural progesterone isn't effective for you, alternative remedies may offer hope. And in fact some of what was once strictly alternative is becoming more mainstream. Natural (biochemically identical) progesterone, for instance, used to be considered unnecessary by most doctors. Now several studies have shown it has benefits over synthetic progestins. Stress-relieving deep breathing may still seem far-out, but research at Wayne State University in Detroit suggests that some women can reduce hot flushes by nearly half.

Other nondrug, non-hormonal alternatives for the menopause include herbs and herbal formulas, nutritional supplements, diet, exercise and several different stress reduction techniques. (You'll find additional or expanded hormone-balancing techniques in Phases 2 and 3 of the Hormone-Balancing Programme, later in this book, beginning on pages 275 and 297 respectively.)

Alternative remedies can work as well as conventional medicine, say doctors who prescribe them. "Many women do very well with just dietary changes, lifestyle changes, herbal supplements, things as simple as vitamin E and flaxseed oil," Dr. Catellani says. "These things control their symptoms to the point where they feel much better and don't feel like they need something more. Plus, they feel like they, not their doctors, are in control of their bodies."

That said, it's always best to work with your doctor when trying alternative remedies, to get the best results and to avoid possible risks or clashes, says Dr. Catellani. (To find a doctor trained in use of alternative medicine for the menopause, see "On the Web & Other Resources" on page 220.)

Here's a sampling of what alternative doctors are likely to have in their menopause medical bag.

## Herbs of Choice for Menopause

Hot flushes, mood swings, insomnia, anxiety and vaginal dryness, among other changes associated with menopause, respond well to either individual herbs or a formulation of combined herbs, Dr. Catellani says. As different people respond to these treatments in different ways, try another route if your first attempts are not successful.

### THE HORMONE ZONE
# THE MENOPAUSE MENU

It's possible to get some effects similar to oestrogen in your body by eating foods that contain phyto-oestrogens, plant versions of oestrogen. For instance, both isoflavones in soya and lignans in flaxseed are rich sources of phyto-oestrogens, says Hope Ricciotti, M.D., an obstetrician gynaecologist at Beth Israel–Deaconess Medical Center in Boston and co-author of *The Menopause Cookbook: How to Eat Now and for the Rest of Your Life.*

Even though isoflavones have been isolated from soya and used to make nutritional supplements that may help alleviate hot flushes, many experts still recommend getting your isoflavones from foods, not supplements. "There's not a lot of data about taking phyto-oestrogens as isolated supplements, and there is some worry that compounds isolated from foods might not work the same as natural sources," Dr. Ricciotti says. "With soya, for instance, it's thought that to get the maximal activity in terms of health protection and symptom reduction, you have to have the whole product, not just isolates or tablets." It may take a few weeks to see an improvement.

Fatty fish, such as mackerel, salmon and tuna, contain fats that help prevent heart disease and reduce tendency for clotting, as well as provide some vitamin D. Low-fat dairy products provide calcium to maintain bones.

Adding certain kinds of food – and subtracting others – targets menopause symptoms such as hot flushes, and it can also help ward off the biggest risk factors for older women: heart disease, osteoporosis, weight gain, arthritis and depression, Dr. Ricciotti says. "Healthy eating does more for overall health and disease prevention than any pill or prescription." More important, a diet high in fruits and vegetables provides the kind of "internal environment" in your intestines that allows phyto-oestrogens to be broken down and absorbed.

# Black Cohosh

The now-outdated but traditional name for this herb, squaw root, reflects its long history as the herb of choice for Native American female problems. It was also one of the main ingredients in Lydia E. Pinkham's Vegetable Compound, a popular herbal formula for "female complaints" during the mid-1800s.

**FOODS TO ADD**

- Silken tofu, firm tofu, soya milk, tempeh, soya beans, soya flour (one 115-g (4-ounce) serving a day)

- Texturised vegetable protein (TVP)

- Red clover tea

- Products made with soya protein isolate (not soya protein concentrate, which does not contain isoflavones)

- Ground flaxseed, 1 tablespoon a day, added to a blender smoothie, hot cereal, or in baking

- Lentils, seaweed, asparagus, squash (contain small amounts of phyto–oestrogens)

- Swiss chard, kale, turnip tops, berries, citrus fruits, winter squash, beans, whole grains, nuts and seeds

- Fatty fish (sardines, mackerel, salmon, tuna and herring), 2 or 3 times a week

- Fat-free milk, low-fat yoghurt and cheese, and other low-fat dairy products (4 or 5 servings a day)

**FOODS TO SUBTRACT**

- Butter, beef, cheese, whole milk, cream

- Hydrogenated fats and trans fatty acids: coconut oil, margarine and palm oil (found in commercial baked goods)

- Grapefruit and grapefruit juice (if you're taking HRT, a compound in grapefruit juice can interfere with your liver's ability to metabolize the hormones, elevating blood levels and causing its effects to linger longer)

## ON THE WEB & Other Resources

The British Menopause Society offers updates on all issues related to menopause. Write to the society at:

**The British Menopause Society**
The Menopause Amarant Trust
22 Barkham Terrace
Lambeth Road
London SE1 7PW
Tel: 01293 413 000
*www.the-bms.org*

BUPA has fact sheets on its Web site on the menopause and osteoporosis. Contact *www.bupa.co.uk/factsheets* which gives lists of hospitals with special units for the menopause and osteoporosis.

Fact sheets are also on the Web site of the Health Education Board, Scotland (HEBS) at *www.hebs.com*

There is a thriving British National Osteoporosis Society. Contact:

**The British National Osteoporosis Society**
Camerton
Bath BA2 0BJ
Tel: 01761 472721
E-mail: *info@nos.org.uk*
*www.nos.org.uk*

Women's Health Concern also has a keen interest in helping women with menopausal problems and osteoporosis. Write to them at:

**Women's Health Concern**
PO Box 2126
Marlow
Bucks SL7 2RY
Tel: 01628 483612

One of the best Web sites for osteoporosis is the BBC. Its site has as much information as women could want, presented very professionally. It is also, of course, independent of any vested interest: *www.bbc.co.uk/health/women/osteo. shtml*

OTHER SOURCES
For up-to-date, detailed information on the HRT–cardiovascular disease controversy, check out the American College of Cardiology's Web site (from the home page, you can search the site for "HRT") at: *www.acc.org*

One of the major components of the national Women's Health Initiative (WHI) study is a hormone replacement therapy intervention that looks specifically at the effects of long-term HRT on coronary heart disease and its effects on fractures as a result of osteoporosis. The study was started in 1991. Final results won't be available until the study ends. For information about WHI, the first randomized clinical trial to examine the relationship between hormones and heart disease and breast cancer, go to: *www.nih.gov/news/nf/womenshealth*

"This is my favourite herb to use for menopausal symptoms. It really does make a big difference," Dr. Catellani says. Studies in menopausal women show that black cohosh alleviates symptoms of hot flushes, night sweats, vaginal dryness, sleep disturbances, nervousness, irritability and depression. Research focusing on a standardized black cohosh extract called Remifemin has found it performs on a par with oestrogen replacement treatment for such menopause symptoms.

Scientists have yet to determine precisely how black cohosh works, but apparently, like soya isoflavones, it modulates both oestrogen deficiency and excess, Dr. Catellani says. Some doctors say it shouldn't be used continually for more than 6 months since its long-term effects have not been studied. But there have been no reported adverse effects from its long-term use, and Dr. Catellani says, "Some women I treat have used it for 3 or 4 years with no problems."

The herb appears to carry no increased risk for cancer. In fact, in Germany, where black cohosh is used regularly, a German drug regulatory agency feels that the herb is safe for use in women with oestrogen-sensitive cancers as well as those with uterine bleeding, liver or gallbladder disease, endometriosis, uterine fibroids and fibrocystic breast disease, all conditions that generally rule out synthetic hormone replacement. Two Asian species of black cohosh also appear to help strengthen bone.

To prevent menopausal symptoms, take one to two 40-milligram capsules or tablets of extract (standardized to 2.5 per cent triterpene glycosides) twice a day. The dosage for standardized extract is ½ to 1 teaspoon (60 to 120 drops) twice a day, says Dr. Catellani. If you are currently taking HRT and would like to switch to black cohosh, you should talk to a health care practitioner, Dr. Catellani says. You may need guidance to cut back gradually on the HRT and to make sure you are taking enough black cohosh to do the trick. Otherwise, you'll have a flare-up of menopausal symptoms.

## Herbal Menopause Formulas

Many of the other herbs used for menopause are sold only in herbal formulas. That's especially true of Chinese herbs, says Frank Scott, a diplomate of Chinese Herbology and Acupuncture (National Commission for the Certification of Acupuncture and Oriental Medicine). Scott, who works with Dr. Catellani at the Miro Center for Integrative Medicine in Evanston, Illinois, sees patients who prefer an Eastern approach to menopause or who want to combine the best of both worlds. Dang gui (also called dong quai),

(continued on page 225)

# Stop Osteoporosis with These Moves

## WIDE LEG SQUAT

Stand about 15 cm (6 inches) in front of a chair that has its back pushed against a wall (so it won't slide). Put your feet a little wider than shoulder-width apart and turn your toes slightly outward. Cross your arms in front of your chest and relax your shoulders. Keep your back, neck and head in a straight line and your chest lifted as you lean slightly forward from the hip. Take a deep breath, then aim your buttocks back and slowly lower yourself onto the chair. Don't move your knees forward (they should remain above your ankles). Pause for a moment in the seated position, then lean forward and slowly stand up. Repeat until you have done 8 wide leg squats. This is one set. Rest for a minute and do a

second set. When you're ready for more, vary the routine by lowering your body almost to the chair, but don't sit. Hold yourself in position for a breath, then rise. When you're ready to add weights, do the exercise holding a dumbbell in each hand, hands crossed over your chest so that the dumbbells rest on the top part of the shoulders.

## STEPUP

Stand close to the bottom step of a staircase and hold the railing lightly for support. Place one foot squarely on the first step so that your toes point forward. Keep your head and torso upright and your eyes focused straight ahead. Make sure the knee of your front leg is directly over your ankle and does not move past your toes. Using the muscles of your front leg to support your weight (don't push off with your back leg), lift your body straight up and tap the toes of your back foot on the first step. Pause for a breath, then slowly return to the starting position. Repeat the move with the same front leg until you have done 8 reps, and then switch legs and do 8 more to complete one set. Rest for a minute and do a second set. When you're ready to increase the intensity of this exercise, start with your front leg on the second step, instead of the first. Or you can cross your arms over your chest and hold a dumbbell in each hand as you do the exercise.

## FORWARD FLY

To get to the starting position, hold a dumbbell in each hand while you sit in a chair with your feet flat on the floor, hip-width apart. Keep your back flat and your spine straight as you bend forward from your hips about 8 to 13 cm (3 to 5 inches). Hold the dumbbells in front of your chest (palms facing each other, elbows slightly bent) so the ends point straight up.

To do the exercise, which will strengthen your shoulders and upper back, pull your shoulder blades together, moving your elbows as far back as possible. Keep your arms slightly bent throughout

the move. Pause, then slowly bring your arms back to starting position. Repeat until you've done 8 reps. Rest and do a second set.

## SEATED OVERHEAD PRESS

Holding a dumbbell in each hand, sit upright toward the front of your chair and plant your feet flat about hip-width apart. To get to the starting position, keep your upper arms at your sides and bend your elbows to bring the weights just in front of your shoulders and parallel to the floor. To begin, slowly press the dumbbells straight up. Extend your arms fully, but don't lock your elbows. The weights should be just slightly in front of your head, not directly above it. Pause, and then slowly return to starting position. Repeat for 8 reps. Rest and repeat a second set of 8 reps.

(continued on page 224)

# Stop Osteoporosis with These Moves (cont.)

## FRONT LUNGE

For balance, lightly hold on to a table or counter with one hand. Take a large step forward with your right foot, landing on the heel and then rolling your foot forward until it is flat on the floor. Keep your body erect as you bend both knees (your hips should drop straight down). Lower your upper body until your front thigh is almost parallel to the floor, and the knee of your back leg approaches the floor (your back heel will come off the floor). The knee of your forward leg should be over your ankle, not past your toes. Pause for a breath, then push back forcefully with the front leg to return to the starting position. To complete one set, alternate legs as you step forward until you have done 8 steps with each leg. Rest for a minute and do a second set.

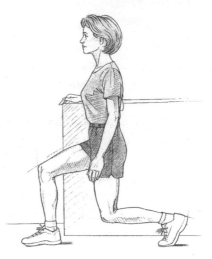

## BACK EXTENSION

Lie face down on a mat with your legs straight and toes pointed. Place your right arm (palm up) down along your side and place your left arm (palm down) straight up above your head.

Raise your right leg and left arm at the same time, as high off the floor as you can in a smooth, comfortable motion; your head and neck will rise, too. Make sure to keep your leg straight as you lift it from the hip, as well as your head and neck in line with your arm. Pause in the lifted position, then slowly return to starting position. For the next lift, raise the other leg and arm. Repeat until you've done 8 reps with both sides. Rest and then do another set. When you're ready to make this exercise more challenging, raise not only your arm but also your shoulder and upper chest as you lift your leg.

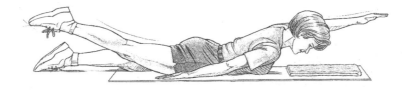

for instance, is blended with other herbs, such as licorice, ginseng and rehmannia. The blend can be "customized" by a Chinese herbalist according to a woman's menopausal symptoms, other health problems, and her "constitutional type," Scott says.

The Chinese menopause formulas you find in health food shops, in contrast, are best avoided, Scott says. They cover a broad range of symptoms, and while they might help one symptom, such as hot flushes, they might not help – or might even exacerbate – another symptom, Scott says. Or they may be so "watered-down" that they're safe but not effective. "If you're really interested in using Chinese herbs safely and effective, get a customized formula, made up specifically for your symptoms, along with good guidance in its use, from a trained Chinese herbalist," Scott says. Word of mouth is probably your best way of finding a good local herbalist.

## Milk Thistle

If you've been taking synthetic hormones and having symptoms related to excess – such as breast tenderness, headaches, or bloating – it may mean your body isn't "clearing" the breakdown products of these drugs, says Dr. Corsello. It's your liver's job to break down these by-products, and to help it out, she recommends milk thistle, or silymarin, a herb that protects the liver against harmful substances and even helps repair and regenerate injured liver cells. Milk thistle is best taken as a standardized extract because it's relatively poorly absorbed, there is no research on milk thistle as a tincture or a tea, and its main constituents do not dissolve easily into water.

The usual dose for milk thistle is 420 milligrams, divided into two to three doses a day, for 6 to 8 weeks, then a reduction to 280 milligrams daily, Dr. Corsello says.

## St. John's Wort

In women who have had hormone-related bouts of depression earlier in life, symptoms may return during menopause, Dr. Catellani says. St. John's wort, long recognized for its ability to fight "melancholy", has been shown to be as effective as some prescription antidepressants. "It's very safe and gentle, but effective for mild to moderate depression," Dr. Catellani says. "It's less likely than prescription antidepressants to cause side effects, such as fatigue, loss of sexual interest, or dry mouth." It may also relieve the anxiety and insomnia that sometimes accompany depression, and physical complaints such as fatigue or aches and pains.

The dosage used in most clinical trials was 300 milligrams in capsule form, three times a day, of an extract containing 0.3 per cent hypericin, one of the active ingredients in St. John's wort. And you may need to use it regularly for 2 to 3 weeks before you see an effect. If symptoms persist, seek immediate help from a qualified mental health professional.

### Ginkgo and Phosphatidylserine

For "mental fogginess" – problems with memory and concentration – Dr. Corsello suggests ginkgo biloba, a herb that improves circulation in the vast network of fine vessels that feed the brain, and phosphatidylserine, a nutritional supplement also used for the treatment of depression and impaired mental function in the elderly. (For details on both of these supplements, see chapter 5.)

## When Your Heart Needs Help

If you have heart disease, current research suggests it might not be a good idea to start on HRT, although if you've been taking it for more than a year with no problems, it should be safe to continue. The usual "alternatives" for heart disease are protective steps most doctors recommend: cut back on saturated fat, lose weight, exercise and eat fish and lots of fruits and vegetables. But you might also ask about either coenzyme $Q_{10}$ (a nutritional supplement) or hawthorn (a herb), says Dr. Catellani.

### Coenzyme $Q_{10}$

Also known as ubiquinone, coenzyme $Q_{10}$ is an essential component of the mitochondria, the energy-producing units of the cells of the body. It's involved in the manufacture of ATP, which is the energy currency – a molecule that cells use to exchange, or pass on, energy – of all body processes. Although the body can synthesize coenzyme $Q_{10}$, deficiency states can exist. And because the heart muscle is one of the most metabolically active tissues in the body, a coenzyme $Q_{10}$ deficiency may affect the heart and, some researchers theorize, lead to heart failure. Supplemental coenzyme $Q_{10}$ can improve energy production in the heart, enhance contractility and reduce blood pressure, and so it is prescribed for people with mild to moderate congestive heart failure, high blood pressure, mitral valve prolapse, or angina. "It's a cardiotonic agent, which means it enhances the function or well-being of the heart," Dr. Catellani says. Because it also acts as an antioxidant and enhances immunity, it's believed to help protect against cancer.

If you have heart disease, you may need to take several hundred milligrams of coenzyme $Q_{10}$ a day. If you're taking it simply as an antioxidant, to protect your heart, a dose of less than 100 milligrams a day is adequate, Dr. Catellani says. And it may be used in conjunction with other cardiac drugs, although after a few months of use your doctor may be able to reduce your dosage of cardiac drugs. Discuss supplementation with your doctor if you're taking the blood thinner warfarin. Coenzyme $Q_{10}$ may reduce warfarin's effectiveness.

## Hawthorn

This herb is a slow-acting but effective cardiovascular tonic that strengthens the heart muscle, improves bloodflow to the muscles of the heart, and enhances overall efficiency of the circulatory system. Research has shown it can have potent therapeutic effects for mild congestive heart failure, mild irregular heartbeat and angina. "I prefer to use coenzyme $Q_{10}$ for these problems, but if someone complains about the price and has no family history of cancer, I will tell them to use hawthorn instead," Dr. Catellani says. "Both have similar activities." Check with your doctor for dosage recommendations.

# Diet and Exercise

Maybe you've heard it so many times before it that no longer registers. But the fact is no pill can improve your health as much as wise eating and regular exercise. No matter what else you do, make these two parts of the programme, Dr. Catellani says.

**Find an activity you can love (or at least like) to do for life.** Women who exercise for at least 30 minutes a day generally have fewer and milder hot flushes – and are more likely to have no hot flushes at all – than women who are sedentary. And regular physical activity is the best way to maintain muscle mass and bone density as you get older, Dr. Catellani says. "Even if you can't do strenuous exercise, studies show that just simply walking every day makes a big difference in staying healthy," Dr. Catellani says. "Anything is always better than nothing."

You don't need to go to a gym every day to exercise. Walk the dog instead of letting it run in the garden, play with your kids or grandchildren, garden, take a stroll around your local area, ask for a treadmill for your birthday, hop on the exercise bike when you turn on the TV, if that's what you can manage.

**Take calcium and vitamin D supplements.** As discussed along with treatment for osteoporosis, you should get 1200 milligrams a day of calcium, including supplements if necessary. (You'll probably have to take about 500 milligrams in supplements.) And if you're 50 or older, get 400 to 800 IU a day of vitamin D. Your body requires vitamin D to be able to use calcium, but lots of women aged 50 or older don't get enough to keep their bones strong, Dr. Cosman says.

**Take a multivitamin/mineral supplement.** Again, this will guarantee that you get enough of all the other nutrients essential to good health: folic acid, vitamins $B_6$ and $B_{12}$, chromium, selenium, magnesium. As we get older, we tend to eat less and absorb less in the way of nutrients, so a multivitamin is often a good idea, Dr. Catellani says. Look for a "souped-up" multi. One that has 100 per cent of the RDA for vitamin C and vitamin B is not good enough, says Dr. Catellani. It should contain 600 per cent to 1000 per cent of the RDA for the B vitamin complex, 100 to 200 milligrams of vitamin C, and a good representation of trace minerals.

**Take extra vitamin E.** Vitamin E is often recommended for hot flushes, but its benefits for hot flushes may be overstated. But it's a lifesaver when it comes to cardiovascular health, Dr. Catellani says. If your multi provides 200 IU or so, take another 200 to 400 IU as a separate supplement.

**Add vitamin C with flavonoids.** In a double-blind, placebo-controlled study, a combination of 1200 milligrams of vitamin C and 1200 milligrams of flavonoids (hesperidin) was found to relieve hot flushes. Flavonoids are compounds found in citrus fruits similar to the isoflavones found in soya, and seem to particularly help strengthen and stabilize small blood vessels, such as capillaries, Dr. Corsello says.

# CHAPTER 12

# Coping with Early or Premature Menopause

**W**omen who go through menopause naturally do so at around the age of 51, give or take a few years. Due to a combination of factors – usually genetics, smoking, or both – about one out of 20 women goes through menopause earlier, between the ages of 40 and 44. Exposure to chemicals that may destroy ovarian follicles – solvents used in some workplaces, environmental chemicals, or some chemotherapy drugs, for example – also causes early menopause.

A few women undergo menopause even earlier, before the age of 40. Premature menopause, also called premature ovarian failure, is rare, however. "Only about 1 per cent of women go through menopause before 40," says Ralph Schmeltz, M.D., an endocrinologist and associate chief of internal medicine at McGee Women's Hospital in Pittsburgh.

Premature ovarian failure tends to run in families. In about half the women affected, the ovaries still function intermittently, Dr. Schmeltz says. "A woman might be diagnosed with premature ovarian failure and then, a few years later, find out she's pregnant," he says. No one knows why the ovaries sometimes seem to spit and sputter like this. The situation is similar to perimenopause, but happens earlier, while a woman is in her thirties.

Not surprisingly, a significant number of women experience fertility problems along with premature ovarian failure. Tests often show that they've developed an immune response to their body's own ovarian tissue, Dr. Schmeltz says. "They have anti-ovary antibodies. Their condition appears to be an autoimmune disease." In simpler terms, they're allergic to their ovaries.

Interestingly, autoimmune diseases – such as type 1 diabetes, thyroiditis and rheumatoid arthritis – may be linked to premature menopause, says Judith Luborsky, Ph.D., a researcher in the reproductive endocrinology and infertility section at Rush Presbyterian–St. Luke's Medical Center in Chicago. Women with type 1 diabetes, for instance, have a higher-than-normal risk for premature menopause. So do women who have autoimmune thyroiditis (Hashimoto's or Graves' disease, both of which are an inflammation of the thyroid gland). The risk for autoimmune disease is also higher if family members have these or other autoimmune diseases, such as Addison's disease (which involves adrenal glands) or rheumatoid arthritis.

More rarely, women turn out to have what's medically termed autoimmune polyglandular type 1 or 2 syndrome (APS I or APS II), which can affect various glands in the body, including the ovaries, parathyroid gland, thyroid gland, pancreas and parietal glands in the stomach.

## Early Menopause Calls to Action

**If you have a family history of premature menopause:** Consider having children sooner rather than later, Dr. Luborsky says. Women with autoimmune premature menopause may experience infertility before their periods stop. "Women with evidence of ovarian autoimmunity (such as ovarian antibodies) have a harder time getting pregnant even with in vitro fertilization methods."

**If you're under 40 and your periods have stopped for more than 6 months, or the pattern of your periods has changed (longer or shorter time between periods, more or less bleeding):** You may be experiencing premature menopause. Dr. Luborsky suggests you get a thorough checkup with a doctor who understands menopause or endocrinology. Menopausal symptoms (hot flushes, night sweats, muscle aches, fatigue, sleep disturbance, depression) may be a sign of declining ovarian oestrogen production.

**If you think you are at risk for premature menopause because you have a family history of autoimmune disease:** You may want to have your oestrogen and follicle-stimulating hormone (FSH) measured annually after the age of 35. FSH is the brain hormone that stimulates oestrogen production by the ovaries. High FSH levels are an early indicator that the ovaries are beginning to fail. As oestrogen begins to decrease, FSH levels in the blood increase. These changes in hormones occur before menstrual cycles stop. "You may have to be persistent, especially if you have symptoms that are diffuse and hard to diagnose, like fatigue," says Dr. Luborsky. Sometimes thyroid dysfunction has the same symptoms. Get a thyroid-stimulating hormone (TSH) test as part of your checkup.

**Consider some form of hormone replacement therapy.** The earlier you go through menopause, the higher your risk for osteoporosis, heart disease and stroke, Dr. Schmeltz says. "All of a sudden, these risks are pushed up by 10 or 15 years." Whether you go through premature menopause by fate or by scalpel, HRT can slash your risk of the effects of dwindling oestrogen. And as with menopause that occurs later, it's also important to pay attention to other risk factors for these conditions, like smoking and calcium intake.

**Avoid environmental toxins.** A long list of chemicals cause ovarian damage in animals, and there's good reason to believe at least some of them affect humans in the same way, says Jodi Flaws, Ph.D., assistant professor of epidemiology and preventive medicine at the University of Maryland School of Medicine in Baltimore. They include certain anticancer drugs such as cyclophosphamide (Endoxana), chemicals used in the manufacture of plastics, pesticides, solvents, heavy metals such as lead and – last but not least – constituents of cigarette smoke.

- *"Know what chemicals are in your workplace and proper precautions against them," Dr. Flaws says. "If you're working with lots of solvents, for instance, wear gloves, masks, and coats to prevent things from getting into your body."*
- *Don't smoke, and don't hang out in smoky bars. "There's pretty good evidence that even sidestream smoke can have an effect on women's ovaries," she says.*
- *At home, follow directions carefully when applying lawn chemicals or pesticide sprays. Wear a mask, closed shoes, and gloves, and change clothes and shower afterwards.*

# CHAPTER 13

# Master Diabetes and Blood Sugar Problems

G lucose (blood sugar) is the fuel your muscles count on to run errands (or a marathon). It feeds your brain when you balance your accounts or do other mental tasks. Playing the piano, knitting, working at your computer, or calling a plumber to fix a leak all require energy. And to use this energy, the hormone insulin must transfer glucose out of the bloodstream and into each of the trillions of cells and organs in your body, including the kidneys, nerves, eyes, and heart and arteries. Insulin is the only substance that can unlock the entry gates of your cells (receptors) and let glucose pour in. Without insulin, cells die and organs fail. It's that simple.

"But the elegance of hormones is not just having them around – hormone regulation is what's so special," says Denise Faustman, M.D., Ph.D., associate professor of medicine and director of the immunobiology lab at Massachusetts General Hospital in Boston.

Between meals or during periods of high activity – say, if you're being walked around the park by your family's frisky new pup – you may not have enough glucose readily available for the energy you need. Your pancreas will then release the hormone glucagon in order to convert back into your bloodstream a storage form of glucose in your liver and fat cells. The pancreas will then release extra insulin to whisk the blood sugar into your hungry cells.

A woman may also require more or less insulin than normal when her reproductive hormones are surging (during pregnancy, for example) or when she produces stress hormones since both types of hormones can raise blood sugar.

More recently, scientists have discovered a previously unrecognized hormone called resistin – produced by fat cells – which prompts tissues to resist insulin. This new hormone may explain why people who are overweight tend to develop diabetes. Researchers believe this discovery will, with more study, lead to new treatments for diabetes.

In order to keep their blood sugar in the healthy range – no lower than 60 and no higher than 120 mg/dl (milligrams per decilitre) – women with diabetes need to understand the interplay among all these blood sugar-regulating hormones.

## Why Blood Sugar Soars

Not all forms of diabetes are alike. With type 1 diabetes, your body cannot produce insulin on its own, typically due to an attack by the immune system on the insulin-producing beta cells of the pancreas. This form of diabetes is not evident until you have lost more than 85 per cent of your insulin-secreting beta cells. Autoimmune attacks appear to have a genetic basis, but the combination of genes is still unknown.

At one time type 1 diabetes was called juvenile-onset diabetes because it most frequently sets in during infancy or early adolescence. More rarely, an adult is diagnosed with type 1 diabetes after damaging her pancreas in an accident or after an illness or medication destroyed her beta cells.

Advancements in insulin-producing cell transplants are being perfected. For now, women with type 1 diabetes need to take insulin for the rest of their lives, to make up for the supply they lack. This is called insulin-dependent diabetes mellitus (IDDM).

Unlike type 1 diabetes, which manifests suddenly as a complete failure of the beta cells' ability to produce insulin, type 2 diabetes is characterized by a gradual decline in insulin's ability to fulfil your body's needs. Two main scenarios cause this, explains Frank Schwartz, M.D., clinical associate professor of medicine, endocrinology and metabolism at West Virginia University School of Medicine in Parkersburg.

In the absence of diabetes, the body produces a burst of insulin the second you start eating. But in a woman with type 2 diabetes, this release is impaired and results in elevated blood sugar immediately after meals. When her beta cells finally put out insulin, she needs extra insulin to compensate for the elevated blood sugar. This defect is called "absent first-phase insulin release".

In the second scenario, insulin receptors are less sensitive or responsive to insulin than they should be. A person is considered "insulin resistant" when she needs to produce extra insulin to make up for her sluggish or faulty receptors. "It's like the receptor is a teenager ignoring the first few times her mother asks her to clean her room. Eventually the room gets cleaned, but it takes more energy on the part of the mother to see that the job gets done," adds Dr. Faustman.

## WHAT'S GOING ON?

Because of its severe symptoms, type 1 diabetes is usually detected within several days of its onset. However, experts estimate that one out of three people with type 2 diabetes – more than 5 million people – don't know they have it.

Many of the serious complications of the diabetes can be avoided by diagnosing diabetes early. So if you have early warning signs, ask your doctor for a fasting plasma glucose test and a complete checkup without delay.

The following quiz will also help you determine if you are at risk for developing diabetes in the future, so you can take preventive action.

**1. Are you a British Asian or Afro-Caribbean?**
These ethnic groups are twice as likely to contract type 2 diabetes as the general public.

**2. Are you overweight or obese?**
Being overweight is the single greatest risk factor for type 2 diabetes. In fact, research by the US Centers for Disease Control and Prevention (CDC) indicates that for every kilogram (2.2 pounds) you are overweight, your risk for diabetes rises about 9 per cent.

**3. Do you seem to urinate more frequently than most people, even at night?**
When there is too much glucose in the blood, you urinate more as your body attempts to remove it from the body. (Over time, the added stress on the kidneys can cause them to fail, requiring kidney transplants or dialysis treatments.)

**4. Are you thirsty all the time, no matter how much you drink?**
Excessive sugar in your blood will suck up your body's stores of water. If you can't drink enough to make it up, you will probably also notice your skin drying out too.

Whether the defect is insulin resistance or impaired first-phase insulin release, the result is usually that your beta cells have to work more overtime than a postal worker at Christmas. The insulin-producing beta cells may completely wear out, making a type 2 diabetic insulin dependent, like a type 1.

Ideally, type 2 diabetes is caught in the earlier stages, when simple dietary changes and exercise may be enough to bring blood sugar under control. There

High enough blood sugar can lead to a life-threatening state of dehydration called hyperglycaemic hyperosmolar nonketotic syndrome (HHNS).

### 5. Do you have an insatiable appetite?
In untreated diabetes, you may be eating plenty, but your cells, in effect, are starving from lack of fuel because there is no insulin to funnel glucose into them. This is why you might also feel fatigued.

### 6. Are you experiencing blurred vision?
When the level of blood glucose is too high, it can alter the amount of water in the lenses of your eyes. Over time high blood sugar can cause retinopathy, a common (but preventable) cause of blindness.

### 7. Do you frequently experience leg cramps, or tingling or numbness in your limbs?
These may be early warning signs of the kind of nerve damage that can lead to permanent damage and loss of a leg.

### 8. Do you have a history of bladder, skin, yeast, or gum infections?
Sugar provides the ideal conditions for bacteria to grow, so high blood glucose can bring increased infections. In addition, excess sugar dulls your immune system by handicapping your white blood cells.

### 9. Have you experienced a recent sudden weight loss, in addition to severe fatigue, blurred vision, or feeling like you have the flu and other symptoms, such as excessive urination, thirst and urination at night?
You may be experiencing the first signs of type 1 diabetes. Call your doctor or visit a casualty department immediately.

are also a number of medications available to override insulin resistance or help your pancreas keep up with the additional insulin needs.

## When Blood Sugar Goes Too Low

When blood sugar takes a slight dip – say, 65 mg/dl rather than your normal 70 – glucagon can handle the job of bringing blood sugar back to normal range. But in the event of a hypoglycaemic episode – that is, if your blood sugar plunges below 60 mg/dl, glucagon signals your autonomic nervous system to

*Escape from* **HORMONE HELL**

# HER "HYPOGLYCAEMIA" IS ACTUALLY DUE TO DIGESTIVE HORMONES

**Q:** My husband and kids can skip meals and it doesn't seem to bother them. But if I don't eat something every 3 hours or so, I get so weak and spaced-out that I feel like I'm going to faint. I try to not leave home without a muesli bar in my bag and a box of biscuits in my glove compartment. It's actually embarrassing when I'm in social situations where I have to stop and eat. Other times, I'm afraid I'm going to pass out.

A friend of mine says it sounds as though I have hypoglycaemia, or low blood sugar. But when I went to my family doctor, she said there's no such thing as hypoglycaemia. I finally convinced her to test my blood sugar, thinking that maybe I have diabetes, but she said my test results were normal on all counts. If so, why do I still feel lousy if I go without eating?

Frank Schwartz, M.D., clinical associate professor of medicine, endocrinology and metabolism at the West Virginia University School of Medicine in Parkersburg, responds: Even though you may feel shaky in between meals, since your blood tests are normal, you don't have to worry about ever becoming unconscious.

I suspect your symptoms aren't due to blood sugar–regulating hormones going haywire when you don't eat. Rather, it's likely that what you eat is having a strong effect on the intestinal hormones in your gut. Some people are sensitive to eating too many simple carbohydrates at once and experience an irritable bowel disorder called postprandial syndrome. With such a big load of carbohydrates to process, the intestines spasm and release an overabundance of hormones that normally regulate the release of digestive enzymes to help release other hormones. When that happens, these hormones – namely adrenaline, cortisol, and growth hormone – play a counter-regulatory role, helping glucagon to free up stored glucose from your liver and fat cells faster than the extra insulin released by the pancreas can whisk it into your cells.

The counter-regulatory hormones also give you the shaky and anxious feeling many women get when they miss a meal. Feeling hypoglycaemic is like smelling the odour of a gas leak – a built-in signal giving you a chance to get out of danger. When a woman with diabetes feels the characteristic

move food through your intestines. These hormones are called cholecystokinin/pancreozymin, pancreatic polypeptide and vasoactive intestinal polypeptide.

When you get a burst of these hormones, it feels similar to how diabetics describe low blood sugar – weakness, nervousness, fatigue, the shakes – so I can see why you'd suspect hypoglycaemia. But your doctor is right. Hypoglycaemia used to be a common diagnosis, but when the esteemed Mayo Clinic studied it in depth, they found that the people who complained of hypoglycaemia had exactly the same sugar levels as everyone else. But these people got the symptoms even when they consumed a form of glucose that your blood doesn't absorb. That's a major reason why we suspect gut hormones rather than a blood sugar problem.

You're on the right track being prepared with snacks between meals. Try to make the meals you do eat small and frequent, like five or six small meals spaced throughout the day, rather than one or two "feasts". But watch that you are not eating purely carbohydrate meals. Avoid simple carbohydrates like white flour-based baked goods. Instead, eat complex carbohydrates, like steamed rice or baked potatoes. The key is to eat "mixed" meals and snacks that contain a balance of protein, fat and carbohydrate, rather than pure carbohydrate, like a box of biscuits.

If you still have symptoms after making these changes, your doctor can write a prescription for an antispasmodic medication, such as dicyclomine (Merbentyl) or hyoscine (Briscopan), used to treat irritable bowel disorders.

symptoms of hypoglycaemia, she is educated to consume 15 grams' worth of readily absorbed carbohydrates – usually sugar – either in the form of a glass of orange juice, 4 teaspoons of sugar, or a large glass of skimmed milk.

"Unfortunately, after a person has diabetes for approximately 5 years, her glucagon-producing alpha cells in the pancreas may fail along with the insulin-producing beta cells," says Dr. Schwartz. Without a glucagon response, often there's nothing to trigger the other counter-regulatory hormones that make you aware of your hypoglycaemia.

If blood sugar falls much lower – to 40 mg/dl, 30 mg/dl, or lower – a woman with hypoglycaemia can experience confusion, drowsiness – or possibly a seizure or a coma, if the brain is seriously deprived of glucose. This can happen when the person takes too much insulin in proportion to too little food or prolonged activity, says Dr. Faustman. In case she becomes unconscious, a diabetic must train her family and friends to administer a lifesaving glucagon injection or make sure they know to call an ambulance at once. Self-tests (using urine strips) can prevent that cascade of events.

People who do not have diabetes rarely experience drastic dips in blood sugar that lead to those kinds of problems. "There was a time when everyone who felt fatigue or anxiety between meals seemed to self-diagnose themselves with hypoglycaemia," says Katherine Williams, M.D., instructor of medicine at the University of Pittsburgh School of Medicine. "But true hypoglycaemia can be confirmed only by a blood test obtained by a doctor under controlled conditions that shows that a person's blood sugar level drops below 40 mg/dl, is associated with symptoms, and relieved with glucose. Most people test negative. What they're experiencing between meals can be treated with a trial of a low-carbohydrate diet or more frequent but smaller meals."

If you do indeed have nondiabetic hypoglycaemia, your doctor will look for another underlying cause, such as a tumour in your pancreas. If other underlying causes have been ruled out or treated, managing hypoglycaemia involves a change in eating habits since hypoglycaemics don't take medication that can compensate for a high or low blood sugar.

And in fact dietary recommendations for hypoglycaemia are stricter than those for type 1 diabetes: "That means eating every 2 to 3 hours and, when you do eat, making sure what you eat contains a mixture of carbohydrate and protein or fat," says Dr. Schwartz.

People prone to hypoglycaemia – diabetic or not – should wear a medical alert bracelet to allow them quick medical help in case they become unconscious or too confused to help themselves, Dr. Williams adds.

# Tighter Control: It's Worth the Effort

Over the course of several years, uncontrolled blood sugar takes a tremendous toll in the body, affecting the kidneys, nerves, eyes, and heart and arteries. At least 190,000 people die each year as a result of diabetes and its complications.

"Don't let the statistics scare you, though," says Anne Daly, R.D., C.D.E., a certified diabetes educator and president of health care and education at the American Diabetes Association in Springfield, Illinois. "Those numbers reflect people who didn't have access to breakthrough blood sugar management tools and techniques now available."

Studies underscore the value of good self-management. The US Diabetes Control and Complications Trial (DCCT) divided 1441 people with type 1 diabetes into two groups. One group took a highly aggressive approach (tight control) to keep their blood sugar as close to normal as possible. The others followed a more conventional protocol, doing just enough to avoid any overt symptoms of high or low blood sugar. After 6½ years, the tight-control group reduced kidney disease by 56 per cent, nerve disease by 57 per cent, eye disease by 76 per cent, and certain heart conditions, like atherosclerosis, by 41 per cent. Intensive therapy effectively delays the onset and slows the progression of these diseases.

In the United Kingdom Prospective Diabetes Study (UKPDS), people with type 2 diabetes enjoyed similar benefits. In fact, for every percentage point that people improved the results of a test that measured their blood glucose levels over the previous 3 months, they reduced by 35 per cent their overall risk of complications.

"The reward of tight control is directly related to the commitment a woman makes to keeping blood sugar in the normal range from hour to hour, day in and day out," explains Lois Jovanovic, M.D., an endocrinologist who specializes in diabetes in women, the director and chief scientific officer at Sansum Medical Research Institute in Santa Barbara, California, and clinical professor of medicine at University of Southern California, Los Angeles.

Technology plays a big role in helping women control blood sugar more easily, and it improves every year. Consider these resources.

**Continuous glucose sensor monitor.** Newly available, this device measures blood sugar every 20 seconds, averages it every 5 minutes, and stores it in a computer for 3 days straight, allowing for more precise monitoring than a few pricks of the skin throughout the day. The sensor, used in hospitals, is inserted in tissue just under the skin, and the monitor (about the size of a beeper) can be worn almost anywhere. "It's a breakthrough in preventing hypoglycaemia or hyperglycaemia," explains Dr. Schwartz.

**Glycosylated-haemoglobin test.** Also known as HbA1c, this shows how you are managing your blood glucose over the long term, giving a percentage of average blood sugar concentration over a 90-day period. "To make changes before high blood glucose takes its toll, book this test every 3 months," advises Dr. Jovanovic.

**Needle-less injections.** Known as jet injectors, these reliable tools actually spray insulin under your skin and are available through a variety of manufacturers with your doctor's prescription. They can help you tolerate frequent insulin doses.

**Insulin pumps.** Battery-operated machines you programme to administer insulin through a tube you wear daily, these help keep blood sugar levels consistent. "They are not the big black boxes they used to be," says Dr. Jovanovic, who sports one herself. "Today's pumps could be mistaken for an everyday pager you clip on your belt or hide under your clothes."

**Diabetes clinics.** In the UK, most practices run their own diabetes clinics with specially trained diabetes nurses attending. Only the more difficult to control cases are referred to the doctor who will refer fewer still to a hospital. In addition to primary care, you will have the advantage of access to diabetes educators, a nutritionist and perhaps an exercise physiologist to design an individualized treatment plan for you, as well as specialists in foot care, optometry and cardiology who work with the rest of your team to resolve complications.

## Syndrome X: An Exaggerated Form of Insulin Resistance

Like those with type 2 diabetes, people with syndrome X (otherwise known as metabolic syndrome) are insulin resistant – that is, they have to produce a higher-than-normal amount of insulin to process blood glucose. The difference is, someone with syndrome X can produce enough extra insulin, or she is not so insulin resistant that her blood glucose levels are in the severely elevated range of a diabetic. She does, however, have glucose levels on the higher side of normal, often hovering between 110 and 126 mg/dl.

Besides controlling blood sugar, insulin's other duty is to help store in fat cells the free fatty acids from the food you eat. But when your cells are insulin resistant, they aren't able to "accept" fat any easier than they are able to accept glucose, and the fatty acids remain in the bloodstream, leading to higher levels of blood cholesterol and triglycerides. The high insulin also increases sodium and water retention, which increases blood pressure.

Making matters worse, the liver responds to extra sugar in the bloodstream by making even more triglycerides. High blood sugar can also impair the flow of blood through the arteries. This constellation of abnormalities explains why heart disease is the leading cause of death among people with diabetes. Heart or blood vessel disease accounts for 80 per cent of the fatalities. Because people with syndrome X also have insulin resistance and elevated blood sugar, the American Heart Association has alerted doctors to recognize syndrome X and offer people so diagnosed the same preventive medicine available to heart patients.

## Preventing Heart Disease in Syndrome X and Diabetes

If you have diabetes, your risk of heart disease is automatically higher. And by the same token, if you have heart disease along with diabetes, both need to be treated.

Both diabetics and syndrome X patients have the following goals:
- *Triglycerides below 200 mg/dl*
- *LDL cholesterol under 100 mg/dl; HDL above 47 mg/dl*
- *Blood pressure under 135/85 mm Hg*
- *Glycosylated-haemoglobin levels (long-term blood glucose) under 7 per cent*

Some measures benefit both your heart and your insulin status. For example, certain lifestyle strategies – losing unnecessary weight, eating a low-fat/high-fibre diet, and improving physical fitness – improve glucose control both directly and indirectly while improving heart health. In fact, normalizing blood sugar may improve results on all five tests mentioned above. In the UKPDS trial, for every percentage point decrease in HbA1c (long-term blood glucose), heart attack risk was reduced by 18 per cent. Tight blood pressure control reduced the risk of stroke by 44 per cent and the risk of heart failure by 56 per cent.

To alleviate insulin resistance (which would indirectly lower blood pressure and lipid profile), even people with syndrome X may benefit from the diabetes medication metformin (Glucophage). However, the other main category of diabetes medication, sulfonylurea agents, may actually increase heart attack risk since they work by encouraging insulin production – dangerous for people who already have high insulin levels in the bloodstream.

If cholesterol and blood pressure don't normalize through glucose-control efforts, experts recommend medications, including a daily dose of aspirin. In fact, some blood pressure medication – such as lisinopril (Carace, Zestril), enalapril (Innovace) and captopril (Capoten) – have proven par-

# A DIET FOR BETTER BLOOD SUGAR CONTROL

How sweet a food tastes is not always the most accurate way to judge how it will affect your blood sugar. What counts is the size of the sugar molecules – something you can't determine without a powerful microscope. Another factor is ripeness or cooking. If you eat fruit that's very ripe, or processed and cooked a lot, it's partially "digested" for you, so it won't take long for the simple sugars to hit your bloodstream.

The glycaemic index is a scientific measure of how powerfully a carbohydrate-containing food alters your blood sugar over time. As a rule, raw foods will be lower on the glycaemic index than the same foods that are cooked, and the softer and fluffier a baked product is, the higher it is on the list. The following examples will help you choose foods that will keep your blood sugar levels more even. A diabetes nurse can provide you with a more comprehensive chart.

**FOODS TO ADD (lower glycaemic index – under 55)**

- Wholegrain pumpernickel, sourdough, or stoneground wheat bread
- Pearl barley and bulgar wheat
- Chickpeas
- Oatmeal
- Whole apple
- Sweet potatoes
- Banana cake
- Low-fat yoghurt

**FOODS TO SUBTRACT (higher glycaemic index – over 70)**

- White bread
- White rice
- Green peas
- Cornflakes
- Orange juice
- Instant mashed potatoes
- Jelly beans
- Pizza

ticularly effective for people with diabetes and have the added benefit of lowering the diabetes-related elevated risk of kidney damage.

While beta-blockers – such as atenolol (Tenormin), metoprolol (Lopressor) and nadolol (Corgard) – are the gold standard for people who already have coronary artery disease, people with diabetes must be aware that these drugs can mask low blood sugar and exacerbate their circulatory problems and fatigue. Experts are beginning to believe that the odds still weigh out in favour of taking a beta-blocker since the next step, heart surgery, threatens dangerous complications for people with diabetes. Cardiologists are currently researching more diabetic-safe surgical methods, but if surgery is necessary, the survival rate for diabetics appears to significantly favour bypass surgery over angioplasty.

## Take Control with Weight Loss and Exercise

If you have diabetes and you're overweight, your first goal should be losing the excess pounds. "Increased body mass means more insulin is needed to run every cell of the body," explains Dr. Faustman. "And since obese people usually consume more calories to maintain their weight, that only kicks up the amount of insulin you need to process the heavy glucose load from a huge meal." In addition, obesity puts extra strain on the already strained pancreas of a person trying to lower out-of-control blood sugar.

You don't have to lose a great deal of weight to benefit. "Losing just 5 to 10 per cent of body weight may be enough to get the blood sugar of a person with type 2 diabetes back to normal – and that's good news. And it's relative. I've seen type 2 diabetics with 13 kg (2 stone) of weight loss be able to come off insulin," says Daly. Gradual weight loss adds up. One to 2 pounds per week becomes 4 to 8 pounds per month.

The obvious benefit of exercise is that it will reduce body mass and thus improve insulin sensitivity in the overweight diabetic. But spending time at the gym actually controls diabetes and its complications in more than one way.

Whether you are flying a kite, perfecting your breaststroke, or stacking heavy tins in the pantry, working your muscles requires a lot of energy. Your muscles will start to pull glucose from your bloodstream to feed its cells. Even 2 hours after you finish your workout, your liver and muscles are still busy clearing glucose out of the blood as they replenish their storage supply.

Better yet, frequent exercise appears to condition your insulin receptors so that less insulin is actually needed to move glucose into muscle cells and other tissues.

As for the type 1 diabetic, even if she doesn't have a problem with obesity or insulin resistance, she can delight in exercise's ability to strengthen her heart and circulatory system.

**Aim for at least 20 minutes of physical activity a day.** Of course, if you start there and gradually increase your time to 40 or 60 minutes, the results also will increase.

**Play it safe.** If you have heart disease or are over the age of 35, ask your doctor for a checkup before beginning a workout programme. If you currently have complications like retinopathy, ask your eye specialist what exercises are safe, says Daly. For example, when you have eye disease, you need to avoid positions that place your heart above your head, and you need to avoid picking up heavy equipment, which will raise pressure in the eyes. Walking is probably the safest option for eye and heart patients, but your doctor can make other suggestions.

**Test blood glucose before, during and after exercise.** The most dangerous thing you can do is have low blood sugar before you even start to exert yourself. If you are habitually in poor glycaemic control, don't set out until your blood glucose level is in the range of 100 to 180 mg/dl, explains Dr. Jovanovic. If it's lower than 100 mg/dl, you have to get it *up* before exercise because at that point it will only go lower.

The harder you exercise, the more glucose the cells in your muscles are going to take up. If you are working out harder than usual, new to exercise, or practising tight control, it's best to test every 20 minutes. Test again when you're finished because it's likely that with all the glucose or sugar you used up, you'll need to lower your dosage of insulin, says Dr. Jovanovic. (Your diabetes nurse or other health care practitioner will teach you how to make changes of insulin dosage based on your self-tests.)

**Always be prepared for a blood sugar plummet.** Whether you're hiking or playing sports, pick a blood sugar booster that's suitable for your activity, and always keep it in a secure place on your body. Handy pickups include a small pocketful of raisins or jelly beans, as well as commercial glucose tablets available over the counter at pharmacies.

**Sweat despite disabilities.** Whatever your limitations, a physiotherapist can suggest *something* that you can do. "I know an endocrinologist who takes all his stroke victims and people with leg amputations, and they meet in his office and practise 'leading the orchestra' or 'directing the choir' with their arms. If you sit down and 'direct the choir' for 20 minutes, you are exhausted, and you got a real aerobic workout," says Dr. Schwartz.

**Let your sport determine where you inject insulin.** Since your muscles are more efficient at using insulin when you exercise, don't inject insulin near a muscle that you are using heavily, or the insulin uptake may be *too* efficient and cause hypoglycaemia, warns Daly. "For example, if you are going to ride a bike, you're better off putting it in your abdomen than your thigh. If you're going to play a tennis match, you'd put it in your leg, not your arm, that day," she says.

**Pay particular attention to central fat.** If you had to pick only one area of body fat to tailor your workout to, it should be your belly, says Dr. Schwartz. Insulin resistance is associated with and contributes to abdominal obesity. Several studies found that losing fat deep in the abdominal region had the greatest effect on lowering blood sugar than losing fat anywhere else. Of course, working *any* muscle will improve insulin's efficiency and losing *any* fat will reduce risks of diabetes complications. Fortunately, aerobic exercise, most known to reduce abdominal fat, will make improvements on all accounts.

**Practise healthy foot care.** People with diabetes often lose sensation in their feet, and any sores they develop heal more slowly and are more prone to infection. Even recreational athletes who are diabetic have to take extra precautions, says Daly. Check your feet every day; keep them clean, and be sure to dry them completely, especially between the toes. Always wear clean socks, making sure the seams are in the right place, accompanied by well-fitting shoes. Shake out your shoes before putting them on since even a small pebble can lead to problems. Get into the habit of inspecting your feet for blisters, corns and callouses that may need attention.

If your feet are calloused or sore, switch to an activity where you don't have to bear weight, such as swimming or using a rowing machine. You may also be able to walk and to ride an exercise bike for short periods (20 minutes) while your feet are healing. But check with your chiropodist first, Daly adds.

## Eating for Insulin Control

A so-called diabetic diet isn't what it used to be, and that's sweet news. Eating to control blood sugar in the 21st century is highly individual and not nearly as restricted as in the past, says Daly.

"There's no need for special diabetic food, and there's no one-size-fits-all eating plan," she says. "Just because you know someone with diabetes who is advised to eat the same thing for lunch every day doesn't mean you will be given a monotonous diet, too."

**Consult a dietitian.** If you've been diagnosed with diabetes, work with a dietitian to develop a plan structured around what your daily schedule is like, your unique food likes and dislikes, how much weight you want to lose, and how sensitive you are to carbohydrates. A dietitian can offer a variety of meal-planning methods to help people meet their goals, Daly explains. "When losing weight is the primary concern, we may get them to count calories; for people working on getting into better glycaemic control, they may focus on counting carbohydrates; and for people who are averse to counting, we would focus on balancing food groups."

**Aim for consistency.** "Even though individual meal plans differ, everyone should always get at least three low-fat, high-fibre meals a day," says Daly. Spacing meals can help regulate blood glucose.

**Keep records.** Periodically record your food intake, along with the results of glucose tests after each meal – especially if you are trying a different diet, a new exercise plan, or a different eating schedule than usual. The idea is to start to see patterns in which foods need to be reduced or increased or which ones warrant medication adjustments. Your diabetes nurse or dietitian can show you different logbooks.

**Try sugar with caution.** While sugar was once considered the white poison of the diabetic world, in recent years the American Diabetes Association liberalized its "no sugar" restriction from its standard guidelines. This liberating decision was based on 12 different studies, all of which showed that the majority of people, after eating sugar, did not experience the dangerous spike in blood glucose once suspected.

"Anyone with blood sugar problems still needs to be very mindful about taking sugar and other carbohydrates into account," says Daly. "But if somebody wants to work dessert into their diet, we can show them how to do it so it's safe." An insulin-dependent diabetic can test her reaction to sweet food and then adjust her insulin dose, a type 2 diabetic will subtract a few more points from her daily "carbohydrate exchange" quota, and the hypoglycaemic learns to always combine sugar-containing foods with protein or fat to slow down digestion.

**Know where your calories are coming from.** For people trying to control diabetes, protein is the only nutrient with a set desired percentage target – 10 to 20 per cent of calories. The remaining 80 to 90 per cent of calories can be split between dietary fat and carbohydrates. While the actual distribution of fat and carbohydrates can vary based on individual nutrition assessment and treatment goals, fewer than 10 per cent of calories from saturated fat is always recommended.

**Double your fibre intake.** People with diabetes need more fibre than the average Westerner consumes. Most Westerners eat between 10 and 16 grams of fibre, but for people with diabetes, 20 to 35 grams a day are recommended, says Daly.

Fibre is important because it is not digested and absorbed like other carbohydrates, such as sugars and starches. When you eat one food with 5 grams or more of fibre per serving, you can deduct the fibre grams from the total carbohydrate count as this amount is considered unavailable for glucose formation, says Daly.

In a University of Texas Southwestern Medical Center study, when people with diabetes bumped up their fibre intake to 50 grams a day, after 6 weeks they lowered blood sugar 10 per cent – as significantly as diabetes medication. All it takes to get this much healthy fibre is a daily goal of 13 servings of fruits, beans, vegetables and grains a day. (Remember to increase your fibre intake gradually so the colon can adjust and you can avoid excess wind.) Some high-fibre foods are muesli (12.8 grams per 230 grams/8 ounces), chickpeas (12.5 grams), oat bran (11.4 grams), oatmeal (9.6 grams), butter beans (9 grams), raisins (6.6 grams), kiwi fruit (6 grams), corn (4.6 grams), oranges (4.3 grams) and blueberries (3.9 grams).

**Set a daily calorie budget.** The American Diabetes Association sets nutrition guidelines for people with diabetes so you get enough calories to stay at a healthy weight. As your body changes, your nutrition needs change throughout your life. Your nutrition specialist can set a calorie budget that's right for you.

To meet your goals, watch calories carefully, says Daly. "Women often live on soups and salad, thinking they're on a low-calorie diet, when in fact they're eating high-calorie cream soups and 1000-calorie salads with dressing. Everything counts, including garnishes and condiments."

**Recognize sugar in disguise.** If you are counting carbohydrates, you need to recognize various forms of sugar by their chemical names so you can account for them in your daily quota. In processed foods, look for sorbitol, xylitol and mannitol, plus any ingredients ending in -*ose*, such as dextrose, fructose (also called levulose), maltose and lactose. Molasses, corn syrup, icing sugar, cane juice and maple syrup all count as sucrose – and therefore need to be counted as part of the total carbohydrates in your meal or snack. If artificial sweeteners don't upset your stomach, you can substitute saccharin, aspartame, acesulfame potassium or sucralose for sugar – they neither add calories nor raise blood glucose.

# "WAKE-UP" HORMONES MAY PUSH UP YOUR BLOOD SUGAR

Growth hormone and cortisol are the hormones that stimulate you to wake up in the morning. Everyone has a mechanism that starts gradually releasing these hormones around 4 a.m. so you have get-up-and-go to roll out of bed when your alarm goes off. But some people get a stronger burst of wake-up hormones than others. Since these hormones are insulin antagonists, a person with diabetes who is a "morning person" might have an increase in cortisol of as much as 20 mcg/dl (micrograms per decilitre) and then wake up with blood sugar higher than 240 mg/dl, known as the "dawn phenomenon", says Lois Jovanovic, M.D., an endocrinologist who specializes in diabetes in women and the director and chief scientific officer at Sansum Medical Research Institute in Santa Barbara, California.

The quick fix is to take higher doses of insulin the next day. But you don't want high blood sugar to begin with, she says. Talk to your doctor: one solution may be switching your long-acting dose to before bed rather than, as is traditional, taking it before dinner, which may coincide better with the release of wake-up hormones. If you still can't prevent the dawn phenomenon, you are a prime candidate for an insulin pump, which you could programme to automatically give you low levels of insulin for the first half of the night and higher levels for the second half, adds Dr. Jovanovic.

It's also a good idea to test your blood glucose a few times around 3 a.m. In fact, some parents of diabetic children *habitually* wake them in the middle of the night and give them juice and get test levels. Once they know they have the pattern, they can go on a pump if they qualify, so they don't have to wake up all the time. The new technology of the glucose sensor, which automatically takes sugar levels every 5 minutes, can be used to avoid having to wake, but not all facilities have this yet.

If your blood sugar is running low, you are only going to get a bigger burst of cortisol and growth hormone to compensate over and above the amount you get as wake-up response. In that case, controlling middle-of-the-night hypoglycaemia by eating fewer carbohydrates at dinner may curb cortisol and growth hormone enough to prevent the dawn phenomenon, says Dr. Jovanovic.

**Cut down on meat.** "If you have diabetes, you should consume around 115 to 170 grams (4 to 6 ounces) of meat for the whole day," says Daly. "This may take some getting used to – the average restaurant portion of beef is 230 grams (8 ounces).

"Rather than meat taking up most of the plate, with a dab of vegetables and starch on the side, make it the other way around," she suggests. "Think of each meal being vegetable-based, with a little meat mixed in. It's also a good idea to plan one entirely meatless supper a week."

**Spice up glucose control.** Since those with diabetes need to curb salt to avoid hypertension, they can still flavour food with spices, such as fennel and turmeric, while lowering their blood sugar to boot. A number of spices appear to actually make fat cells more responsive to insulin, with cinnamon wowing the most researchers. The Agricultural Research Service (a branch of the US Department of Agriculture) found that cinnamon increases glucose metabolism twentyfold. Its chemical constituents may even offer the added advantage of lowering blood pressure, according to the research.

## Menstrual Cycles and Menopause Play a Big Role, Too

With so much focus on insulin, you may not have given much thought to the role of oestrogen and other reproductive hormones in controlling diabetes. Yet both oestrogen and progesterone are considered insulin antagonists – that is, they interfere with insulin's ability to normalize blood sugar. Progesterone in particular is linked to high blood glucose. It appears to weaken insulin's binding ability at cell receptor sites, causing temporary insulin resistance or worsening existing resistance.

Since both reproductive hormone levels are highest in the week before menstruation, insulin-antagonizing effects are most noticeable then. "An insulin-dependent woman with tightly controlled blood sugar levels may need as much as 20 per cent more insulin at this time," says Dr. Jovanovic.

In contrast, she can expect her insulin needs to *decrease* as she approaches the menopause, when levels of reproductive hormones drop. Honouring these decreased needs is essential in order to avoid hypoglycaemic episodes. Of course, if you go on HRT, you'll need the same amount of insulin as you did when you were menstruating.

The justification for HRT is higher in women who don't have their blood glucose under control. High blood sugar brings on calcium wasting, where the mineral leaches from the bones and increases the risk of fracture. Since plummeting reproductive hormones also encourage osteoporosis, HRT can control the damage, Dr. Jovanovic says.

If you have diabetes, consider these other distinctly female concerns.

**Increased facial and body hair.** Either extreme insulin resistance or chronically taking too much insulin over a lifetime irritates the outer coating of the ovaries, causing them to pump out more testosterone than normal. In women with diabetes, this can lead to masculine features such as facial hair and a lower voice. "Doctors joke that they can identify a diabetic woman on the subway by her moustache, but that's an exaggeration," Dr. Jovanovic says. At menopause, when the diabetic woman's female hormones are already low, the extra testosterone can bring out the male features. "Generally, the extra testosterone would cause noticeable male feature changes in only diabetic hyperinsulinaemic menopausal women who aren't taking any oestrogen to counterbalance the testosterone also coming from the ovaries," explains Dr. Jovanovic. Fortunately, HRT has been shown to decrease the levels of male sex hormones in women with diabetes. If you develop hirsutism (excessive growth of hair) but aren't menopausal, ask your doctor to screen you for polycystic ovary syndrome, which is accompanied by obesity and irregular menstrual cycles or infertility (see "Polycystic Ovary Syndrome on the Rise" on page 150 for more information). Otherwise, consider other hair-removal methods while you get insulin under control. (For details, see Upper Lip and Facial Hair on page 335.)

**Find your unique premenstrual insulin requirements.** "On average, an insulin-dependent woman should carefully increase her overnight dose by 3 per cent a day (1 to 2 units per night) for the 5 days before her period. On the day she gets her period, she should go back to the original dose because at that point oestrogen and progesterone have dropped back down to their lowest level," says Dr. Jovanovic.

Check with your doctor on that strategy. Each woman may differ in the threshold of progesterone she reaches, as well as in her vulnerability to hypoglycaemia, so the formula is not set in stone. Dose adjustments should be based first and foremost on the results of your self-tests, which will also compensate for any changes in eating or activity that may occur just before menstruation.

**Normalize sex hormones with birth control pills.** Whether you're premenopausal or simply can't manage the insulin fluctuations caused by your monthly cycle, you're a good candidate for birth control pills if you have diabetes, says Dr. Schwartz. But make sure they are *low-dose* pills, with only 10 to 20 milligrams of progestin. All diabetics should avoid Depo-Provera, which releases sustained levels of high-dose progestin – and can raise blood sugar the same way your own internal insulin-antagonizing progesterone surges do, says Dr. Jovanovic.

**Get PMS under control.** If a woman is extremely agitated or is struggling with the physical pain of cramps, her stress hormones will soar, exaggerating the anti-insulin effects of her soaring progesterone. Another dangerous scenario is when a woman who already has high blood sugar gives in to her cravings and eats an entire packet of chocolate chip cookies. The multiple hormone effects can cause uncontrolled PMS to make the blood sugar level more difficult to control, says Dr. Schwartz. For strategies to help cope with the emotional side of PMS, see chapter 3. For details on managing physical symptoms, see chapter 7.

**Don't retire from activity.** A metabolic slowing down at menopause combined with a slower-paced life at retirement is a dual threat to good blood sugar control. An unchecked tendency to gain weight will only worsen insulin resistance and raise an already elevated risk for heart disease.

"People often view retirement as a time to treat themselves to work-saving machines or hiring helpers to do mundane work," says Daly. "But if you have diabetes, the only things you are treating yourself to are worse glucose control and compounded risk for osteoporosis." If at all possible, continue to do your own house painting, gardening, car washing and errand running.

**Get your thyroid tested yearly.** Thyroid problems become more prevalent in menopausal woman, and if you're diabetic, they will also interfere with your glucose control. "If you become hyperthyroid (overactive thyroid), your blood sugar levels may go higher since your body is more metabolically active, and if you become hypothyroid (underactive thyroid), you may gain weight, which can also make blood sugar levels rise," explains Dr. Williams. Make sure your doctor prescribes an annual thyroid screening, and ask for one if you have symptoms described in "Is Your Thyroid Underactive – Or Overactive?" on page 64.

## Pregnancy for the Insulin-Dependent Woman

If you have diabetes and you get pregnant, you'll have to step up your self-care strategies. The protocol for a pregnant woman with type 2 diabetes is nearly identical to that of a woman with gestational, or pregnancy-induced, diabetes. For details, see "When Pregnancy Triggers Diabetes" on page 152.

Some women erroneously assume that type 1 diabetes rules out pregnancy.

"By following the extra steps of tight control, even a type 1 diabetic woman can expect the same chances of delivering a normal, healthy baby as a non-diabetic woman," says Dr. Jovanovic.

"As long as insulin-dependent women pass certain tests, I give them clearance to safely get pregnant," Dr. Jovanovic says. They include:
- *Ophthalmological checkup confirming stable eye status*
- *Normal blood pressure*
- *Normal 24-hour urine test for kidney function*
- *Normal gynaecological examination*
- *Normal HbA1c tests*

Just like a pregnant woman with non-insulin-dependent diabetes, an insulin-dependent pregnant woman must set strict mealtimes and count carbohydrates more so than usual. "If she isn't already testing her blood sugar levels five to 10 times a day, she will be because the blood sugar standards I give to a diabetic mum-to-be are even lower than the general public," says Dr. Jovanovic. "She must keep her blood sugar levels in the absolute lowest side of normal without getting hypoglycaemia, which is between 55 and 70 mg/dl premeal, and under 140 mg/dl 1 hour after eating."

Keeping low blood sugar levels will even eliminate the chances of delivering an oversize baby, which results when too much sugar passes into the placenta, she adds.

Like someone with gestational diabetes, a woman with type 1 diabetes who gets pregnant will still be considered high risk – which means working intensely with her doctor and diabetes experts before, during and after delivery. In addition to the care those professionals provide, consider these self-care guidelines recommended by Dr. Jovanovic.

**If you get hypoglycaemic, don't overcompensate.** Spikes in blood sugar over 140 mg/dl are the leading cause of birth defects for the babies of diabetic women. The worst-case scenario is if you become unconscious and whoever intervenes gives you so much glucagon that you go from 20 to 600 mg/dl, says Dr. Jovanovic. Let your caretakers know that if you become unconscious while you're pregnant, they should administer only half of your usual, prepregnancy glucagon injection amount, wait 10 minutes, and then, if you're still unconscious, administer the second half of the dose. If, after the glucagon dose, you are unresponsive, instruct your caretaker to call for help. Also, if your caretaker lets a paramedic intervene in an emergency, make sure he or she is told that you are pregnant and should get only half the dose.

As always, when treating your own low blood sugar, make sure you don't take more than the recommended 15 milligrams of sugar, she adds.

**Adjust insulin if you breastfeed.** An insulin-dependent woman can breastfeed since her insulin does not affect the baby. She does, however, need to protect herself from hypoglycaemia by lowering insulin doses after each breastfeeding, particularly if she breastfeeds late at night when she won't be taking a meal until morning to bring her blood sugar back up. And since the infant takes in more of the mother's sugar as he grows, mothers can expect insulin requirements to gradually decrease over time.

**Take care of postnatal moods.** "After delivery, all mothers can expect emotional highs and lows as their reproductive hormones adjust. The diabetic woman also has the sugar roller coaster to contend with as her blood sugar-controlling hormones are compromised by shifts in her reproductive hormones," says Dr. Jovanovic. Knowing that it's normal to feel like you were in a train crash for a few weeks after delivery may help calm your nerves.

For details on managing postnatal moods, see "Beyond the Baby Blues: Postnatal Depression" on page 154. But if you're having the added stress of finding the right insulin doses from hour to hour, you need to chart all the foods you consume, times of nursing, emotions, your sleep patterns, and your six to eight daily test results. Then review your records with the most experienced diabetes experts on your health care team.

## Relieve Stress, Control Blood Sugar

Cortisol – one of the body's most powerful hormones – stimulates you when you're under stress. It also functions as a counter-regulatory hormone to help raise blood glucose if a woman with diabetes takes too much insulin. The liver, however, doesn't care why cortisol is released; it just knows that cortisol is its signal to send out blood sugar. So even if your blood sugar level is already high, the liver will release stored glucose into the bloodstream when you experience physical or emotional stress.

Cortisol's antagonistic effects on diabetes control are clear. Dr. Jovanovic observes that her patients have some of their historically worst glucose control during the week they submit their tax return. Practitioners also note poor HbA1c test results the month after a death in a family. And all diabetes nurses warn their patients to check blood glucose levels more carefully during illness.

Keeping careful watch over emotional and physical stressors that might increase cortisol – and blood sugar – is an essential part of diabetes management.

And when a person is under duress, she is more likely to slack off on her exercise and good eating habits, which in turn will only worsen glucose control.

If you can't unwind well or smooth out distressed moods on your own, don't wait to get professional help, says Dr. Williams. Depression – which is even more common in diabetics than the general population – is associated with an increased risk of diabetic complications and may worsen insulin resistance.

Diabetics respond well to treatment for emotional distress. In a Washington University School of Medicine study, when type 2 diabetics added cognitive behavioural therapy to their normal diabetes education management, more than 70 per cent went into remission from depression and also brought down, or improved the results of, their HbA1c tests. In contrast, those who didn't use therapy actually increased their HbA1c levels, and the majority stayed depressed. And although older antidepressants were suspected of raising blood sugar, the newer class of SSRI antidepressants, such as fluoxetine (Prozac), have been shown to slightly *decrease* blood sugar while improving depression in more than 60 per cent of depressed diabetic people. See chapter 3 for more information on mood problems.

## Learning to Adjust

If you have diabetes, experts offer these additional tips for caring for your mental and physical wellness.

**Give yourself a year.** When someone is diagnosed with diabetes, she must undergo the same five stages of grieving as a person who has lost a loved one: disbelief/denial, anger, depression/withdrawal, recovery, acceptance. In addition, both high blood sugar and low blood sugar increase anxiety and are to be expected while you learn to employ the right management strategies. "It can take about a year for your emotions and your blood sugar to stabilize when you're newly diagnosed. Allow yourself this adjustment period and know that it's not going to last for ever," advises Dr. Jovanovic.

**Ask questions.** It's perfectly understandable to be fearful and devastated if you believe that all people with diabetes go blind, die, or rely on kidney dialysis machines, or that you can never eat ice cream for the rest of your life. (For the record, these beliefs are unfounded.) Don't let your imagination run wild. Instead, express your fears to your health care team, advises Daly. They will be able to separate myths from reality, and give you a step-by-step plan to avoid any future complications.

**Integrate relaxation into your lifestyle.** When Dr. Jovanovic and her

## ON THE WEB & Other Resources

If you've just been diagnosed with diabetes, Diabetges UK is the definitive organization to supply you with information, keep you abreast of advancements, and further expand your knowledge of all aspects of diabetes management. Some years ago, diabetologists throughout the United Kingdom came together to form one organization to help people with diabetes, and the result is a very efficient body with wide interests that will cover all that anyone with diabetes wishes to know. There are local offices of Diabetes UK in every district, often based in local district and general hospitals, and who work together with family doctors. You can contact the organization at:

**Diabetes UK**
10 Parkway
London NW1 7AA
Tel: 0207 424 1030
E-mail: *info@diabetes.org.uk*
*www.diabetes.org.uk*

Also good for support and discussion:
*www.diabetes-insight.info*

peers taught relaxation techniques to people with diabetes, they found a 20 per cent decrease in insulin requirements in order to maintain glucose levels in the normal range. Meditation, imagery, progressive relaxation, yoga, biofeedback and massage all work. Experiment to find what suits you.

**Choose a role model.** Focus on people like multi-medal winning oarsman Sir Steve Redgrave. This type 1 diabetic hero is able to monitor glucose and manage insulin with an active, exciting life. You may also benefit from finding someone in your own community who proactively manages her diabetes and ask her to be your mentor. A good place to meet such a person is a support group for those with diabetes, which you can locate through your local hospital. (See "On the Web & Other Resources" on page 255.)

**Take extra care during illness.** Having flu or a bad cold and other threats to your immune system are accompanied by hormones that suppress insulin, including cortisol. So people with diabetes are prime candidates for annual flu injections. If you have an injection and catch flu anyway, test your blood sugar at least five times a day, and adjust your insulin according to your doctor's instructions, advises Dr. Williams.

Remember that you still have to eat to prevent hypoglycaemia. If you are vomiting, call your diabetes health care team for advice, says Daly. Also remember that over-the-counter remedies are available sugar-free for people with diabetes. Be prepared in advance by asking your doctor about any over-the-counter medications that you have in your medicine chest and getting approval for your favourite "sick foods".

## PART THREE

# The Hormone-Balancing Programme

A Three-Phase Plan to Restore and Maintain
Your Hormone Levels and Customize
the Programme for Your Personal Needs

# Phase 1:
## Jettison the "Bad" Hormones

**W**orried that synthetic hormones like recombinant bovine growth hormone (rBGH) might fuel the development of breast cancer, more and more women, particularly in America where the routine use of hormones is much more extensive than it is in the UK, are on the hunt for hormone-free milk and meat when shopping for themselves and their families. Concerned about pesticides that raise their oestrogen levels – and perhaps their risk of breast and ovarian cancers – more women buy organically grown fruits, vegetables and other groceries. Hearing reports that clingy plastic wrap may release hormone-disrupting chemicals, some consumers switch to nonplastic cling film.

Governments say that hormonally active agents, or HAAs (chemicals in the environment that mimic our own natural hormones) – also known as xeno-oestrogens – are safe. Women – and men – concerned about their hormone health aren't so sure. Researchers studying the health effects report potentially serious effects.

Other research shows that everyday substances such as cigarettes, alcohol and caffeine also have the potential to mess up our hormones. All may or do cause serious consequences: cancer, osteoporosis, infertility and birth defects.

No hormone-balancing programme would be complete without taking into account the effect of hormonally active agents in the environment – whether they're swallowed or inhaled, voluntarily or involuntarily. While there's evidence to suggest that some of these substances can potentially harm our hormonal health, there's no conclusive proof that they do. Still, in the light of current evidence, some researchers advise going the "better safe than sorry" route and taking steps to reduce your exposure to these potentially harmful substances. There are lots of ways you can protect yourself and those you love from these potentially hormone-disrupting substances. And most are surprisingly simple. You can start with any step you like, and proceed in any order, or simply continue taking measures that are already part of your lifestyle.

# Week 1: If You Smoke, Quit

Between 1974 and 1994, lung cancer deaths among women increased 150 per cent, compared with only 20 per cent among men. Emerging research suggests that there may be genetic or hormonal reasons.

In one study, for example, women were three times more likely than men to carry a genetic mutation known as K-ras. A marker for a particularly aggressive form of lung cancer, K-ras, researchers think, may spur tumour growth in response to some of the body's own hormones, especially oestrogen.

Might this mutation – or other genetic factors – account for women's apparent higher vulnerability to smoking? At this point, there are still more questions than answers. But researchers know one thing for sure: smoking drains our levels of oestrogen – both the natural oestrogen we make before menopause and the supplemental oestrogen we may take after menopause.

That can increase our risk of developing conditions linked to lower oestrogen levels, says John G. Spangler, M.P.H., M.D., associate professor in the department of family and community medicine at Wake Forest University School of Medicine in Winston-Salem, North Carolina. And that's regardless of whether we smoke three cigarettes a day or 20.

For example, those of us who smoke – and are draining our oestrogen stores – are thrust into menopause 1 to 2 years earlier than our nonsmoking sisters.

Further, "when a woman smokes while on oestrogen replacement therapy, she's throwing away the benefits of that oestrogen," says Dr. Spangler – specifically, the lower risk of heart disease and osteoporosis.

Even when we're premenopausal, "throwing away" our natural oestrogen gradually erodes the sturdiness of our bones. In fact, studies have shown that women who smoke have from two to four times the risk of breaking a bone due to osteoporosis that those who don't.

As explained elsewhere in this book, osteoporosis occurs when there's an imbalance between bone cells that build bone – called osteoblasts – and those that break down bone, called osteoclasts.

"Oestrogen seems to affect the balance between osteoblasts and osteoclasts," says Dr. Spangler. "In osteoporosis, the osteoclasts tend to get the upper hand."

Many studies also link smoking with increased risk of breast and cervical cancers, although the evidence is far from conclusive. "But it's clear that cigarette smoking is carcinogenic," says Dr. Spangler, "and not just to our lungs."

If you don't smoke, skip ahead to Week 2.

## To Quit for Good, Work with Your Hormones

It's estimated that up to 304,000 smokers successfully quit every year with the help of over-the-counter stop-smoking products such as the nicotine gum and patch.

And one of those ex-smokers can be you.

One programme – developed by a physician at JL Pettis Veterans Affairs Medical Center in Loma Linda, California, and used in several university-affiliated smoking-cessation programmes throughout the United States – seems particularly effective.

One year after 4,000 smokers tried the programme, 40 to 60 per cent remained smoke-free. That's compared with the 10 to 15 per cent success rate for nicotine-replacement products alone.

With your doctor's help, you can try this approach. It combines the non-nicotine smoking-cessation drug bupropion (Zyban), a nicotine-replacement product such as the patch, and counselling to explore the reasons why you smoke.

**Start this or any smoking-cessation programme during the first half of your menstrual cycle.** Researchers at the University of Pittsburgh School of Medicine found that women who quit smoking between the first and 14th days of their cycle had fewer tobacco-withdrawal symptoms such as depression, anxiety and irritability.

"Quitting produces withdrawal symptoms that are often similar to premenstrual symptoms," says Kenneth A. Perkins, Ph.D., professor of psychiatry at the university. "Giving up smoking during the second half of the menstrual cycle would have additive effects that could make the experience more difficult."

**Begin taking the bupropion 1 to 2 weeks before your quit day.** Most people take a 150-milligram pill for the first 2 to 3 days, then a lower-dose pill for 6 to 12 weeks. Bupropion is thought to stabilize the same brain chemistry nicotine stimulates, but it isn't addictive. And it's nicotine-free, so you won't have withdrawal symptoms when you stop using it. *Caution:*

tell your doctor if you have a seizure disorder. This drug may increase the risk.

**Pick a nicotine-replacement product.** Your choices include the patch, nasal sprays, oral inhalers and nicotine gum. Your doctor can help you choose the one that's right for you.

**Get counselling.** Aim for four to seven sessions over a 2-month period – ideally, with a clinician who specializes in treating addictions.

# Weeks 2 and 3:
## Reduce Your Caffeine Intake

Whether we're talking about coffee, tea, or caffeinated soft drinks, low doses of caffeine typically make us feel energetic, alert and self-confident. At higher doses, it can leave us anxious, irritable and unable to sleep.

That's because caffeine affects a brain chemical (neurotransmitter) called adenosine. Caffeine blocks the "receivers" on the surface of brain cells – called receptors – that "listen" for adenosine. Normally, adenosine slows the activity of other neurotransmitters. And typically, when lots of adenosine interacts with adenosine receptors in the brain, we get drowsy.

But caffeine is an adenosine "impersonator".

Even though caffeine "fits" adenosine receptors, like the right key fits a lock, caffeine doesn't slow down the brain. Caffeine speeds it up – by blocking the actions of adenosine.

This means that neurons, the cells that transmit nerve impulses, keep firing, and firing and firing. This uncontrolled firing of neurons causes your brain to go into overload.

It causes the pituitary gland, located in the brain, to secrete ACTH (adrenocorticotropic hormone), which signals the adrenal glands to pump out the stress hormone cortisol. The resulting activation of the sympathetic nervous system causes the release of two more stress hormones, epinephrine and norepinephrine.

These neurotransmitters activate the fight-or-flight response, the body's automatic reaction to physical or emotional danger. So in effect, we may react to too much caffeine the way we would an oncoming lorry in our path: our hearts speed up. Our breathing turns to panting. Our skin turns cold and sweaty.

What's more, imbibing lots of java in the morning stresses our bodies all day – and may raise our risk of heart disease, according to research conducted at Duke University in Durham, North Carolina.

Researchers got 72 men and women to drink 500 milligrams of caffeine in the morning on two separate workdays. (That's about four 180-millilitre (6-fluid ounce) servings.)

They found that these people's levels of norepinephrine and epinephrine rose significantly. So did their blood pressure – by two to three points. And the numbers *stayed* high into the evening.

Researchers are also homing in on exactly why too much caffeine too close to bedtime can leave us staring at the alarm clock until it's time to get up.

One theory: in addition to its effects on adenosine, caffeine can also reduce levels of melatonin, says Kenneth P. Wright Jr., Ph.D., D.Ph., associate neuroscientist and instructor in the circadian, neuroendocrine and sleep disorders section, division of endocrinology-hypertension at Harvard Medical School and Brigham and Women's Hospital in Boston.

Melatonin is a light-sensitive hormone produced by the pineal gland, located in the brain. Each night, the biological clock in our brains signals our melatonin levels to rise, making us drowsy. Melatonin levels remain high all night and are very low during the day.

Studies conducted by Dr. Wright and researchers at Bowling Green State University in Ohio have found that caffeine – along with bright light – reduces night-time melatonin levels.

This is good news for shift workers, who must remain awake and alert at a time when their bodies are primed to sleep. But if you're a 9-to-5 type, abstain from caffeine for up to 6 hours before bedtime – and dim the lights at least 1 to 2 hours before you turn in, advises Dr. Wright.

## The Caffeine-Cutback Plan

Whether you want to reduce your intake of caffeine or stop consuming it entirely is up to you, depending on how sensitive you are to its effects on hormonally related functions.

To cut back on coffee:

**Make one cup of coffee at a time, rather than a whole pot.** Do this even if you use an automatic coffeemaker.

**Buy yourself an exquisite coffee cup or dainty teacup . . .** And pack away your jumbo café au lait mugs.

**Consider purchasing a percolator.** One 180-millilitre (6-fluid ounce) cup of percolated coffee contains 75 milligrams of caffeine, compared with 105 milligrams for the same amount of filter coffee.

**Switch to instant.** This makes it easier to make one cup at a time. Plus, instant contains quite a bit less caffeine – 60 milligrams per rounded teaspoon.

**To ease withdrawal symptoms, cut back gradually over the period of a week or two.** If you usually imbibe three cups a day (about 300 milligrams of caffeine), drinking as little as 30 or 50 millilitres/1 or 2 fluid ounces (25 milligrams) can help, says Roland Griffiths, Ph.D., professor in the department of psychiatry at the Johns Hopkins University School of Medicine in Baltimore. That's the amount in demitasse cups customarily used for espresso.

## Sugar Causes Tooth Decay, But Not Diabetes

The idea that eating too much sugar "causes" diabetes has been around for a long time – and it's a myth.

Truth is, the most important risk factor for type 2 diabetes isn't how much sugar you eat. It's how much extra padding you have. Weighing too much and moving too little make our cells more resistant to the hormone insulin, which regulates our bodies' use of glucose, or blood sugar.

When cells resist insulin's efforts to move glucose out of the blood and into the cells – where it's needed for energy – blood sugar stays high. Which is the hallmark of diabetes.

So losing weight and breaking into a sweat – rather than swearing off sugar – is the best way to reduce your risk of diabetes.

Nor are sugary foods off-limits to those who already have diabetes. Experts once believed that simple carbohydrates, such as white sugar, were digested and absorbed into the blood more quickly than complex carbohydrates, such as bread and potatoes.

Studies have since shown that simple carbohydrates don't raise blood sugar any higher or faster than other, complex carbs.

But this doesn't mean that you now can scoff sweets or pastries with impunity. Sugar-laden foods don't offer much in the way of nutrients. On top of that, they're often high in fat and calories, which can cause weight gain. So, count carbohydrate grams, not sugar grams.

To quit coffee completely:

To save yourself the agony of quitting coffee cold turkey, follow this 2-week strategy.

**Days 1 to 5:** Make coffee with a mix of three-quarters caffeinated to one-quarter decaffeinated.

**Days 6 to 9:** Mix half caffeinated coffee with half decaffeinated.

**Days 10 to 13:** Mix one-quarter caffeinated coffee with three-quarters decaffeinated.

**Day 14 and beyond:** Make 100 per cent decaffeinated coffee.

To make these 2 weeks a little easier:

- *Instead of regular decaf, consider trying herbal coffee, available at health food shops or in the health food section of your supermarket. It's brewed just like coffee, and connoisseurs say it has the same deep, rich flavour and aroma.*
- *Start the programme during a quiet weekend or relaxing holiday – a time when you're neither busy nor stressed. Brew some camomile tea – often used to ease stress – and take lots of warm baths, walks and naps to get you through the first few days.*

If you're a cola-holic:

- *Switch from caffeinated soft drinks to those that are caffeine-free. You may follow the same tapering guidelines as those given for coffee.*
- *Better yet, drink good-for-you beverages such as water, hot or iced caffeine-free herbal teas, or fruit or vegetable juices.*
- *To save calories, dilute fruit juice with water, sparkling water or soda water. (Large bottles of fruit juice, which often contain two or more servings, pack up to 240 calories in a 600-millilitre/1 pint bottle.)*

# Week 3:
## Protect Yourself from Pesticides

When you pile your plate with fruits and vegetables, you get a load of vitamins, minerals, and plant chemicals that help protect against heart disease and cancer. But most likely, you also get pesticides – chemicals used to protect crops from all manner of creepy crawlies, including bugs, rodents, mould and bacteria.

If you use pesticides on your lawn and garden, or to protect your pets from fleas and ticks or to rid your home of bugs or rodents, you're exposed to even more pesticides. Altogether, about 350 different pesticides are used on foods, in or around homes, or on pets.

There's no denying the benefits of pesticides: they've increased food production and dramatically reduced the incidence of diseases such as malaria, carried and transmitted by mosquitoes. But pesticides are potent – and potentially toxic – chemicals.

At high doses, they can cause birth defects and cancer. People who are routinely exposed to pesticides – farm workers, pesticide applicators, people involved in the manufacture of pesticides – are at the greatest risk.

Pesticides shown to be toxic to humans, such as DDT (dichlorodiphenyl-trichloroethane) and chlordane, were banned years ago. Unfortunately, these pesticides stick around, both in the environment and in our bodies, where they're stored in fat and tissue, says Gerald A. LeBlanc, Ph.D., professor and assistant department head in the department of environmental and molecular toxicology at North Carolina State University in Raleigh.

During times of stress, our tissues and fat release these chemicals, freeing them to circulate in our bodies, says Dr. LeBlanc. "Stress" is defined as any situation in which our metabolism rises and we use fats for energy – during pregnancy and breastfeeding, weight loss, or times of extreme emotional stress.

And researchers express mounting concern that even low exposure to pesticides may lead to cancer, reproductive problems and changes to our delicate hormonal systems.

## The Pesticide/Hormone Link

Some pesticides are just one type of substance known as hormonally active agents (HAAs), or xeno-oestrogens. These man-made chemicals – also found in some plastics, household products and industrial chemicals – alter hormonal function. They "impersonate" female and male sex hormones (oestrogens and androgens, respectively), block their effects, or alter the production and breakdown of our own, natural hormones.

Research has linked HAAs to a variety of health problems in wildlife and laboratory animals. And there's evidence that they affect people, too, says Dr. LeBlanc.

In women, HAAs – including some pesticides – mimic our own, natural oestrogen. And high oestrogen levels have been linked to cancers fuelled by oestrogen, such as some forms of breast cancer.

## THE HORMONE CONNECTION

# HORMONES SEEM OUT OF WHACK? CHECK YOUR MEDICINE CABINET

Drugs that are commonly prescribed to treat depression, allergies and asthma, high blood pressure and infections can alter hormonal balances. Here are a few examples.

**Fluoxetine (Prozac)** Used to treat major depression, obsessive-compulsive disorder, and panic disorder, this widely prescribed drug has been shown to raise blood levels of corticosterone, a "stress hormone" that is produced by the adrenal glands.

Common side effects include nervousness, drowsiness, anxiety, sleeplessness, difficulty concentrating and sexual problems.

**Methylprednisolone (Solu-Medrone, Depot-Medrone)** A steroid drug used to treat inflammatory diseases such as arthritis, allergic reactions and asthma, methylprednisolone mimics the effects of the body's natural steroid hormones. These include the stress hormones cortisol, norepinephrine and epinephrine, made from cholesterol by the adrenal glands.

Common side effects of methylprednisolone include increased blood pressure, weight gain, fluid retention and increased appetite.

**Ketoconazole (Nizoral)** Used to treat serious fungal infections, ketoconazole may interfere with the body's use of oestrogen and testosterone when taken long term in tablet form. Women may stop menstruating; men may have trouble getting and maintaining erections.

**Spironolactone (Aldactone)** Used to treat high blood pressure and congestive heart failure, this drug increases blood levels of oestradiol, the most abundant and potent form of the female sex hormone oestrogen.

Common side effects of spironolactone include nausea, vomiting and increased hair growth.

Ask your doctor about the potential effects your medication may have on your hormonal health. And if, after beginning a new medication, you experience symptoms such as the growth of facial hair, a waning sex drive, or changes in your menstrual cycle, be sure to bring it to your doctor's attention.

"Evidence clearly indicates that exposure to high doses of HAAs can harm our health. But scientists don't know whether low concentrations can, partly because they don't completely understand how these chemicals behave at very low doses," says Dr. LeBlanc.

In recent years, environmental groups – including the US Environmental Protection Agency (EPA) – have tried to direct research into classes of pesticides used now. These include the pesticide and fungicide vinclozolin, as well as other fungicides called imidazoles, which are used extensively on crops and in home lawn care products.

There have also been some preliminary studies on the effects of pesticides in people. Some of their findings:

- *A multicentre study, conducted in Canada, of women with and without breast cancer found that women diagnosed with breast cancer who had the highest blood levels of organochlorines were more likely to have large breast tumours that had spread to surrounding lymph nodes. This research suggests that organochlorine exposure may influence the growth or aggressiveness of breast cancer, rather than initiate breast cancer.*
- *Mice who had been fed high amounts of the pesticide atrazine developed more mammary tumours than those who hadn't.*
- *Research conducted in Italy found that women exposed to atrazine had a higher risk of ovarian cancer.*
- *The breakdown product of the pesticide methoxychlor significantly lowered the production of testosterone in laboratory animals. This raises the possibility that it may also reduce testosterone levels in men, reducing their fertility – a potential concern if you and your husband hope to have children.*

## Your Pesticide Protection Plan

The US EPA concedes that pesticides can cause health problems. That's why it evaluates them for a wide range of negative health effects in laboratory animals – from eye and skin irritation to cancer and birth defects – and regulates every one of the 865 active ingredients registered as pesticides. But starting this week – today – you can take steps to protect yourself from unnecessary pesticide exposure. These surprisingly simple strategies can help.

**Rinse – don't soak – fresh fruit and vegetables.** Running water's abrasive effect helps to remove pesticide residue from the surface of produce.

**Consider peeling fruits and vegetables.** Doing so removes surface residues.

**Trim the fat from meats.** Some pesticides collect in animal fat.

**Eat a wide range of fruits and vegetables.** Specific pesticides are used for specific food crops, so eating a variety of produce can help prevent you from eating too much of any given pesticide.

**Better yet, consider buying organically grown food.** More and more supermarkets sell fruits, vegetables and other plant foods grown and processed without the use of synthetic fertilizers or pesticides. In fact, according to one survey, 23 per cent of the shoppers polled use organic products twice a week or more – and 69 per cent are extremely concerned about pesticides in foods.

Specifically, look for organically grown strawberries, peppers, spinach, cherries, peaches, melons, celery, apples, apricots, green beans, grapes and cucumbers. Based on data from the EPA and the Food and Drug Administration (FDA), the Environmental Working Group (EWG) in Washington, D.C., has found that depending on their country of origin (United States, Mexico, or Chile), these fruits and vegetables consistently contain the most pesticide residues.

**Use home, lawn, and garden pesticides sparingly, and only when absolutely necessary.** And follow to the letter the directions for use.

**If you play golf, wash your hands thoroughly afterwards.** Golf courses use large amounts of pesticides.

# Week 4: Use Plastics Safely

We take plastic food wrap and soft drinks bottles for granted and use them daily. But a growing number of scientists are concerned about the safety of these products, along with tin cans and dental sealants.

Evidently, some substances in certain plastics used to make various products have been shown to be HAAs. And researchers are studying the possible adverse effects they may have on our hormonal health.

One such chemical is bisphenol-A, used in the manufacture of reusable bottles, food and drink containers, the linings of food and drink cans, dental sealants and baby bottles. Bisphenol-A has been found in liquids from food cans as well as in saliva – the chemical had leached from dental sealants.

No one knows how bisphenol-A affects people. But in animal tests, bisphenol-A has been shown to have oestrogen-like effects.

Researchers at the University of Missouri in Columbia exposed pregnant mice to the same levels of bisphenol-A that we're typically exposed to. They found that the chemical caused the offspring of the mice to grow faster after birth and to enter puberty earlier than normal.

Other research has shown that yet another common plastic product – cling film – may also pose health risks.

Some cling films made of a type of plastic called polyvinyl chloride (PVC) contain plasticizers – chemicals that lubricate the film and make it more pliable. The plasticizer used in PVC cling film, di (ethylhexyl) adipate, or DEHA, is in the plastic film that supermarkets use to wrap cheeses and meats. It's also found in at least one brand of household cling film. Check the packaging before you buy.

Some animal studies suggest that DEHA is an endocrine disrupter. Other research has shown that DEHA can leach into food wrapped in plastic.

The US FDA says that there's no evidence that DEHA is an HAA. But the US EPA has begun to screen thousands of chemicals, including DEHA, to target possible HAAs for further study.

## What You Can Do Starting Today

Until we know more about the effects of common plastics on our health, use these commonsense strategies to protect yourself.

- *Use plastic wraps and plastic cookware made of polyethylene, which don't contain plasticizers. Check for a consumer information phone number or Web site on the product's packaging and contact the company directly to ask if plasticizers are used if the packaging doesn't make it clear.*
- *When you reheat or cook food in a microwave oven, don't allow the plastic wrap to touch the food.*
- *Immediately remove cling wrap from cooked meats and cheeses and transfer them to a plastic bag or container.*
- *Better yet, ask the person on the deli counter to wrap your cooked meats and cheeses in paper.*
- *If you buy hard cheeses wrapped in plastic, use a cheese slicer to shave off a layer of the surface. Shaving can help remove DEHA.*
- *Cook only in containers labelled for use in the microwave.*
- *Don't reuse the plastic trays that come with frozen microwave dinners.*
- *Before you defrost meat, poultry, or fish in the microwave, remove it from its tray and cling film.*
- *Don't microwave food in margarine tubs or dairy food containers (such as yoghurt containers). They aren't heat-tested and could allow chemicals to leach into food.*

# Week 5: If You Eat Meat, Buy Organic

The use of all hormones for growth promotion purposes is banned in the EU. However, the situation in the US is different, so much so that it's caused an international "meat war" that's kept hormone-treated beef from the United States from being sold in Europe since 1989.

Beef, poultry and farm-produced fish in the US are likely to include a variety of hormones, plus other substances. Could the hormones farmers give to beef cattle and dairy cows – and the antibiotics given to them and to many other animals – adversely affect health?

## Natural and Synthetic Hormones

More than 90 per cent of all the beef cattle in the United States receive a combination of up to three naturally occurring and three manmade hormones: oestradiol, progesterone, testosterone, trenbolone acetate, zeranol and melengestrol acetate. No, the cattle aren't suffering hot flushes or going through menopause. Rather, beef cattle given hormones gain weight more quickly, which makes their meat more tender and flavoursome. The faster cattle fatten up, the less money farmers must spend feeding and caring for them – and the less we pay for meat at the supermarket.

The US FDA maintains that eating hormone-treated beef poses "no measurable or adverse health effects".

Some researchers (and the EU) disagree.

According to Carlos Sonnenschein, M.D., professor in the department of anatomy and cellular biology at the Tufts University School of Medicine in Boston, eating hormone-treated beef may be one reason why girls in the United States reach puberty earlier than in the past. In the mid-19th century, the average girl began to menstruate at 15. Today a girl's first period arrives 2 to 3 years earlier. Dr. Sonnenschein also believes that by increasing their lifetime exposure to oestrogen, eating hormone-treated beef may increase girls' future risk of breast cancer.

What's more, contrary to FDA and USDA assurances, administration of natural and/or synthetic sex hormones to cattle results in high residues in meat. It has been known for decades that these hormones induce breast and other reproductive cancers in a wide range of animal studies, says Samuel S. Epstein, M.D., professor of environmental and occupational medicine at the University of Illinois School of Public Health in Chicago. "These carcinogenic effects are substantially increased when the hormone is given in the cattle's infancy or when two or more hormones are administered simultaneously, as is the practice in many feedlots," he adds.

## Recombinant Bovine Growth Hormone (rBGH)

Most dairy cows in the United States are now injected with rBGH, administered to increase their milk production.

There's evidence that rBGH also increases the levels of insulin-like growth factor-1 (IGF-1) in cow's milk. This hormone, or growth protein, regulates cell growth, division and differentiation. Over the past decade, converging lines of evidence have clearly implicated IGF-1 as a major risk factor (increasing risk by up to sevenfold) in the promotion of breast cancer, as stated in articles published by Dr. Epstein in peer-reviewed medical journals.

The potential hazards are not limited to women. Dr. Epstein has additionally published articles stating that that an elevated blood level of IGF-1 is a major risk factor for colorectal and prostate cancers in men.

## Antibiotics

For many years beef and dairy cattle, chickens and even farmed fish have been routinely treated with antibiotics everywhere, both to keep them healthy and to step up their weight gain. Forty per cent of all antibiotics used in the United States are fed to animals raised for food. However, the EU is working to reduce all levels of feedstuff additives to protect consumers of livestock products.

As far as anyone knows, antibiotics don't have a hormonal effect. And antibiotics given to animals don't harm us directly. The problem is that the antibiotics given to animals give rise to strains of bacteria that are resistant to lifesaving antibiotics we sometimes need when we're sick, perhaps eventually making them less effective – or not effective at all. According to a study from the US Centers for Disease Control and Prevention, for example, fewer than 1 per cent of salmonella microbes were resistant to antibiotics in 1980. By 1996, nearly 34 per cent were resistant. Consequently, many US cattle farmers who decline to use growth hormones tend to also avoid using antibiotics on their animals.

Based on the evidence accumulated so far, Dr. Sonnenschein recommends buying organic meat and fish, which is becoming increasingly widely available. The term organic is defined by law and all organic food production and processing is governed by a strict set of rules. Animals and fish are reared without the routine use of drugs common in intensive livestock farming.

# Week 6: Drink Lightly or Not at All

If you don't drink alcohol, move on to Phase 2 of the Hormone-Balancing Programme on page 275, which discusses positive ways to deal with stress and blunt its potentially deleterious effect on your hormones.

But if you do drink, you'll want to know how alcohol can protect your health. Or damage it.

If you enjoy a nightly glass of wine with dinner, you're golden. Research links moderate drinking – defined as one drink per day for women of any age – to a reduced risk of heart disease. (A "drink" equals one 350-millilitre (12-fluid ounce) can of beer, one 150-millilitre (5-fluid ounce) glass of wine, or a mixed drink containing 44 millilitres (1.5 fluid ounces) of 80-proof alcohol.) But when women drink much more than that, alcohol's health benefits vanish. Chronic, heavy drinking among women can:

**Raise breast cancer risk.** Six studies of more than 300,000 women evaluated for up to 11 years found that women who drank approximately two to five drinks a day increased their risk of breast cancer by 41 per cent. A recent study shows that even one drink a day raises breast cancer risk.

So far, no one knows for sure exactly how alcohol and breast cancer are related; however, alcohol appears to increase a woman's blood and urine levels of oestrogen, known to encourage hormone-fuelled cancers such as breast cancer. In fact, some studies have found that alcoholic women have higher oestrogen levels than those who drink moderately or not at all. It may be these women secrete more of this hormone – or that their bodies aren't able to eliminate excess oestrogen as well.

**Weaken our bones.** Bone isn't "dead". It's dynamic, living tissue, and large amounts are constantly being formed and "torn down" in a process called remodelling. Two hormones play a role in this process: parathyroid hormone (PTH), produced by the parathyroid glands, and calcitonin, produced by the thyroid gland.

Studies link heavy drinking with bone loss. Alcohol appears to weaken bone by disrupting the remodelling process – particularly the rebuilding of bone by osteoblasts. This suppression of osteoblast function results in less bone being built than is "torn down".

**Cause fertility problems and birth defects.** Women who drink heavily may have irregular periods, menstruate without ovulating, or stop menstruating altogether. All can be caused by alcohol's interfering directly with our reproductive hormones, particularly oestrogen.

**ON THE WEB** & Other Resources

For up-to-date information on all food-related topics in the UK contact the Food Standards Agency:
**Food Standards Agency**
Aviation House
125 Kingsway
London WC2B 6NH
Tel: 0207 276 8000
*www.foodstandards.gov.uk*

To find out more about organic food production, contact the Soil Association:

**The Soil Association**
Bristol House
40–56 Victoria Street
Bristol BS1 6BY
Tel: 0117 929 0661
E-mail: *info@soilassociation.org*
*www.soilassociation.org*

For information and advice on a wide variety of environmental concerns, see:
**The Environmental Agency**
*www.environment-agency.gov.uk*

In pregnant women, heavy drinking during pregnancy can cause foetal alcohol syndrome, a group of birth defects that include abnormal brain size, developmental delays, behaviour problems and distinctive facial features. And while moderate drinking doesn't appear to be associated with birth defects, it may be linked to lower birth weights. Since no safe threshold has been set, some health authorities in the UK advise pregnant women to abstain from alcohol completely.

**Interfere with blood sugar control.** If you're diabetic, having an occasional drink won't significantly impact your blood sugar levels. But consuming alcohol regularly – even in moderation – interferes with blood sugar control and increases the risk of nerve and eye damage.

Chronic heavy drinking is especially dangerous for anyone with diabetes. In people with diabetes who are well-nourished, long-term alcohol use can lead to excessive blood sugar levels. But many heavy drinkers don't eat well – or at all. And heavy drinking in these "noneaters" can cause life-threatening declines in blood sugar.

Experts aren't sure why alcohol affects blood sugar so dramatically, nor have studies been conducted on the effects of heavy drinking on insulin secretion or insulin resistance.

## Get Help for Alcohol Abuse

If you've thought more than once about getting help for your drinking, its effects on your hormones might prompt you to do something about it, starting this week.

Alcoholics Anonymous (AA) is the best-known group (although its "members" maintain strict anonymity). Organized in 1935, AA is an informal society of more than 2,000,000 recovering alcoholics across the world. Women make up 35 per cent of the total membership.

AA is nondenominational, anyone can be a member, and meetings can be found virtually anywhere, even in the smallest towns. The cornerstone of the AA recovery programme is the Twelve Steps, which describe the experience of the earliest AA members.

You'll find a listing for AA in the Yellow Pages. If you're online, contact AA on the Internet at www.alcoholicsanonymous.org.

Britain is well served by many other organizations set up to help people with alcohol problems and their families (AA does not work for everyone), so that there are many alternatives. Their phone numbers are listed here in alphabetical order. Their titles suggest their main interest. Feel free to get in touch with any of these:

**Al-Anon Family Groups.** 0207 403 0888, www.hexnet.co.uk/alanon

**Alcoholics Anonymous.** 01904 644 026

**Alcohol Concern.** 0207 928 7377, www.alcoholconcern.org.uk

**Alcohol Problem Advisory Service.** www.apas.org.uk

**Alcohol Recovery Project.** 0207 940 0623

**Institute of Alcohol Studies.** 01480 466 766

**National Association for Children of Alcoholics.** 0117 924 8005

**TACADE** (The Advisory Council on Alcohol and Drug Education). 0161 745 8924

# Phase 2:
## Crank Up the "Good" Hormones

Once you've tackled all the dietary and lifestyle factors that trick your hormones into behaving badly, the next step is to make other positive changes that put your system into balance and keep it there.

"Simple things like getting enough sleep, eating a good diet, and reducing the stress in your life can have dramatic effects on your hormonal health," says Connie Catellani, M.D., of the Miro Center for Integrative Medicine in Evanston, Illinois.

Many of the hormone-balancing tactics you'll read about here have long been known to protect us against disease. But you're also in for a few surprises.

Other, less well-known strategies also have a direct and significant impact on our hormones and our health.

This phase of the Hormone-Balancing Programme benefits virtually all women, regardless of age. Each week, you'll learn a new way to keep levels of crucial hormones from inching up into the danger zone or to encourage levels of "feel good" hormones to rise. Naturally. (You can start with any week and take longer at each step, if you need to.) In Phase 3, which follows, you'll learn how to customize this basic programme to fit your particular health concerns, from allergies to hot flushes, urinary tract infections to cancer.

## Week 1: Relax!

If you're like many women, you've got a demanding job, a family who needs you, and a to-do list as long as John Grisham's last novel. No wonder you feel tired or depressed, anxious or irritable. Or perhaps you can't sleep (although you have no problem eating). Sex – or at least good sex – is a distant memory.

All are hallmark symptoms of chronic stress – the cumulative load of minor, everyday annoyances or frustrations that are all too commonplace.

Unrelenting stress can launch the female body into major hormonal action. The chemical and electrical dance among the brain, various glands, and the sympathetic nervous system activates the fight-or-flight response, the body's involuntary response to a threat. When we're emotionally excited or find ourselves in danger, it's this response that makes our hearts pound, our breath turn to pants or gasps, and our skin turn cold and clammy.

The hypothalamus, a grape-size structure tucked in the centre of the brain, sounds the first alarm. Under stress, the hypothalamus releases CRH (corticotropin-releasing hormone). This chemical races down the stalk that connects the hypothalamus to the pea-size pituitary gland.

Primed by the hypothalamus, the pituitary releases another hormone, ACTH (adrenocorticotropic hormone). This secretion of ACTH prompts the adrenal glands – the small, pyramid-shaped glands perched above the kidneys – to release the top gun of all stress hormones, cortisol.

Meanwhile, our adrenal glands are pumping out norepinephrine and epinephrine, the hormones that activate the fight-or-flight response.

But it's cortisol that has the most potential to damage our health.

Norepinephrine and epinephrine have short-acting effects, lasting only as long as a toddler's attention span. But cortisol promotes more long-lasting responses to stressors. And the longer it runs through your veins, the more damaging its effects.

Cortisol "overload" suppresses your immune system, making you more vulnerable to colds and infections. It increases your risk of heart disease and high blood pressure. It's even linked with insulin resistance, a risk factor for type 2 diabetes.

Chronic stress also affects your brain, particularly a tiny area called the hippocampus, which controls "fact" memory – your recall of names, faces, words and dates. Indeed, in one study, women and men given the prescription drug cortisone – which our bodies convert to cortisol – were less able to memorize and recall words.

The hippocampus is loaded with tiny "traps" that latch on to cortisol. Over time, too much cortisol suppresses the mechanisms in the hippocampus and other parts of the brain that control memory.

Chronic stress can actually kill cells in the hippocampus that generate and transmit nerve impulses, perhaps ageing our brains before their time.

# Stress-Defusing Strategies

To help reset your internal stress-o-meter to normal levels – and perhaps reduce stress-related hormonal changes – experts recommend the following strategies.

When you're stressed *right now*:

**Talk some sense into yourself.** Silently repeat a soothing word or phrase, such as "peace" or "This, too, shall pass," while taking slow, deep breaths through your nose, says Ellen Toby Klass, Ph.D., associate professor of psychology at Hunter College in New York City.

**Put photos in your personal "stress zones".** Choose shots that transport you back to a perfect moment in your life, suggests Tim O'Brien, director of The Institute for Stress Management in Tallahassee, Florida. Clip to your sun visor a photo from your anniversary trip to Paris to calm you when you're stuck in traffic. Place in your work area beautifully framed pictures of your children as chubby-cheeked, innocent infants. When stress closes in, turn to those images. Recall in vivid detail what you saw, heard, smelled and felt in those moments. Change the photos often to stimulate soothing memories.

At least 15 minutes a day (or more):

**Schedule regular play periods into your diary.** Whether it's piecing together a 1000-piece puzzle or going sledging with your kids, play distracts us from our worries, providing a temporary refuge from stress, says Lenore Terr, M.D., clinical professor of psychiatry at the University of California, San Francisco, and author of *Beyond Love and Work: Why Adults Need to Play*.

We should dedicate at least 1 per cent of our lives to play, says David Earl Platts, Ph.D., founder of David E. Platts and Associates, a personal coaching and counselling firm in Knaphill, Woking. "In practical terms, that's 15 minutes a day, or less than 2 hours once a week."

Once or twice a day, for 10 to 20 minutes:

**Just say "Om". Or repeat "one", "love", "peace", or "calm."** Or a phrase rooted in your belief system ("Hail Mary, full of grace" if you're Catholic, "Our Father who art in Heaven" if you're Protestant, "Sh'ma Yisrael" if you're Jewish, and so forth). Whatever word or phrase you choose is the crux of the relaxation response.

The following simple exercise, from *The Relaxation Response*, was formulated more than 25 years ago by Herbert Benson, M.D., founding president of the Mind/Body Medical Institute at Beth Israel Deaconess Medical Center in Boston.

And it works! Research shows that when performed regularly, the relaxation response can reduce the fight-or-flight response and its resulting cascade of stress hormones. It also has been shown to reduce high blood pressure and is commonly recommended to treat heart conditions, chronic pain and other health conditions. Here's how to do it.

## When Women Are Stressed, "Peacekeeping" Hormones Kick In

For decades, behavioural scientists have assumed that women cope with stress the way men do – with the fight-or-flight response, the body's automatic response to danger that readies it for either battle or retreat.

But researchers at UCLA challenge that view.

After analysing thousands of human and animal behavioural studies, they identified an alternative response to stress exclusive to women: "tend and befriend".

The males of most species tend to react to stress with aggression ("fight") or withdrawal ("flight"), they argue. But females of most species are prone to nurture their children or to seek comfort and support, especially from other females.

Hormones – particularly oxytocin, released by the pituitary gland – appear to play a key role in the tend-and-befriend response, says lead researcher Shelley Taylor, Ph.D., professor in the psychology department of the University of California, Los Angeles.

Oxytocin, responsible for the "letdown" reflex in nursing mothers, has been studied largely for its role in breastfeeding. But stress, too, gets the oxytocin flowing. "Animals and people with high levels of oxytocin are calmer, more relaxed, more social, and less anxious," says Dr. Taylor.

Both men and women secrete oxytocin during stress. But its calming effects appear to be muted by testosterone, which is higher in males. What's more, oestrogen (a predominantly female hormone) pumps up the stress-reducing effects of oxytocin.

We may still experience the *physiological* fight-or-flight response – the pounding heart and tense muscles – that results from the body's outpouring of stress hormones. But the tend-and-befriend system may in some ways protect women against the harmful physical consequences of stress, says Dr. Taylor. "It may provide insight into why women live an average of 7½ years longer than men."

1. *Pick a word, short phrase, or prayer that is rooted in your belief system.*
2. *Sit quietly in a comfortable position.*
3. *Close your eyes.*
4. *Relax your muscles, starting from your feet and moving to your calves, thighs, abdomen, shoulders, head and neck.*
5. *Breathe slowly and naturally, and as you do, say your focus word silently to yourself as you exhale.*
6. *Don't worry about "doing it right". When other thoughts come to mind, simply say to yourself, "Oh, well," and gently return to your repetition.*
7. *Continue for up to 20 minutes.*
8. *When you're done, continue to sit for a few minutes and allow other thoughts to return.*
9. *Open your eyes and sit for another minute or so before you stand up.*

# Week 2: Laugh It Up!

For more than 20 years, Lee S. Berk, M.P.H., Dr.P.H., has studied the effect of mirthful laughter and humour on our hormones and immune systems. But his findings are anything but silly.

"If we put what we currently understand about laughter's effects on the neuroendocrine and immune systems into a pill, it would require FDA approval," says Dr. Berk, associate research professor at the Loma Linda University School of Medicine and Public Health in California and associate director for the university's Center for Neuroimmunology.

Dr. Berk's research has found that laughter triggered by humour (rather than, say, hostility) causes significant changes in our levels of stress hormones. And when they go south, our immune systems rev up.

In one study, Dr. Berk and his colleagues got six healthy young men to watch an hour-long humour video, which they chose themselves. They instructed a second group of six men to sit quietly for the same amount of time.

Blood tests showed that the video watchers had 30 per cent less cortisol in their blood during and after the tape than the sitting-quietly group. The video-watching group's levels of another stress hormone, epinephrine, also declined significantly.

"This is important because cortisol and other stress hormones suppress the immune system," says Dr. Berk. "When we reduce those stress hormones, we allow for the immune system to optimize itself. These results may apply to women as well."

Dr. Berk's studies show that mirthful laughter activates key immune system components. Specifically, it increases the activity of natural killer cells, immune cells that go after cells infected by viruses or those that cause some cancers. It also increases a specific antibody called immunoglobulin A (IgA) – located in the mucous membranes, which protect against upper-respiratory infections, such as colds – and gamma interferon, an immune system hormone that fights

## Balance Stress Hormones with Visualization

You can dramatically reduce your stress by tapping into your most powerful inner resource: your imagination, says Martha Davis, Ph.D., a psychologist at the Kaiser Permanente Medical Center in Santa Clara, California, and lead author of *The Relaxation and Stress Reduction Workbook*. Here's a sample visualization for dissipating stress hormones. Record it on an audiocassette. Then lie down, get comfortable, close your eyes, and follow the directions.

In your mind's eye, walk slowly to a quiet, peaceful, safe place, inside or outside. Picture yourself unloading your worries. Notice the view in the distance. What do you smell? What do you hear? Notice what is before you. Reach out and touch it. How does it feel? Smell it. Hear it. Make the temperature comfortable. Be safe here. Look around for a special spot, a private spot. Find the path to this place. Feel the ground with your feet. Look above you. What do you see? Hear? Smell? Walk down this path until you can enter your own quiet, comfortable, safe place.

You have arrived at your special place. What is under your feet? How does it feel? Take several steps. What do you see above you? What do you hear? Do you hear something else? Reach and touch something. What is its texture? Are there pens, paper, paints, nearby, or is there sand to draw in, clay to work? Go to them, handle them, smell them. These are your special tools to reveal ideas or feelings to you. Look as far as you can see. What do you see? What do you hear? What aromas do you notice?

Say an affirmation such as "This is my special place. I can come whenever I wish."

Open your eyes and spend a minute or two savouring your inner calm.

viruses and "switches on" specific components of the immune system.

All things to smile about.

### Raise Your "Ha-Ha Ratio"

Kids laugh about 400 times a day; we grownups, about 15. The plan below can help you strengthen your humour "muscles", says Paul McGhee, Ph.D., an early pioneer in humour research and president of The Laughter Remedy in Wilmington, Delaware.

Every day:

**Keep alert for inadvertently funny newspaper headlines, ads, or public signs.** One of Dr. McGhee's favourites, posted in a restaurant in Mexico City: "The water served here has been personally passed by the manager."

**Look for the humorous in everyday life.** While at the supermarket, Dr. McGhee was stumped by how to swipe his debit card through an unfamiliar machine. The cashier said, "Strip down and face towards me." Dr. McGhee laughed. The cashier blushed.

Every week:

**Lighten up your commute.** Alternate your favourite tunes with a cassette or CD of your favourite comedian or a humorous book on tape.

**Get thee to a video store and head to the comedy section.** Sample everything, from classic *I Love Lucy* episodes to modern fare such as *The First Wives Club* or *Absolutely Fabulous*.

Regularly:

**Wear or carry something guaranteed to amuse people.** Your "prop" might be a clown nose, an office toy, a funny T-shirt, even a weird piece of jewellery. Steven Sultanoff, Ph.D., president of the American Association of Therapeutic Humor in Phoenix, uses a wristwatch – featuring the Disney character Goofy – that runs backwards. "I long for people to ask me what time it is."

# Week 3: Treat Yourself to Massage

Regular rubdowns aren't frivolous indulgences – they can benefit your hormone levels in measurable ways. Deep-pressure massage reduces blood levels of norepinephrine, epinephrine and cortisol, jump-starting your immune system's ability to activate infection-fighting immune cells, says Tiffany Field, Ph.D., director of the Touch Research Institute at the University of Miami School of Medicine.

In one study conducted at the Touch Research Institute, 20 women with breast cancer got a massage twice a week for 5 weeks. All the participants in the study reported reduced anxiety and improved mood and quality of life. Blood tests revealed lower stress hormone levels and improvements in their immune systems.

In other studies, of women with fibromyalgia and ME, full-body massage also lowered cortisol levels – along with participants' stress, anxiety and depression.

Massage stimulates pressure receptors in our skin, says Dr. Field. These receptors signal our brains to "turn on" the vagus, one of the 12 nerves that originate in the brain. Among its other job functions, the vagus helps regulate heart rate, breathing, and digestion, all of which are influenced by stress. And when the vagus revs up, says Dr. Field, heart rate and breathing slow and cortisol levels go down.

But massage doesn't just shore up the immune system. It also brightens mood and reduces perception of pain. That's because massage causes levels of two brain chemicals, serotonin and dopamine, to rise almost immediately. Both have hormone-like effects and play a role in the regulation of mood. Low serotonin levels are thought to cause depression, while dopamine has been nicknamed "the feel-good hormone". That's why, after a massage, we tend to feel refreshed, relaxed and alert.

## Get Rubbed the Right Way

As if you needed more incentive to wheedle a massage from your mate: many of the benefits of massage, including lowered cortisol levels, occur during and immediately after a massage. If you can't partner up for a massage, let your *own* fingers do the walking. This massage mini-guide will cover the basics.

Any time you feel tense:

**Tame tension in 10 minutes or less.** Give yourself a head and scalp massage, says Maureen Moon, president of the American Massage Therapy Association in Evanston, Illinois. Use the pads of your fingertips in a gentle yet firm circular motion. Use firmer pressure on spots that feel especially tense. Here's how.

*1. Rub your hands together to warm them. Place them over your face for 30 seconds.*

2. *Starting at the nape of your neck, work your fingers around your scalp until you've covered every inch. Repeat six times.*
3. *Massage between your eyebrows, moving up along your forehead, then down to your temples. Repeat three times.*
4. *Massage your cheeks, chin, jaw and nose, and around your mouth. Repeat three times.*
5. *Return to your forehead, and massage along your eyebrows and below your eyes.*

Repeat three times, two to three times a week.

You'll find books and videos on dozens of massage techniques, from traditional Swedish massage to Oriental forms of bodywork such as shiatsu. But no matter which form you choose, share massages with your partner, following the guidelines below.

**Use deep pressure.** It stimulates the vagus, says Dr. Field. "If there's not enough pressure, you don't get the benefits." Rule of thumb: the area being massaged should turn slightly whiter. Of course, if you're wincing in pain, ask your massage therapist or partner to ease off.

**Choose soothing, sensual surroundings.** Take your massage in a warm room on a firm, comfortable surface, such as a futon or mat. Play soft music and enjoy your massage by candlelight.

**Use a light oil or lotion that smells divine.** The scents of lavender and clary sage promote feelings of relaxation.

**Now give your partner a massage.** He deserves it. You'll benefit, too. Dr. Field's research has shown that people who *give* a massage reduce their own levels of stress hormones.

# Week 4: Put Poor Sleep Habits to Bed

Do you pride yourself on your ability to function on 5 hours of sleep a night?

It's a dubious achievement. In fact, you may be taxing your hormones – and ageing yourself before your time.

"Chronic sleep loss has a profound effect on metabolism and hormonal function," says Eve Van Cauter, Ph.D., professor in the endocrinology section at the University of Chicago Medical Center. "Ongoing research suggests that the effects of chronic sleep loss may be as profound as the lack of physical activity."

Getting too little sleep – usually defined as less than 8 hours a night –

affects two mechanisms that regulate sleep and wakefulness. The first: circadian rhythm, better known as our biological clock. Controlled by the hypothalamus, circadian rhythm not only tells us when to sleep (hopefully at night) but tells our bodies to release or stop releasing specific hormones, particularly cortisol.

Sleep deprivation also impacts sleep–wake homoeostasis, which regulates how long we stay awake and how much we need to sleep. It, too, regulates the stop-and-go release of hormones – particularly growth hormone, which influences muscle strength and the ratio of muscle to fat.

To study this phenomenon on humans, Dr. Van Cauter and her colleagues spent 16 consecutive nights restricting and then extending the sleep of 11 healthy young men.

The first three nights, the men were allowed to sleep 8 hours. The next six nights, they were allotted 4 hours. The last seven nights, they spent 12 hours per night in bed.

At the height of their sleep debt, the men took 40 per cent longer than normal to regulate their blood sugar levels after a high-carbohydrate meal. Further, their bodies' ability to secrete insulin dropped dramatically – an early symptom of diabetes.

The sleep-deprived men also had more cortisol in their blood. Elevated evening cortisol levels, which are typical of older people, have been linked to various different age-related problems such as insulin resistance and memory loss.

"What we found suggests that these young men had metabolic and hormonal profiles that, in some ways, resembled those of men in their sixties," says Dr. Van Cauter. "When they were allowed to sleep 12-hour stretches, everything returned to normal, or better than normal." Similar studies have yet to be done on women.

## Sleep Tricks That Work with (Not Against) Your Hormones

Whether you have trouble falling or *staying* asleep, this "bye-bye, insomnia" programme can help you unpack those bags under your eyes – for good.

Every day:

**Get at least 30 minutes of natural light a day.** Natural light helps reset our inner alarm clocks so we'll want to fall asleep at the right time, says Joyce Walsleben, Ph.D., director of Sleep Disorders Center at New York University in New York City and author of *A Woman's Guide to Sleep: Guaranteed Solutions for a Good Night's Rest.*

**Take a walk . . .** In one study of more than 700 people, those who took daily walks were one-third less likely to have trouble sleeping until their normal wake-up time. Those who walked *briskly* slashed the risk of any sleep disorder by half.

**. . . at the right time.** Because natural light is so critical to our sleep/wake cycle, Dr. Walsleben "prescribes" walking time depending on the sleep problem. If you can't fall sleep before 2 a.m., consider walking early. Really early. "Walking in the first morning light within 15 minutes of awakening will help strengthen normal circadian rhythm," says Dr. Walsleben. If you tend to doze off in the early evening only to pop awake in the wee hours, walk in the late afternoon.

To promote regular, restful sleep:

Some of the tips in Phase 1 of the Hormone-Balancing Programme automatically help with insomnia: reduce or eliminate your intake of coffee and other caffeine-containing foods and beverages, such as tea, cola drinks and chocolate, and cut back on nicotine and sugar before bed. (All are stimulants and can interfere with falling or staying asleep.) Also, avoid alcohol, which is sedating but disrupts sleep. The following sleep-well strategies may help, too.

**Make your bedroom as dark as possible.** Darkness stimulates the pineal gland, causing it to produce more melatonin, a light-sensitive hormone produced by the tiny pineal gland, located in the brain. Some evidence suggests that supplementing with this hormone can help remedy insomnia. Take only under the supervision of a knowledgeable medical doctor. To manipulate this hormone naturally, invest in thick, heavy curtains, or simply don an eye mask.

**Exercise early in the day, when possible.** Regular exercise is a drug-free sleep aid because it alleviates stress. It also raises body temperature, which primes us for slumber. Just don't work out close to bedtime. Exercise tends to increase levels of cortisol and make it harder to fall asleep. Late afternoon is ideal, says Dr. Walsleben.

**Make sleep a must.** In a US National Sleep Foundation poll, 45 per cent of those surveyed said they would sleep less to get more done. This popular attitude exasperates Dr. Walsleben. "Do we go without water on a hot day because we're too busy to drink it?" she asks. So no matter how harried your life, reserve 8 solid hours of it each night for sleep – and let no last-minute "emergency" keep you from slumber.

# Week 5: Make Love – It's Good for You

David Weeks, Ph.D., consultant clinical neuropsychologist at the Royal Edinburgh Hospital believes that making love – often – extends our youth.

If anyone knows, he should. Over a 10-year period, Dr. Weeks studied 3500 women and men, most in their forties to their sixties, to find out why some looked younger than others. He published his findings in a book, *Secrets of the Superyoung: The Scientific Reasons Some People Look 10 Years Younger Than They Really Are – And How You Can, Too.*

As you might expect, Dr. Weeks's research found that people in the younger-looking group watched their diets and exercised regularly. But they also spent a lot of time in bed. Not necessarily sleeping.

When visually rated for youthfulness, those who had sex three times a week

## DHEA: Not a Magic Hormone

From time to time, you'll read or hear claims that supplements of dehydroepiandrosterone (DHEA) burn fat, build muscle, crank up the sex drive, and slow ageing – in addition to warding off heart disease, cancer, type 2 diabetes and Alzheimer's disease.

The adrenal glands make DHEA, and the body uses it to make the sex hormones oestrogen and testosterone. Blood levels of DHEA skyrocket during puberty, peak in early adulthood, and decline with age. Those of us who are peri-menopausal, for example, have only 50 per cent of the DHEA we had in our twenties and thirties.

Emerging research hints that taking supplements of DHEA may well help delay the process of ageing.

Some researchers speculate that there's some link between the decline in DHEA levels as we grow older and the ailments associated with ageing – and that supplementation may help counter them.

Animal studies of the effects of DHEA are intriguing. In one study, mice given the hormone performed better on learning tasks. Another found that mice that were treated with DHEA lived longer than those that weren't.

Studies of DHEA supplementation in *people*, however, have been few – and small. Until recently. A large study conducted in France has produced some provocative – if still preliminary – results. In this large study, called the DHEAge study, 280 healthy men and women aged from

or more looked from 10 to 12 years younger than their actual age – the result of "significant reductions in stress, greater contentment, and better sleep," says Dr. Weeks.

Not only did the younger-looking folks have 50 per cent more sex than an equal number of people in a control group, but their lovemaking lasted three times as long.

Dr. Weeks speculates that, in part, increased levels of endorphins account for the "superyoung" group's youthful appearance. These "neuro-hormones" – chemicals released in the brain during exercise and, yes, after sex – are natural painkillers and also help to alleviate anxiety. (Endorphins are also responsible for the so-called runner's high – that feeling of elation the long-distance runner feels as she pounds along path or track.)

60 to 79 were given either 50 milligrams of DHEA or a dummy pill for 1 whole year.

After 6 months, those who had taken DHEA had levels of that hormone that approached – and sometimes exceeded – those of a young adult. After a year, the levels had declined, but stayed within the young-adult range.

Women over 70 appeared to reap substantial benefits from DHEA. Researchers found measurable improvements in bone density, and the women reported that their interest in sex had increased. And, regardless of their age, women who took DHEA had measurable improvements in their skin's texture and thickness.

While this study is encouraging, there's still not enough evidence to warrant taking DHEA to ward off ageing – or any other condition, says Frank Bellino, Ph.D., administrator of the endocrinology programme in the Biology of Aging Program at the National Institute on Aging in Bethesda, Maryland. "At this point, we just don't know enough about DHEA," he says.

When you consider that DHEA's short-term side effects include acne, aggressive behaviour and (yuck) increased body hair – often on the face – there's ample reason to wait for further proof that this "miracle" supplement is worth the risk.

For now, treat DHEA as a promising but unapproved drug, and use it only under a doctor's supervision.

The more we make love, the more endorphins our brains release, says Dr. Weeks. So that classic, endorphin-fuelled "afterglow" may help explain why more sex, more often, helps keep the wrinkles away.

## Start Your (Sexual) Engines

If you've enjoyed a healthy, happy sex life in the past, this programme can help restore the twinkle in your eye and the tingle in your loins.

Every day:

**Look for quiet moments – before bed, after a nice dinner out, during your daily walks – to clue your partner in to how you're feeling.** And gently encourage him to do the same. "Most women consider an emotionally intimate discussion, in which both partners disclose their fears and vulnerabilities, to be an aphrodisiac," says Jean Koehler, Ph.D., A.A.S.E.C.T., certified sex therapist and clinical instructor in the department of psychiatry and behavioural sciences at the University of Louisville in Kentucky.

**Wear Dolly Parton's undies.** Or, rather, slip into the lingerie you *think* she'd wear. Whether you're a size 8 or 18, slipping into an exquisite lace bra-and-panty set or a silk baby-doll nightgown will remind you that you're a woman with *needs*, not merely the disseminator of clean sheets and lunch money.

Every week or frequently:

**Have a pillow fight.** "Physical activity can be sexually stimulating," says Dr. Koehler. "I'll sometimes encourage couples to wrestle with each other. It's a playful activity that gets your body revved up and your sexual juices flowing."

**Watch romantic-yet-spicy "couples" videos.** Rest assured – there *are* videos that won't make you want to hide under the sheets. Dr. Koehler suggests the *Better Sex* video series or another series, *Ordinary Couples, Extraordinary Sex.* Both feature real couples exploring creative ways to enjoy loving sex. "They're likely to be more appealing to women than the typical sex video, which is geared toward men's fantasies," says Dr. Koehler. Both are available by mail order. Write to The Alexander Institute, 15030 Ventura Boulevard, Suite 400, Sherman Oaks, CA 91403.

Three times a week:

**Work it on out.** Exercise and physical fitness can contribute positively to your sex drive, says Dr. Koehler. Staying in shape is one of the best things you can do to help you feel good about yourself and your body. When we have an improved body image, an improved sex life often follows.

If boredom doesn't seem to be behind your lack of desire, see a doctor or therapist to rule out a physical or emotional cause, says Dr. Koehler.

Hormonal problems (such as hypothyroidism or, during menopause, waning levels of oestrogen or testosterone), illness, marital problems, or depression can dampen a woman's ardour.

# Week 6: Eat for Hormonal Health

Cheese puffs or wholewheat crackers? Barbecued spare ribs or grilled chicken? One thing's certain: as discussed in Phase 1, whatever finds its way into our mouths can have a significant impact on our hormones.

One example: taking in too much saturated fat (the kind found in abundance in meat and dairy products) can raise oestrogen levels in the blood. In premenopausal women, too much oestrogen can lead to menstrual cramps, PMS, or more frequent or severe hot flushes.

On the other hand, a healthy diet "can have a dramatically positive effect on hormone levels," says Dr. Catellani.

The basic plan? A diet that's loaded with whole grains, fresh fruits and vegetables, low- or no-fat dairy products – and that contains less red meat and processed foods, which tend to be high in unhealthy saturated fats. (This is assuming you've jettisoned food with sugar, growth hormones and other ingredients that adversely affect your hormone balance.)

The diet should also include specific foods research has shown to protect our health – and affect levels of specific hormones – fibre, foods high in essential fatty acids (such as grains and nuts), and foods high in phyto-oestrogens (such as soya beans or legumes).

## Fibre: the Blood Sugar Regulator

From the perspective of hormonal health, "it's crucial to keep your blood sugar stable," says Julie M. Wiener, N.D., a naturopath in private practice in Framingham and Brookline, Massachusetts. This is a point too often overlooked as a principle to a healthy endocrine system. One area of irregularity in the endocrine system could in turn have an effect on the other systems of the body, says Dr. Wiener.

A high-fibre diet can help keep your sugar levels stable. Whole grains are packed with fibre. Not so, foods made with refined grains, such as white bread, white pasta and white rice.

These "white foods" contain no bulk to slow them down as you digest them, so they speed through the digestive tract. This rapid breakdown triggers a flood of insulin, the hormone that ferries the body's primary source of fuel, blood sugar, into the cells.

Shortly thereafter, blood sugar levels drop precipitously – which signals the adrenal glands to release more cortisol.

By contrast, beans, brown rice, and whole grain cereals take hours to digest. So insulin levels rise gradually, blood sugar levels remain steady, and cortisol levels don't skyrocket.

Fibre also helps bind oestrogen and carry it out of the body, reducing the levels that circulate in the blood, says Fred Pescatore, M.D., founder of The Center for Integrative and Complementary Medicine in New York City. That's good news for those of us who are premenopausal because both breast and endometrial cancers are fuelled by high levels of circulating oestrogen.

## "Smart Foods" with Omega-3 Fatty Acids

Cold-water fish – such as salmon, tuna, rainbow trout, anchovies, sardines, and mackerel – are good sources of omega-3 fatty acids, "good" fats that can help put the kibosh on conditions that produce painful inflammation, such as severe menstrual cramps and rheumatoid arthritis. So are flaxseed, flaxseed oil, walnuts, walnut oil, and dark green leafy vegetables. They blunt the body's production of hormonelike substances called prostaglandins, which regulate its response to inflammation.

## Soya Foods: Get Your Oestrogen from Plants

Certain plant chemicals in soya, called phyto-oestrogens, are weaker versions of our own, natural oestrogen. It's thought that phyto-oestrogens attach to "traps" on the surface of cells, called oestrogen receptors. In effect, phyto-oestrogens steal natural oestrogen's "parking spaces".

Blocking the more potent natural oestrogen may reduce the risk of developing types of cancers fuelled by excess oestrogen, such as breast and endometrial cancers.

But phyto-oestrogens are multitalented. They can also supplement a woman's natural oestrogen – a possible boon for women in menopause, when declining levels of oestrogen and progesterone can cause hot flushes and night sweats.

Readily available soya products include tofu, soya milk, soya cheese, vegetarian burgers and sausages, soya protein powders. soya beans, soya desserts, flavoured drinks and ice-creams. They are all excellent sources of phyto-oestrogens.

# Church: The Newest "Wellness Centre"

If you regularly attend church or synagogue, mosque, monastery, or other place of worship, you may benefit in ways that balance your hormones – and prolong your life.

Michael McCullough, Ph.D., associate professor of psychology at Southern Methodist University in Dallas, and his colleagues reviewed 42 studies – involving nearly 126,000 people – that examined the link between religious involvement and health. ("Religious involvement" was defined as regular attendance at houses of worship and praying.)

Those who reported having been more involved in religious activities were 29 per cent more likely to be alive when researchers recontacted them than those who had been less involved.

Being spiritually minded may help short-circuit the impact of stress on physical and mental health, says Dr. McCullough. "Religion provides people with a meaning system that helps explain why they encounter hard times, and helps them see those stressful events as temporary and fleeting. As a result, it's easier for them to cope with stress."

Religious involvement also gives us a sense of connection with others. "It puts people in touch with people who care about them and who provide emotional resources in times of crisis," says Dr. McCullough. "They may also feel that their relationship with God is another kind of social support – another person, so to speak, who's on their side, rooting for them."

Religious involvement enhances our physical health in specific ways. For example, researchers at Duke University Medical Center in Durham, North Carolina, found that elderly churchgoers had lower blood levels of interleukin-6 (IL-6). Research suggests that blood levels of IL-6 rise with age and that elevated levels are found in a wide variety of ageing-related diseases, such as osteoporosis, rheumatoid arthritis, and Alzheimer's.

In a study of 3,963 people 65 and older, also conducted at Duke, researchers found that those who attended religious services at least once a week tended to have lower blood pressure than those who attended less than once a week.

So if you've considered attending worship but have been putting it off, this could be one more reason to stop procrastinating.

## The Hormones-in-Harmony Eating Plan

This easy-to-follow, good-for-you plan will "nourish" your hormones and lower your risk of a slew of health conditions, such as high blood pressure, diabetes and cancer.

As a bonus, you may even lose some weight on this 1500-calorie diet. Which delivers a hormonal benefit: it can help the body better respond to insulin, vital for those of us with diabetes or a family history of the disease.

Every day:

**Eat 9 servings of fruits and vegetables (4 fruit, 5 veggies).** One serving equals 2–3 tablespoons chopped fruit or 2 tablespoons cooked vegetables or 1 small dessert bowl of salad or raw greens; 1 small glass (150 ml/5 fl oz) fruit or vegetable juice; 1 medium piece of fruit.

---

### Under Stress? See About C

If there's one vitamin that can help counteract the deleterious effects of stress hormones, it's vitamin C. Large doses have been found to boost the immune systems of stressed-out lab rats. And it may well confer the same benefit on women, too, helping to protect us from stress-related health problems such as heart attacks and cancer.

"Vitamin C may indirectly bolster the immune system, reducing the debilitating physical effects and illnesses associated with chronic stress," says P. Samuel Campbell, Ph.D., chairman of the biological sciences department at the University of Alabama in Huntsville.

To see whether vitamin C would dampen hormonal responses to stress, Dr. Campbell and his colleagues completely immobilized lab rats for an hour a day (a safe form of stress for the rats). Some rats were given 200 milligrams of vitamin C, while others weren't.

After 3 weeks, the rats given vitamin C were producing significantly less corticosterone. Normal levels of these stress hormones, produced by the adrenal glands, help the body cope with everyday stress. But chronically high levels can weaken the immune system, affecting resistance to disease.

The RDA of vitamin C is 40 milligrams. To reduce cortisol and cortisone production in times of chronic severe stress, people would probably need to take at least 1000 milligrams a day, says Dr. Campbell – an amount well within safe limits.

**Eat 3 to 6 servings of whole grains.** One serving equals one slice of wholemeal bread or 200 g (7 oz) of a cooked whole grain or whole wheat pasta. To ensure you're really getting wholegrain bread or cereal (not a blend, or wheat bread with caramel colouring), look for the word "whole" on the label and a fibre content of 2 or 3 grams per slice. If the first ingredient doesn't include the word "whole", pass it by. It's made primarily with white flour.

**Consume 2 to 3 servings of high-calcium food.** One serving equals 200 ml (7 fl oz) of skimmed milk, 1 pot of fat-free or low-fat yoghurt, 30 g (1 oz) of reduced-fat cheese (preferably free of growth hormones), or 40 g (1½ oz) of calcium-fortified cereal, or 200 ml (7 fl oz) orange juice or soya milk. Lactose intolerant? Opt for dairy products that are lactose-free.

Every week:

**Eat at least 5 servings of beans (including soya milk or soya beans).** One serving equals 145 g (5 oz) cooked, dried beans or lentils. (To reduce the exorbitant sodium content of most tinned beans, opt for the low-sodium variety. Or drain the liquid from regular tinned beans and rinse them before use.)

**Eat 5 servings of nuts.** One serving equals 30 g (1 oz), chopped. Store nuts in the refrigerator to keep them from turning rancid.

**Eat 2 servings of fish.** One serving is 90 g (3 oz), cooked. If you don't regularly cook fish for dinner, simply eat a tuna sandwich a couple of times a week. Or snack on tinned sardines, mackerel, or herring.

# Week 7: De-Fang Stress Hormones with Herbs

Chronic stress may brutalize our bodies, but the Earth has blessed us with natural stress "shields": herbs called adaptogens help our bodies adapt to various physical stresses such as infections, sleep deprivation and extreme altitudes, as well as fortify us against the physical effects of emotional stress, says Douglas Schar, Dip.Phyt., M.C.P.P., a practising herbalist in Washington, D.C.

Basically, adaptogens help the body achieve balance, says Schar. Scientists call this "balance" homoeostasis – the body's ability to maintain internal equilibrium even as the outside environment changes.

We need adaptogens now more than ever. "We don't live in balance today, and that's not going to change," says Schar. "And when life wears you out, your immune system craps out. Your nervous system shorts out. You get sick more.

"Adaptogenic herbs have a strengthening effect that seems to make us less prone to the effects of a not-so-great lifestyle," says Schar.

Research has found that adaptogens boost the workings of several components of the immune system. For example, they appear to step up the activity of infection-fighting white blood cells and stimulate the production of interferon, a protein that assists white blood cells in their fight against viruses and bacteria.

Exactly how adaptogens perform these feats remains a mystery, says Schar. But one theory is that they give the adrenal glands a helping hand, increasing the body's ability to resist stress-related damage.

But as helpful as adaptogens can be, they're not once-per-day vitamin pills, says Schar. Use them to get through a period of intense, unremitting stress, such as when a work deadline disrupts your normal, healthy sleep and dietary habits. Or to beef up your immune system against colds and flu, start taking them a month before cold or flu season in the doses listed below or suggested by your health practitioner. "Adaptogens are very subtle herbal remedies; they lack that instant 'kick' you might get from a cup of coffee," says Schar. "However, people usually notice they feel less run-down after taking them for 2 weeks or so."

## Once-a-Day Herbal Hormone Helpers

Schar recommends the adaptogens licorice, Siberian ginseng and astragalus to help reduce the hormonal mayhem caused by stress. Take *one* of the herbs below, following the dosages given.

Every day for no longer than 3 months:

**Licorice.** One of its constituents, glycyrrhizin, is structurally similar to cortisol, and herbal healers often prescribe licorice to strengthen the adrenal glands. Dried root: two 500-milligram tablets three times a day. Tincture: 1:1 strength: 20 drops, twice a day; 1:5 strength: 1 teaspoon, twice a day. (See caution about licorice on page 450.)

**Siberian ginseng.** This herb appears to reduce the response of the adrenal cortex, the part of the adrenals that pump out cortisol. Dried root: two 500-milligram tablets three times a day. Tincture: 1:1 strength: 20 drops, three times a day; 1:5 strength: 1 teaspoon, three times a day.

**Astragalus.** Both ancient Chinese healers and modern-day herbal healers have used the root of this herb to counteract the debilitating effect of stress on the immune system. "I give it to people who feel generally run-down or who catch cold after cold," says Schar. Dried root: two 500-milligram tablets three times a day. Tincture: 1:1 strength: 20 drops, three times a day; 1:5 strength: 1 teaspoon, three times a day.

# Week 8: Move That Body

Why is it that, as much as we may dread hitting the gym, we usually leave feeling rejuvenated?

One word: endorphins.

While most research on endorphins and the so-called runner's high has been conducted on long-distance runners, there's strong anecdotal evidence that moderate exercise – a brisk walk, a 45-minute "date" with the Nautilus machines – also triggers the release of these "pleasure chemicals," says Beth Braun, Ph.D., a physiologist at the Miro Center for Integrative Medicine in Evanston, Illinois.

Exercise has also been shown to reduce symptoms of depression. Perhaps that's because, along with endorphins, working up a good sweat also activates the "feel good" neurotransmitters dopamine and serotonin.

Regular workouts also enable the body to more effectively use the hormone insulin. This is a boon to those of us who are overweight because extra pounds make us vulnerable to developing insulin resistance.

People with this condition produce enough insulin, which transports energy, in the form of blood sugar, to our cells. Problem is, the insulin doesn't work effectively. So blood sugar doesn't make it into the cells. It just backs up in the blood and eventually becomes toxic. Insulin resistance and high blood sugar are the hallmarks of type 2 diabetes.

Studies of women and men with diabetes have shown improvements in blood sugar control after only 1 week of aerobic exercise – and just one bout of exercise boosts insulin sensitivity for 16 hours or longer.

Exercise may even confer some protection against breast cancer by limiting our lifetime "exposure" to our own oestrogen. (As mentioned, high levels of oestrogen circulating in the blood can instigate the growth of hormone-sparked cancers.)

In the Nurses' Health Study, which has followed a group of more than 120,000 nurses since 1976, women who exercised for 7 hours a week or more were nearly 20 per cent less likely to develop breast cancer than their more sedentary sisters.

Here's an oddity: exercise actually *increases* cortisol levels.

That shouldn't really be surprising. After all, the body releases cortisol to help cope with physical stress.

Moreover, in and of itself, the release of cortisol is not necessarily good or bad. As long as cortisol levels return to normal in a relatively short time, as they do after exercise, the body doesn't suffer the ill effects of the cortisol glut associated with chronic stress.

## Your Exercise "Prescription"

Generally speaking, most experts recommend 30 to 60 minutes of exercise three to six times a week. But your exercise routine will depend on your general health and any health conditions you may have, such as diabetes or heart disease. So don't start an exercise programme until you talk to your doctor.

Most of us start an exercise programme with no trouble. It's deciding what kind of workout suits us – then sticking to it – that often trips us up. Here's how to make that decision – and how to make exercise a habit.

**Find your passion.** You'll be more likely to stick with an exercise programme if you actually *enjoy* it, says Dr. Braun. Yet many of us don't choose workouts that mesh with our temperaments. Before you pick your workout, consider your personality. Do you feel more comfortable exercising in a group or by yourself? If you're in the latter group, exercise classes may not be for you. Do you thrive on or dislike routine? While running or lifting weights is a joy for some of us, it's pure tedium for others.

**Make – and keep – "sweat dates".** When we break an appointment with a friend at the last minute with no explanation, we usually feel guilty. So make a date to walk or lift weights with a friend, neighbour, or colleague. You'll be less likely to miss your workouts when you know someone else depends on you for motivation, says Dr. Braun.

**Get back in the saddle.** Don't allow one missed workout to derail your fitness programme. Besides, missing one workout – or even several – doesn't undo all the good you've done, says Dr. Braun. If you're working out three times a week, you'll still be okay if you miss no more than two to four times in a month, she says.

# Phase 3: Customize Your Hormone-Balancing Programme

Your body contains nearly 200 hormones and hormone-like substances, affecting major organs and microscopic cells alike. Once you've cut back on outside agents that negatively affect your hormones and taken steps to optimize production of hormones that protect your health, you can fine-tune your health further.

In this section, you'll learn how to fix any of 28 specific health problems, from hot flushes to snoring, by taking into account the effects of hormones in your life.

For example, you probably know that the loss of oestrogen that comes with the menopause can make your skin more prone to wrinkles. But did you know that hormone changes can also cause your hair to get thinner? Hormone changes can also contribute to bladder control problems, chronic fatigue syndrome, urinary tract infections . . . a whole host of irritations and problems, up to and including vision problems. Hormone fluctuations during puberty, pregnancy and periods have even been shown to be a factor in gum disease, of all things.

Here you'll find out what the experts recommend, and you'll find out where to go for state-of-the-art updates in research and treatment methods. In some cases, there's much that you can do on your own.

But if you do need to seek medical help – as is often the case with hormone-related problems – doing your "homework" ahead of time will help you get the most out of your appointments with your doctor and solve the problem together more effectively.

# Hot Flushes

Although practically synonymous with the menopause, hot flushes can strike anywhere between the ages of 18 and 80. Some premenopausal women experience hot flushes with other symptoms of premenstrual syndrome (PMS). In one study, more than 80 per cent of women with either PMS or other menstrual cycle-related symptoms reported that they had 5 to 10 hot flushes a month.

That said, hot flushes are most common among women entering the menopause or during perimenopause, the 8 to 10 years before and 1 year after the menopause.

During a hot flush, blood surges to the surface of the skin on your chest, neck, and head. The increased bloodflow heats up your skin by about 4.5°F (2.5°C). Your heart rate accelerates, and you breathe a little faster. Some women also have heart palpitations, headaches, dizziness, and feelings of weakness or anxiety. As your body heat dissipates, your core body temperature drops, and so you may feel cold and clammy afterwards.

Most hot flushes – sometimes called "flashes" – last 2 to 5 minutes. Some women have only occasional flushes; others have more than a dozen a day. And they can recur for anywhere from a few months to decades. Untreated, hot flushes decline gradually – by about 20 per cent within 4 years after the onset of menopause – and eventually stop on their own.

No one knows exactly what causes hot flushes, but they are most likely triggered by fluctuations in oestrogen levels. "Those changes somehow stimulate the part of the brain that controls body temperature, throwing off its normally finely tuned control," says Robert Freedman, Ph.D., director of behavioural medicine at Wayne State University in Detroit. As a result, the brain signals the body to dissipate heat – to flush and sweat. The hot flush follows a slight increase in core body temperature. "Women who have hot flushes seem to be intolerant of even a slight increase in core body temperature," Dr. Freedman says.

If your hot flushes don't bother you, you don't have to do anything about them. If they are driving you bonkers, you may be able to reduce their intensity enough to put up with them without using drugs, says Ann Webster, Ph.D., director of the Menopause/Perimenopause Program at the Mind/Body Center for Women's Health at Beth Israel Deaconess Hospital in Boston. " You don't have to get rid of them completely to get substantial relief," she says.

# Hormonal Strategies

Because it restores oestrogen and progesterone levels to premenopausal levels, hormone replacement therapy (HRT) pretty much eliminates hot flushes. Either natural micronized progesterone or oestrogen – or a combination of both – seems to do the trick. Chances are, your doctor will recommend whatever she's most familiar prescribing. To help determine what's best for *you*, consider these guidelines.

## Short-Term HRT

If you're postmenopausal, hormone replacement therapy will cool down your hot flushes, pretty much guaranteed, within a week or less. In fact, that's the main reason women use HRT short-term. (It even works for men having hot flushes after hormonal therapy for prostate cancer.) And if you're taking HRT for other reasons – say, to protect your bones – then consider relief of hot flushes a bonus.

If you stop taking it, though, even if you've taken it for years, you'll tend to have hot flushes for a while, says Connie Catellani, M.D., director of the Miro Center for Integrative Medicine in Evanston, Illinois. You may need to taper off your dose, or switch to a herb, such as black cohosh (discussed shortly).

If you're going through surgically induced menopause (you've had your uterus and ovaries removed), studies indicate that you can relieve hot flushes better if you use a combination of oestrogen and progesterone rather than oestrogen alone. And both transdermal and oral HRT are equally effective at relieving hot flushes.

## A New Use for the Pill

If you're perimenopausal but your periods haven't yet stopped, and you don't smoke, your doctor will probably suggest oral contraceptives, rather than HRT, for hot flushes. Hormone therapy in perimenopause does not stop ovulation and can lead to irregular bleeding. Birth control pills do help to relieve hot flushes, and for a few women they may relieve PMS symptoms, says June LaValleur, M.D., assistant professor of obstetrics and gynaecology at the University of Minnesota and director of the Mature Women's Center, both in Minneapolis. Plus, birth control pills provide contraception, still needed during this time, and they regulate menstrual cycles very nicely, so there's less worry about irregular cycles or endometrial overgrowth. A number of brands are available for women aged 35 or older. Ask your doctor which one is best for you.

## Progesterone Alone

If you can't or prefer not to take HRT or oral contraceptives, taking prog-esterone without oestrogen can relieve hot flushes in perimenopausal women, Dr. Catellani says. Progesterone cream is available in the US, in many European countries and online, but it's important to buy one that actually delivers the goods. Natural progesterone creams based on wild yam are also available. In one study, after a year of using a progesterone cream, more than 80 per cent of women reported an improvement in their hot flushes, com-pared with fewer than 20 per cent of those using a placebo. You can also take oral progesterone, available by prescription only.

## The Patch

Women who have hot flushes only during or shortly before their periods can wear an oestrogen patch during that time to stop hot flushes, Dr. LaValleur says.

# Non-hormonal Strategies

If you experience serious hot flushes but simply can't use hormone supplements in any form, you have other options. A number of drugs approved for treat-ing conditions as diverse as epilepsy, depression and high blood pressure have been shown in studies to also relieve hot flushes, so they can be a godsend for women seriously bothered by hot flushes. The antidepressants fluoxetine (Prozac), venlafaxine (Efexor) and paroxetine ( Seroxat), for instance, cool hot flushes in women being treated for cancer. Gabapentin (Neurontin), an anti-seizure drug sometimes also used to treat migraine headaches, can also help hot flushes. So can the blood pressure-lowering drug clonidine (Catapres).

# Cool Down Naturally with Herbs and Supplements

Not all women need hormones or drugs to stop hot flushes. In fact, many women do well with non-hormone remedies, Dr. Catellani says. "You may need to do more than one strategy – diet and herbs, for instance. These reme-dies don't work as fast as hormones. But they're generally safe, and some have additional health benefits."

## Black Cohosh: The Right Dose

This herb has a reputation for stopping hot flushes. Research focusing on stan-dardized black cohosh extract has found it performs as well as oestrogen replacement treatment for such menopause symptoms. The dosage for stan-

# CHILL HOT FLUSHES WITH FOODS, NOT PILLS

Foods that contain nitrites (hot dogs and some salamis) or sulphites (some wines and dried fruit) or even red pepper may induce hot flushes. So can alcohol in general.

On the other hand, several studies show that isoflavones – plant oestrogens found in soya and in red clover (used as a tea; look for the dried flowers at health food stores) – can help cool hot flushes. Right now, research using isolated isoflavones (products such as Promensil and Estroven) is limited, but it suggests these products do help you chill out. (They are available online in the UK – www.healthstore.co.uk)

Some researchers, however, contend you get the best health benefits, especially cardiovascular and bone protection, from eating whole foods. Some studies have shown the need for as much as 90 milligrams of isoflavones a day to see an effect on bone loss. (The evidence for their use with hot flushes is less conclusive. But if you try soya foods and feel cooler, stick with them.)

The average Asian consumes soya foods with 30 to 50 milligrams of isoflavones (one to two servings of soya foods) a day, so experts say that's a commonsense level to aim for, until we know more about isoflavones.

Don't take isoflavone supplements if you are taking hormone replacement therapy, tamoxifen (Nolvadex) (used for the prevention and treatment of breast cancer), or raloxifene (Evista) (used for the prevention of osteoporosis) without checking with your doctor first. All of these drugs have effects similar to isoflavones in the body.

You can also snack on flax. Flaxseed contains substances called lignan precursors that your body turns into weak oestrogens. Added to your own dwindling supply, this may help balance your shifting hormones, says Connie Catellani, M.D., director of the Miro Center for Integrative Medicine in Evanston, Illinois. Try 1 tablespoon of ground flaxseed on your cereal or salad. Grind it right before eating.

**FOODS TO ADD**

- Soya milk, soya beans, tofu, soya nuts, soya cereal, soya burgers, soya protein bars
- Soya dessert, ice cream, and drinks
- Ground flaxseed

**FOODS TO SUBTRACT**

- Hot dogs and salamis containing nitrites
- Dried fruit with sulphites
- Alcohol (especially wine)

dardized extract is 40 drops, twice a day. However, because brands vary, follow the label instructions.

Black cohosh apparently works by modulating both oestrogen deficiency and excess, Dr. Catellani says. In Germany, where the herb is used regularly, a German drug regulatory agency considers black cohosh safe for use in women with oestrogen-sensitive cancers as well as in uterine bleeding, liver or gallbladder disease, endometriosis, uterine fibroids and fibrocystic breast disease – all conditions that rule out synthetic hormone replacement. The herb appears to carry no increased risk for cancer. Two Asian species of black cohosh – *Cimicifuga heracleifolia* and *Cimicifuga foetida* – also appear to help strengthen bone.

If you are currently taking HRT and would like to switch to black cohosh, talk to a health care practitioner, Dr. Catellani says. You may need guidance to cut back gradually on the HRT and make sure you're taking enough black cohosh to do the trick. Otherwise, you may have *more* hot flushes, not fewer.

### Try This Vitamin Mix

Vitamin E is often recommended as a remedy for hot flushes, and it might help some over the long run. Doctors usually recommend 400 to 800 IU a day, says Dr. Catellani. In studies using only 50 to 100 IU a day, vitamin E was no more effective than placebos. In a carefully controlled study, women taking 1200 milligrams of vitamin C and 1200 milligrams of a flavonoid, hesperidin (which has a chemical structure similar to oestradiol), had relief from hot flushes.

## Other Personal Cooling Tactics

If you're like most women with hot flushes, you've instinctively learned to turn down the heat and crank up the air conditioning, or seek shade or water when you're outdoors. "Keeping the ambient temperature cool really does help," Dr. Freedman says.

Other helpful strategies:

**Spritz yourself cool.** Fill a 120-millilitre (4-ounce) spritz bottle with water, and add 6 to 8 drops of essential oils, using geranium (*Pelargonium graveolens*) or rose (*Rosa damascena*), suggests Jane Buckle, Ph.D., an instructor in the holistic nursing programme at College of New Rochelle in New York and author of *Clinical Aromatherapy in Nursing*. Carry the bottle with you and simply spray it on your face, neck and shoulders whenever you feel the need to chill. It's wonderfully cooling and beneficial.

**Breathe to destress.** In one study, women who had been having 20 or more hot flushes a day reduced that number by half with the help of deep breathing, Dr. Freedman says. "The technique seems to reduce the arousal of the central nervous system that normally occurs in the initial stages of a hot flush," he says.

Sit up straight and loosen the clothes around your waist so your belly can move freely. Begin by exhaling through your nose longer than you normally would. Then inhale through your nose slowly and deeply, filling your lungs from the bottom up while keeping your belly relaxed. When your chest is fully expanded, exhale slowly and deeply, as if sighing. Continue this pattern of inhaling and exhaling until the hot flush subsides.

**Strip down as needed.** Clothes that trap heat against your body can raise core body temperature, causing hot flushes. So dress accordingly. Turtlenecks are out; plunging necklines are in. Wear layers of moisture-wicking clothes made of cotton or linen that you can peel off or unbutton.

**Hit the road, Jackie.** Walk, run, bike, or swim. Choose whatever type of pulse-accelerating exercise you like, but do some form of moderate-intensity exercise three times a week (or more) for 30 minutes at a stretch. No one understands just how exercise reduces perimenopausal problems, only that it does, says Dr. LaValleur.

**Head 'em off at the pass.** After they've had a couple of hot flushes, most women can sense one starting. Taking measures at the very beginning to cool yourself down, before things really heat up, can make a hot flush less severe, Dr. LaValleur says. Fan yourself, loosen or remove clothes, splash your face and hands with water, or guzzle down a glass of iced water. Also, avoiding alcohol can help prevent hot flushes.

## Maybe the Real Problem Is Your Medication

If you have hot flushes for no obvious reason – or if neither hormone therapy or natural remedies seem to relieve the problem – check your medication. Vasodilating drugs – such as glyceril trinitrate (Suscard, Sustac) for angina, calcium channel blockers (Procardia) for high blood pressure, bromocriptine (Parlodel) for infertility, tamoxifen (Nolvadex) for breast cancer, and buserelin (Suprecur) for endometriosis – cause hot flushes in some women.

Ask your doctor about the drugs you're taking – you may be able to switch to a similar drug less likely to cause flushes.

# Night Sweats

For many women, hot flushes are no big deal. Night sweats are a different story – they're like hot flushes on steroids. Some women wake up drenched and dazed, and have to change their wet nightclothes – maybe the sheets, too – before returning to bed.

"Night sweats are very disruptive to sleep, and can contribute to memory and mood problems some women experience around this time," says June LaValleur, M.D., assistant professor of obstetrics and gynaecology at the University of Minnesota and director of the Mature Women's Center, both in Minneapolis. Sleep deprivation is a well-known form of torture. "When you're not sleeping well, your whole body suffers," she says.

## The Cool, Deep Night

The same hormone-balancing tactics that chill down hot flushes, such as oestrogen supplements or black cohosh, can quell night sweats. In addition, try these "no sweat" tactics.

**Chill out at bedtime.** Keep your bedroom cooler than the rest of the house. One expert recommends setting the thermostat at 20°C (65°F), by either turning down the heat or cranking up the air conditioner. "Simplistic as it may sound, it's solid advice," says Robert Freedman, Ph.D., director of behavioural medicine at Wayne State University, in Detroit. "Anything that raises body temperature even a little bit, such as being in a too hot room, can trigger a hot flush." If you feel *too* chilly at first, use enough blankets to keep

## Aromatherapy for Night Sweats

The fragrant scents of some essential oils may help you relax and sleep. "You can add them to your bathwater, make up a cooling spritzer, or simply put a few drops on a cotton ball that you place on your pillow," says Jane Buckle, Ph.D., an instructor in the holistic nursing programme at College of New Rochelle in New York and author of *Clinical Aromatherapy in Nursing*. Try sweet marjoram, frankincense, or ylang-ylang to help you get back to sleep. One drop of each used together is a magic combination, she suggests. To reduce heat, spritz with rosewater and 1 drop of peppermint, which may improve your hormonal balance.

yourself comfortable – you can always throw off blankets as needed.

**Keep your feet cool.** "There's actually been a study showing that if you keep your feet cool, you have fewer night sweats," Dr. LaValleur says. So kick the covers off your feet, and never wear socks to bed.

**Try a cooling soak.** Before you go to bed, run a comfortably warm bath and soak in it long enough for the water to cool – about 20 minutes. "This may make night sweats less frequent and less severe," says Connie Catellani, M.D., director of the Miro Center for Integrative Medicine in Evanston, Illinois. Hot soaks can make things worse.

**Beware the nightcap.** Alcohol only makes sleeplessness worse. While it may help you drift off sooner, it disrupts normal sleep patterns. It also causes you to flush even when you aren't in a state of hormonal flux. Alcohol can trigger hot flushes. "A nightcap simply isn't the answer to night sweats," Dr. LaValleur says.

# Vaginal Dryness and Irritation

For a woman, nothing dampens the pleasure of sex quite the way pain does. Feel sore enough, often enough, and before long, you might just find yourself making all sorts of excuses to avoid making love.

Lots of things can cause vaginal dryness and irritation – stress, a lack of foreplay, membrane-drying decongestants, antidepressants, even oral contraceptives. Breastfeeding often causes vaginal dryness because prolactin – the hormone that stimulates breast milk production – also suppresses the production of oestrogen, the hormone that keeps the vagina moist, elastic and healthy.

The dryness associated with age-related decreases in oestrogen starts earlier than some women might suspect. Some notice it by their late thirties, well before menopause. Some women may notice it if they enter a new sexual relationship at midlife, says Connie Catellani, M.D., director of the Miro Center for Integrative Medicine in Evanston, Illinois. "They try to have intercourse and realize things are not the way they were when they were younger," she says. "Some women tell me it's more and more difficult to have a regular sex life." More often, however, women suffer in silence. They're reluctant to discuss the problem with their doctors, and their doctors don't ask about it.

Oestrogen maintains the health of the vagina and neighbouring structures in two ways. It promotes pelvic bloodflow, which ensures that nutrients and moisture reach the tissues. And it creates an environment inside the vagina that promotes the growth of friendly bacteria, called lactobacilli, which produce the lactic acid that keeps the vagina slightly acidic and inhibits the growth of E. coli and other faecal bacteria that can cause vaginal and urinary tract infections.

While vaginal dryness can occur in perimenopause, or within a few years after the start of menopause, a woman's vagina shrinks and loses muscle tone. Its normally thick walls become thin and delicate, and can eventually become inflamed, a condition called atrophic vaginitis that's often accompanied by a greyish discharge. Vaginal secretions lessen and become less acidic, setting the stage for infection. Sometimes the urinary tract is also affected, and a woman may need to urinate more frequently, have a sense of urgency, and need to get up and go at night.

Fortunately, none of these changes need be inevitable. Here are the details.

## Hormones to the Rescue

Taken orally or applied topically, oestrogen virtually reverses the process of vaginal atrophy, and a few versions of vaginally applied oestrogen are remarkably safe. So-called local vaginal oestrogen therapy also significantly reduces the prevalence of urinary tract infections in postmenopausal women. (See also page 309.)

Here are your options.

**Try oestriol cream.** Your body makes three kinds of oestrogen – oestradiol, oestrone and oestriol. Oestriol is the type that specifically targets the mucous membranes of your vagina, keeping it moist and supple, and some alternative doctors also think it is protective against cancer. Some alternative doctors treat vaginal dryness by prescribing a cream that contains oestriol, Dr. Catellani says. The cream needs to be made up by a chemist, in any strength your doctor prescribes. (The usual dosage is a 0.05 or 0.06 per cent concentration of oestriol in a cream base.) "If the only symptom a woman is concerned about is vaginal dryness, or if hot flushes are managed by soya or black cohosh, then she can use this cream," Dr. Catellani says. "Once the vagina has recovered some of its resiliency and pliability from using the cream once or twice a day for a week or two, then she can use a maintenance dose of two or three times a week."

There's no need to insert the cream vaginally, so it's not messy. "It's so concentrated, just rubbing about ¼ teaspoon on the outside affects the entire vagina," Dr. Catellani says. And unlike with oral hormone therapy or other vaginal hormone creams, you don't need to use progesterone along with this treatment, to counter oestrogen's growth-promoting effects on the uterine lining. Oestriol does not promote endometrial overgrowth.

**Ask your doctor about Estring.** If vaginal dryness is your sole complaint, the prescription Estradiol vaginal ring, or Estring, is likely to be a choice among traditional doctors. Introduced a few years ago, Estring is a soft, flexible silicone ring, about 5 cm (2 inches) in diameter, inserted into the vagina, that slowly releases oestradiol for a period of 90 days. It's then removed and replaced. (You can do that yourself. You can also remove it during sex if you want.)

Blood levels of oestrogen are slightly elevated for 3 days after initial insertion, then return to postmenopausal levels. "Estring provides the least systemic exposure to oestrogen of any hormone treatment available for vaginal dryness," says June LaValleur, M.D., assistant professor of obstetrics and gynaecology at the University of Minnesota and director of the Mature Women's Center, both in Minneapolis. "We even use it in some of our breast cancer patients (with their oncologists' consent) and women who've had Stage I endometrial cancer. It's so effective, some women say it's worth its weight in diamonds. It restored their ability to have intercourse again."

With Estring, so little oestradiol is absorbed that you don't need to take progesterone to counter oestrogen's growth-promoting effects on the uterine lining. "Vaginal oestrogen creams, such as Premarin (Prempak), on the other hand, are highly absorbed and can lead to abnormal bleeding and endometrial overgrowth," Dr. LaValleur says. If you use a vaginal cream other than oestriol cream, you will have to also take progesterone.

## Non-hormonal Help

If you prefer not to take hormones – or can't for medical reasons – other simple strategies may help relieve your symptoms.

**Try a vaginal moisturizer.** This is a product you use any time, usually several times a week, to restore vaginal moisture. (You can also use it during sex if you want to.) They include Replens, K-Y Long-Lasting Vaginal Moisturiser Gel, Moist Again Vaginal Moisturising Gel, and Vagisil Intimate Moisturiser Lotion. These products contain ingredients that help retain moisture for long periods of time. However, they don't help counter vaginal thinning and atrophy the way oestrogen does, says Dr. Catellani.

**Use vitamin E oil.** This can reduce the dryness, irritation and burning of atrophic vaginitis, Dr. Catellani says. Simply pop open a capsule, squeeze the oil on your finger, and rub it in where it's needed. Do this twice a day, or whenever you need relief. Alternatively, you can get beeswax cream with vitamin E.

**Always use a lubricant when you have sex.** Even if you use a vaginal moisturizer or vitamin E oil, you may still require lubrication during sex. Use an unscented, colourless, water-based lubricant such as K-Y jelly. "K-Y jelly is very acceptable, has a natural feel to it, and is easily available," Dr. Catellani says. Apply the lubricant at the vaginal opening and to the penis.

Never use petroleum jelly or other petroleum-based products as a sexual lubricant. Same goes for cocoa butter, ordinary butter, or baby oil. These types of lubricants remain in the vagina and harbour yeast and other infection-producing microbes. They can do the same in the urethra, the urinary tract opening.

**If you're using condoms, opt for lubricated.** They cut down on friction and irritation. If you add more lubricant, make sure it's water-based. Oil-based lubricants weaken latex and increase the chance that a condom will break.

**Try the same herbs used for other menopausal symptoms.** Both black cohosh and chasteberry (vitex) can help eliminate vaginal dryness, along with hot flushes, irregular bleeding, and other symptoms of the menopause, Dr. Catellani says. But it may take months before the herb's effects are realized, so in the meantime you may want to use oestriol cream or some of the other strategies.

For black cohosh, a common dosage is 40 drops of standardized tincture twice daily, added to water or juice. However, because strengths vary, follow the instructions printed on the bottle label. Black cohosh is most effective when used as a liquid extract, tablet, or capsule, rather than as a tea, says Dr. Catellani.

As for chasteberry, clinical trials have shown it lowers levels of prolactin,

---

## Don't Confuse Irritation with Infection

A low-grade yeast infection can cause irritation during intercourse, but it will usually also cause some itching and a whitish discharge. If you've been diagnosed with yeast infections before and know what to look for, an over-the-counter antiyeast cream or suppositories can usually knock the infection out in 2 or 3 days. Use as directed. If your symptoms persist, see a doctor. You may have some other kind of infection.

the "nursing" hormone, which causes vaginal dryness. Chasteberry can be taken as a tincture, capsule, tablet, or tea. In clinical trials, the dosage used was 40 drops of standardized extract, taken once a day. For capsules or tablets, take one 650-milligram capsule up to three times a day; for tincture, 40 drops added to liquid up to three times a day. For tea, drink one cup two to three times a day, adds Dr. Catellani.

**Refrain from douching.** Commercial douches contain astringent ingredients that dry out vaginal tissues. "If you already have vaginal dryness, a douche is likely to make your problem even worse," says Leslie Shimp, Pharm.D., associate professor of pharmacy at the University of Michigan in Ann Arbor. "I don't ever recommend them."

**Slow down and savour the moments.** It takes time to get ready physically to have sex, and the older you are, the longer it can take, says Barbara Bartlik, M.D., clinical assistant professor of psychiatry in the department of psychiatry at Weill Medical College of Cornell University in New York City. "Remember those long, romantic Sunday afternoons or evenings you had when you were young, maybe before you even started to have sex? When you spent hours just petting? Try doing that again," she suggests. Just enjoy yourself, with no goal in mind. (For more on sex and hormones, see chapter 8.)

# Urinary Tract Infections

t's amazing how long some women will put up with urinary tract infections (UTIs) before getting help.

Take Lorene Williams. At 88, she's had UTIs since she was in her thirties – sometimes as often as every other week. Her discomfort and urinary frequency got to the point where it was interfering with her sleep. Finally, she got fed up, dumped her doctor, changed her lifestyle, and started oestrogen replacement therapy.

The results are stunning. Williams no longer endures the predictable and painful symptoms of chronic lower urinary tract infections (also known as cystitis).

Almost half of all women will contract a urinary tract infection in their lifetime. And many of those women – between 10 to 15 per cent – experience chronic problems after they turn 60.

But experts say too many women, especially those who are postmenopausal, are like Williams. They stoically endure pain merely because they're not seeking or getting the medical care they need. And yet most UTIs can be eliminated or reduced through some simple behavioural and medical changes.

"While urinary tract infections are very pervasive, they're also very avoidable," said Wulf H. Utian, M.D., executive director of the North American Menopause Society in Cleveland. "There's no reason for women to suffer."

## A Cascade of Causes

The usual cause of cystitis is the growth of bacteria in the bladder. The bacteria then produce chemicals and toxins that make the bladder lining swollen and inflamed, causing pain and burning.

The most common scenario for cystitis is when bacteria from the bowel spread from the anus and perineum into the urethra. There, the bacteria gain entry into the bladder and then proliferate.

At first, a woman will feel a need to urinate frequently, sometimes as often as every 5 to 15 minutes. She may also feel pain in her lower abdomen.

When women are younger, they often experience urinary tract infections as a result of overindulgence: frequent sex (prompting the name honeymoon cystitis), overconsumption of alcohol, or a steady diet of rich food. But when women are menopausal, they must also contend with physical changes that make it easier for the bacteria to spread. For example, the drop in oestrogen levels during menopause can cause significant changes in a woman's pelvic health. The hormone is responsible for keeping bladder, urethra and vaginal walls supple as well as keeping vaginal pH levels acidic, all useful in preventing urinary tract infections. Without oestrogen's influence, the walls can grow thinner and the urogenital area can have a higher (less acidic) pH, which allows "bad" bacteria to flourish.

At the same time, the pelvic floor is weakening, often the result of childbirth, a lack of exercise, and obesity. When that happens, the uterus, bladder and rectum drop, closing the distance between the source of bacteria and the bladder.

Other problems related to ageing also contribute to UTIs. For example, as women get older, they may experience both urinary incontinence and constipation, which can lead to a frequent urge to urinate and staining of underwear or adult pads, thus providing a breeding ground for bacteria. (Chronic constipation can result in a compressed bladder and a frequent urge to urinate.) These ailments often coexist.

At the same time, a woman may find she can no longer relax as she urinates

– instead, she finds she has to force things along. "This just pushes the urethra wider – allowing bacteria a better opportunity to enter the bladder," says Niall T. M. Galloway, M.D., medical director of the Emory Continence Center and associate professor of urology at the Emory School of Medicine in Atlanta.

In women with diabetes, the excess glucose in their urine is an ideal meal for bacteria. Cutting out sugar and getting more exercise such as swimming and walking can help, says Dr. Galloway.

## Don't Assume It's a UTI

If you have pain on urination, frequent urge to urinate, lower-back pain, or other symptoms and think you may have a UTI, see your doctor immediately to confirm the diagnosis.

"Any time they get a lower-back pain or a frequent need to void urine, women think they have an infection," said Jay M. Kulkin, M.D., an obstetrician gynaecologist in private practice in Atlanta and a member of the American Association of Health Plans' Women's Task Force. "But the simple fact is, the cause may be related to something else."

"A woman can have an irritable colon, which may mimic a UTI," says Dr. Utian. So you can't assume an infection is to blame.

In Lorene Williams's case, for example, many of her alleged episodes of cystitis turned out to be tied to constipation, not infection. Her previous doctor had not considered bowel problems but had simply kept Williams on a constant regime of antibiotics, which can cause diarrhoea and an overgrowth of yeast.

Her new physician – Dr. Galloway – discontinued the antibiotics and instead recommended she take natural laxatives, such as two capsules of fish oil after her evening meal, to loosen her stools. (Two capsules of flaxseed oil are also effective.) He also put her on a mild over-the-counter laxative and recommended she increase her intake of water. That greatly helped her symptoms, allowing her to sleep through the night.

As a result, she felt much better.

Dr. Galloway also prescribed Williams a topical cream, Vagifem vaginal cream, containing oestradiol (a form of oestrogen) to help protect her urethra from infection, as well as Macrobid, an antimicrobial, or much milder version of an antibiotic. By using Macrobid on an as-needed basis, Williams has been able to stop any UTI before it becomes painful.

Urinary tract infections always have the potential to become serious, spreading to the kidneys and possibly requiring hospitalization.

"So treat a UTI like you would treat a fire in your home," says Dr. Galloway. "Don't let it get out of control before you start doing something."

---

*Escape from* **HORMONE HELL**

## SHE LINKS UTIs TO A HYSTERECTOMY

**Q:** I'm 52 years old and I'm in great shape. I play tennis three times a week and eat responsibly. But ever since I had a hysterectomy, I've had three serious urinary tract infections. Doctors tell me the infection might have been originally linked to the catheter during surgery. Each time, I've been treated with antibiotics – first Septrin, then Ciproxin. Neither one worked. I'm now being treated for the fourth time. But I want to prevent these from happening again. What can I do?

Niall T. M. Galloway, M.D., medical director of the Emory Continence Center and associate professor of urology at the Emory School of Medicine in Atlanta, replies: First, remove from your diet anything that might be on the dangerous list of "bladder irritants" – things like alcohol, anything with caffeine, fruit sugars and artificial sugars, spicy foods, and milk products.

Then you create a bowel-management programme. Start by taking 60 ml (2 fl oz) of milk of magnesia, to clean your colon. Then take one scoop of a soluble fibre agent, like Fibogel, Isogel or Regulan, with water every day.

Next, start to acidify your urine by taking 500 milligrams of vitamin C three times a day, for a total of 1500 milligrams. Void urine every 2 hours, whether you need to or not, during your waking hours.

In addition to tennis, add half an hour of steady exercise, such as aerobics or dance exercise, to your daily regime, to help keep your bowels moving regularly. Bowels function best on a consistent schedule.

Last, talk to your physician about a standing prescription for a mild antimicrobial, such as Macrobid. The standard routine is to take it for 3 days if you get a hint of any symptoms that have not responded to these strategies.

If you're feeling better, with no signs of infection, start to slowly add back foods you cut out. That way, you will be able to determine what your body can tolerate and enjoy life without the pain of a urinary tract infection.

## Take Action ASAP

If you do indeed have a UTI and not something else, Dr. Galloway and others recommends taking these simple steps to stop the infection in its tracks.

- *Immediately cut out all sugar and fruit juices, as well as any liquids other than water.*
- *Increase your intake of vitamin C up to 500 milligrams, two to three times a day, to start acidifying your urine.*
- *Drink unsweetened cranberry juice. (Sweetened juice is probably not going to have much effect.) If you find the taste overwhelming, you can dilute the juice with water. But be sure to drink only one 240 ml (8-fl oz) glass per day, as even unsweetened juice still contains sugar, says Joy Hewitt, R.N., a certified continence nurse at the Emory Continence Center in Atlanta.*
- *Try to urinate every 2 hours, whether you feel like it or not – taking care not to force it, however.*
- *Walk regularly, to help prevent constipation, she adds.*
- *Do not use deodorant or perfumed soaps on anything that may come in contact with the genital area – it may irritate the genital tissue, says Hewitt.*

## Prevent UTIs

To keep trouble from starting, Hewitt offers the following tips:

- *Drink at least six to eight glasses of water a day, and a couple of glasses after sex.*
- *Urinate before and after having intercourse.*
- *Wipe gently from front to back after urinating or having a bowel movement.*
- *Don't use coloured toilet paper, bubble bath, perfumed soaps, or deodorant tampons or sanitary pads.*
- *Take showers, not baths. If you must sit in the tub, limit yourself to no more than 10 minutes.*
- *After showering or bathing, use a hair dryer set on cool to dry the skin in the urogenital area.*
- *If you wear incontinence protection, change pads at least twice a day.*

## Hormones Are Not Always the Answer

An occasional case of cystitis doesn't necessarily call for oestrogen hormone replacement. But several studies indicate that the application of oestrogen

– especially in the form of a vaginal ring, Estring – is helpful in reducing uro-genital problems. A vaginal ring is a soft, flexible silicone ring, about 5 cm (2 inches) in diameter, inserted into the vagina, that slowly releases oestradiol for a period of 90 days. It's then removed and replaced.

"I only recommend it when there is clear indication that it might help, such as in recurrent or persistent chronic UTIs," says Dr. Utian. "But if the

---

THE HORMONE ZONE

# A BLADDER-FRIENDLY DIET

Doctors say that women prone to chronic urinary tract infections may be able to head off future episodes if they cut down on foods that act as "bladder irritants."

You don't necessarily have to give up all these foods. Simply keep a food diary and try eliminating them one at a time to see whether avoiding certain ones leads to fewer infections.

Pay attention to your choice of juice: While juices are acidic, many contain fructose – and other sugars, if they're sweetened – which provides UTIs a gourmet meal of nutrients.

### FOODS TO ADD
- Warm broth
- Light herb teas instead of coffee
- White chocolate instead of normal chocolate
- Water (six to eight glasses a day)
- Unsweetened cranberry juice
- Cranberries and blueberries
- Bran

- Wholemeal breads
- Oats
- Vegetables in their skins
- Popcorn

### FOODS TO SUBTRACT
- Alcohol in any form (spirits, wine, wine spritzers, beer)
- Caffeine (coffee, tea, including "decaffeinated" versions, caffeinated fizzy drinks)
- Dark chocolate
- Very acidic fruit or fruit juices (oranges, grapefruit, lemon, lime, mango and pineapple)
- Spicy foods (Mexican, Thai, or Cajun cuisine)
- Milk products (milk, cheese, cottage cheese, yoghurt, ice cream)
- Sugar (corn sweeteners, honey, fructose, sucrose, lactose in packaged foods)
- Artificial sweeteners (saccharine, aspartame)

woman seems to be fine most of the time without it, we try to make other adjustments first. And I always leave the final decision to the woman."

# Wrinkles

Wrinkles are like a scrapbook of our lives, visible reminders of late nights with little sleep, and summers at the seaside. Perhaps your furrows bear a family resemblance to your mother, aunts, or grandmothers.

While some degree of wrinkling is inevitable as you age, others are avoidable. Environmental factors – especially sun exposure, cigarette smoke and pollution – account for 98 per cent of wrinkles, says Richard Glogau, M.D., clinical professor of dermatology at the University of California, San Francisco. Women who smoke tend to enter menopause earlier, depriving skin of oestrogen sooner than nonsmokers – but smoking also ages skin prematurely, directly causing wrinkles.

Other, less preventable contributors include:

**Smiling or frowning.** Over time, the muscles we move when displaying emotions create visible creases in the skin surface.

**Sleep patterns.** Sleeping with your face against the pillow in the same way every night can create surface lines.

**Gravity.** It pulls on the skin and muscles as we stand or sit upright.

**Intrinsic ageing.** Simply put, the skin wears out.

## Oestrogen and Testosterone: Anti-Wrinkling Hormones

Just about every organ in your body contains oestrogen receptors. Oestrogen receptors, in fact, have been found throughout the various layers of our skin, and even in the blood vessels that feed the skin, helping to maintain skin tone and structure.

"After menopause, skin holds less water, so it's drier," says Dr. Glogau. "Also, the dermis – the skin's bulky, collagen-rich underlayer – shrinks. And elastin – fibres that give the skin youthful elasticity – subtly changes." As a result, skin becomes thinner, less elastic, and less efficient in retaining the moisture that makes skin feel young and supple.

Intriguingly, oestrogen-related effects on ageing skin occur at the same time as changes seen in the bones. Just as one-third to one-half of bone loss is blamed on oestrogen deficiency at menopause, skin loses about 30 per cent of its collagen, the fibrous protein that helps to form the scaffolding for the skin, in the first 5 years after menopause. After that, the decline in collagen levels slows to about 2 per cent a year.

Staying out of the sun, and not smoking, can go a long way to minimize wrinkling due to non-hormonal influences. But even if you lived your life shaded by hats and parasols, your face would begin to show some crinkling and wrinkling after menopause. Years of smiles and frowns create hyperactive muscles, leaving furrows between your brows and crow's-feet at the corners of your eyes. And by midlife, you lose much of the underlying fat that gives the face a healthy, rounded look associated with youth.

Women's relatively low levels of testosterone also contribute to wrinkles, says Jean Carruthers, M.D., clinical professor of ophthalmology at the University of British Columbia in Vancouver, and an aesthetic ophthalmologic surgeon. "Men's beard hair is stronger and denser, helping to support their skin and stop the wrinkling," she says. "That's why women and men age similarly right around the eyes, but men don't get wrinkles around the mouth that bother women so much."

## A Welcome Benefit from HRT

Oral oestrogen therapy has been proven to plump up skin thinned from a lack of oestrogen. It has the potential to build collagen fibres within the dermis and even prevent collagen loss. This is significant because collagen is responsible for the bulk of skin thickness: the down of the duvet, if you will. Preliminary research has also found that women who take oestrogen are better able to retain moisture in the stratum corneum, the uppermost layer of the epidermis.

Preventing wrinkles shouldn't be your overriding reason to take hormone replacement therapy (HRT). But if you and your doctor decide that oestrogen replacement would help to manage symptoms of menopause, you may find that HRT provides pleasant side benefits for your skin.

## Coverups, Creams and Peels:
## The Non-hormonal Route

No matter what else you do, your first step in wrinkle prevention should be wearing a daily sunscreen cream or moisturizer with both UVA and UVB protection. If you don't do this already, start now.

"If you do nothing else to control wrinkles but use sunscreen, your skin will look better in a year," vows Dr. Glogau. And of course, if you smoke, it makes sense to quit. Otherwise, any attempt to control wrinkling is a waste of time and money.

You can always do what women have always done for wrinkles: cover them with makeup. Do it right, though, or you'll end up making wrinkles more noticeable, not less. To soften facial lines, apply moisturizer first, then use a base foundation with white undertones and a pearled base so it will sit on top of wrinkles. A light, reflective powder will also minimize wrinkles. For lips, start with foundation or a lip-setting cream to hold your lipstick where it belongs, not sneaking up or down the vertical lines that surround your mouth. You can also use a lip pencil, to draw a boundary beyond which you don't want lipstick to go.

Other efforts to counteract the effect on your skin of declining oestrogen, the environment and ageing will depend on how extensive your wrinkles are, how much time you have, and how much you want to spend. Some are available over the counter, some by prescription. Whatever you decide to try, follow label instructions precisely and give your skin at least 4 months to see results.

**Vitamin C creams.** There is no question that the antioxidants naturally found in fruits and vegetables – including vitamin C, glutathione, and vitamin E – help to prevent wrinkles. When consumed as food, they neutralize free radicals that are generated by metabolism – or in skin – by harmful rays of the sun. The problem is that cosmetic scientists have had a tough time duplicating the tricky chemistry involved in converting these antioxidants into useful agents when applied to the skin surface.

Vitamin C, for example, is a profoundly unstable molecule. In order to be effective in the skin, it must be formulated to a pH of 3.5 or lower or it won't penetrate the skin, says Sheldon Pinnell, M.D., professor of dermatology at Duke University in Durham, North Carolina. The vast majority of products on the market do not meet this requirement. Moreover, vitamin C makes products discolour over time. Manufacturers have tried to overcome the problem by using substances derived from vitamin C, but these derivatives don't work in the skin like vitamin C.

The exception may be ascorbyl palmitate, according to Nicholas Perricone, M.D., assistant clinical professor of dermatology at Yale University School of Medicine and author of *The Wrinkle Cure*. A vitamin C derivative with a neutral pH, ascorbyl palmitate neutralizes free radicals, stimulates collagen and minimizes fine lines without triggering inflammation, as seen with l-ascorbic acid, he asserts. Vitamin C creams are available without a prescription through dermatologists, pharmacies and salons.

**Vitamin E.** A product label may list vitamin E among its ingredients, but if the source is tocopherol acetate or tocopherol succinate, your skin won't ben-

---

*Escape from* **HORMONE HELL**

# WRINKLES ARE RUINING HER PEACE OF MIND

**Q:** I'm worried about my best friend from college. We're both entering menopause, plucking grey hairs and suffering a few hot flushes. But while I'm fairly content with growing older, even welcoming the crinkles I call my "wise lines," she is becoming obsessed about her appearance. Even though she's as beautiful as ever, she seems to dwell on every new wrinkle. She's thinking about laser surgery or a face-lift. She can afford them, but I wonder if that's her only option. Most of all, I'm concerned that her problem is more than skin-deep.

Cori Baill, M.D., director of the Menopause Center in Orlando, replies: some women think of their wrinkles as signs of maturity and character, that they're hard-won and worth having. Others really feel that wrinkles prevent them from looking their best. What I would want to know about your friend is how she is feeling in general. Is she sleeping well? Taking care of herself? Or is she suffering mood swings, irritability, and a feeling of desperation that may be driving her concern about her appearance? In the latter case, I would want to explore whether a lack of oestrogen is causing both her wrinkles and her anxiety. If hormone replacement therapy is not an option, there may be other alternatives that would help.

Once the medical issues were resolved, I would counsel your friend to be her own person, not to be manipulated by the ads that try to sell the 1.8 million American women a year who enter menopause on the notion that youth alone equals femininity.

If your friend is doing what she can to prevent premature wrinkles – drinking lots of water, not smoking, wearing sunblock outdoors – but still thinks she would look more vibrant minus a few lines, there's nothing wrong with trying something more ambitious. I'd advise her to start with the less expensive options – a few chemical peels at the dermatologist. That may be all she needs.

efit. Both forms are converted to vitamin E when consumed from food sources, but not if you put them on your skin, says Dr. Pinnell. Researchers at Duke University have been developing technology to combine active vitamins C and E to work synergistically to protect and rejuvenate skin cells. This product is available online as Primacy C + E from SkinCeuticals.

**Coenzyme $Q_{10}$.** A powerful antioxidant found in all cells and newcomer on the skin scene, coenzyme $Q_{10}$, found over the counter in pharmacies, has only recently been used as a topical solution for ageing skin. A number of dermatologists believe it has potential for reducing sun damage and thereby minimizing wrinkles.

**Alpha lipoic acid.** Dr. Perricone has conducted extensive research on this lesser-known antioxidant. Alpha lipoic acid is water soluble, like vitamin C, and fat soluble, like vitamin E; it also aids in energy production in the cell. So he thinks it has a unique ability to protect both the cell membrane and the cell's interior. According to Dr. Perricone, alpha lipoic acid alone reduces facial lines and improves the appearance of scars. He uses it in combination with DMAE, 2-dimethylaminoethanol, to reduce inflammation and mediate free radical damage. You can find products containing alpha lipoic acid and DMAE where over-the-counter health and beauty products are sold.

**Hydroxy acid products.** Ever since Cleopatra, women have used potions derived from fruit acids, sour milk and other natural products to rejuvenate their skin. Modern women can buy creams, lotions and gels containing alpha hydroxy acids or beta hydroxy acids. These products work by breaking apart the glue that holds rough, dry cells on the surface of the skin.

Over-the-counter hydroxy acid products are generally too weak to produce a lasting effect on wrinkles, says Patrick H. Bitter Jr., M.D., a dermatologic surgeon and researcher in Campbell, California. Women who use them may notice their skin feels smoother and looks rosier, but wrinkles are likely to show no more improvement than they would with a mild prescription-strength glycolic or alpha hydroxy acid peel (discussed below).

**Tretinoin (Retin-A acid).** Known as retinoids, vitamin A acids have been subjected to intense scientific scrutiny. Sold by prescription as Retin-A, Acticin and (with an antibacterial) Aknemycin Plus, Retin-A products have been proven to diminish fine lines and even reduce the appearance of larger wrinkles (although it will not make them disappear). Retin-A products are, in fact, the only agents proven to repair sun-damaged skin under the surface at a molecular level as well as in the skin's layers, where they bulk up the dermis and thicken the epidermis. They may even prevent further wrinkling, perhaps by blocking enzymes that can break down collagen and elastin.

Be forewarned: Retin-A may be irritating to the skin as well as drying, especially at first, so be patient. The changes induced by tretinoin occur slowly, perhaps not fully appreciated for months.

**Retinol.** Many over-the-counter wrinkle creams list retinol, a form of vitamin A, among the ingredients. But the retinol concentration in these products is highly variable and unregulated. If you don't see impressive results in 4 to 6 months, you may be paying a premium price for a product that is really no more than a moisturizer.

## Advanced Wrinkle Control

If you've got money to spare and your wrinkles really bother you, a qualified dermatologist can undo some of the wrinkling that graces us all at midlife, especially if HRT isn't an option.

### THE HORMONE CONNECTION
# DOES STRESS REALLY CAUSE WRINKLES?

Chronic stress – and the hormones released in response to it – takes its toll on the immune system. But does chronic stress show on your face? Does workplace stress, financial strain, or family strife contribute to wrinkles?

The connection between stress and wrinkles is not clearly understood, says Patrick Bitter Jr., M.D., a dermatologic surgeon and researcher in Campbell, California. "Stress overwhelms the skin and the body's ability to protect against free radical damage, producing cellular damage and death and accelerating the ageing process," he says. But the precise effect on the skin of stress hormones like cortisol and epinephrine is uncertain.

Stress definitely produces muscle tension, which clearly contributes to frown lines between the eyes, forehead lines, and wrinkles around the mouth.

Finally, stressed people also tend to take shortcuts on their general health: they are more prone to sleeping poorly, eating fast food on the run, and robbing themselves of relaxation time. They tend to develop dark circles under their eyes and lose the robust appearance of healthy skin, and these accentuate the appearance of wrinkles in the face, says Dr. Bitter.

So relax – you'll look younger.

**Chemical peels.** Performed in a beauty clinic, chemical peels remain one of the most popular ways to eradicate fine wrinkle lines, says Dr. Glogau. Glycolic acid or trichloroacetic acid is used in combination with other chemicals to loosen the outer layers of your skin. The initial sensation is one of tingling and stinging, and over time the skin will peel away in sunburn layers, like when you get sunburn. You'll use skin creams to help heal and moisturize your skin until new, firm skin appears. Chemical peels aren't pretty, and it takes a couple of weeks before you're presentable again. But if you're determined to turn back the clock, they're a time-honoured choice for many.

**Botox injections.** Without question, the most revolutionary advance in cosmetic dermatology in the past several years has come from a highly unlikely source: botulinum toxin, a deadly natural poison. Used in minuscule concentrations, botulinum toxin type A (found in the product Botox) can temporarily freeze the muscles responsible for deep furrows between the eyes, crow's-feet at the edges of the eyes, and forehead lines.

Even the most conservative physicians are impressed by the results and the unblemished safety record botulinum injections have achieved over the past 5 years. To date, the only side effects reported for Botox are associated with the injection of too much. An eyelid might droop temporarily, for example.

Many physicians recommend that patients apply ice prior to the injections, to numb the area, but no other anaesthetic is required. You may not see the full effect of a botulinum injection for several days, and it will last for about 4 months to a year.

**Tissue augmentation (wrinkle fillers).** Dermatologic surgeons call them marionette lines or Howdy Doody lines – creases that extend from the corners of your nose to the corners of your mouth and then may continue downwards toward your chin. No amount of cream or lotion will help. Nor will Botox. Filling the crease with fat or collagen may be the best way to fill these lines and smaller, troublesome creases surrounding the lips or even the eyes.

Designed to sit under the skin's surface, sometimes within the dermal layer, this fills up the crevasses we see as wrinkles, says Melvin Elson, M.D., a dermatologist and researcher in Nashville. Some dermatologists and plastic surgeons harvest fat from your thighs or buttocks, perhaps during liposuction, and inject it into areas of your face that could do with some plumping up. Such fat transfers aren't permanent, but they can be repeated.

If you're allergic to beef products, you may have to move out of the line for bovine collagen. Physicians perform skin tests on any patient considering collagen injections just to ensure against allergic reactions, delaying the procedure for several weeks. The good news is that injectable bovine products are quite safe – they've been used in more than 2 million people – and may be mixed with an anaesthetic so that the procedures are virtually painless, according to Dr. Elson. However, the newer injectable fillers, derived from human tissue, do not have anaesthetic mixed with them, but there are procedures that can be done to minimize discomfort, he adds.

None of the injectable fillers are permanent, so anticipate getting touchups every 4 to 6 months unless you want to undergo surgery to implant a permanent tissue filler shaped to augment thin lips or slide into that Howdy Doody crease. Done properly, implantation with permanent fillers – made from Gore-Tex and other materials – can achieve nice results, but there are risks. Some may generate inflammatory reactions, for example, and their removal can be traumatic as well as disfiguring.

## High-Tech Skin Resurfacing

Nowhere is the power of harnessed light energy more alluring than in the beauty world. To be sure, the procedure called laser resurfacing, or laser rejuvenation, has a powerful potential to remodel the skin, both at the surface and deep within the dermal collagen. But laser resurfacing, which amounts to burning the skin, can be painful and expensive.

"What it boils down to is, there's no free lunch," says Dr. Glogau. "You can get significant changes with the deeper injury associated with the carbon dioxide ($CO_2$) laser, but you have to be willing to assume more risk."

The $CO_2$ laser penetrates deep into the skin layers, destroying the epidermis in the process. Healing takes weeks as the skin regrows, and side effects such as redness may last for months or even a year. One upsetting complication involves a whitening of the skin, called hypopigmentation, which may be permanent. Still, the results are amazing, making even deep wrinkles around the mouth, eyes and cheeks disappear. New collagen tightens the skin as well, not so much as a face-lift but often enough to make one unnecessary.

Because women have been wary of what is involved in $CO_2$ laser surgery, the search has begun for less radical options. From this quest came the Erbium:YAG (Er:YAG) laser, a beam that works at a different wavelength, produces less damage, and speeds healing. Although the jury is still out on results, some physicians and their patients feel the Er:YAG produces enough smoothing of their wrinkles to make them happy, with fewer risks. Recent research, reports Dr. Glogau, has suggested that using the two lasers together may achieve better results than the Er:YAG but with an easier recovery than is possible with $CO_2$ laser resurfacing.

Another exciting advance involves various methods of cooling the skin prior to each blast of the laser beam. The aim is to protect the epidermis while allowing the force of the beam to reach below the skin's surface, creating collagen improvement without destroying the epidermis.

Finally, researchers are looking across the spectrum of light to find even less invasive methods of treating wrinkles. Dr. Bitter, for example, uses intense pulsed light during sequential treatments to smooth fine wrinkles. "Greater degrees of wrinkles and loose skin at the present will still benefit most from surgery (either laser surgery or plastic surgery)," says Dr. Bitter. "But in the future? I believe that we will have very effective nonsurgical and nonlaser options."

## Do You Need a Lift?

Wrinkles caused by sun exposure can often be minimized by topical solutions, fillers, or laser surgery and related procedures. Wrinkles caused by expression lines in the upper face can be smoothed with Botox injections. But none of these options will fix gravity's strong pull on the muscles and skin of the face, which results in droopy eyelids, bags under the eyes, saggy cheeks and flabby jowls.

These problems are still best corrected by plastic surgery, which often can be done endoscopically today. Necessitating only tiny, hidden incisions, insertion of the eye of the endoscope allows the surgeon the same clear view as seen with a long incision. Plastic surgery tightens and removes excess skin from above or below the eyes or from the whole face. It's probably the most expensive wrinkle treatment available, but it produces the most dramatic results for very deep lines.

# Acne

Just the word "acne" conjures up memories of school reports, sleepovers, and other hallmarks of teenage life we expected to leave behind in adolescence.

Not always.

"Acne is not just a high school-age problem," says Kathy Fields, M.D., a clinical instructor of dermatology at the University of California, San

Francisco. In some, acne flares around the age of 34 and can continue erupting into a woman's sixties, when she expect wrinkles, not zits, to be her top skin concern.

The reason is hormones. While acne can be a result of pore-clogging makeup or even genetics, often the key triggers – just like when we were teenagers – are hormones. "All acne is hormonally driven," Dr. Fields says.

## Hormonal Surges at Fault

The acne grownup women get differs in important ways from teenage skin trauma. As adults, we tend to break out more on the chin, lower cheeks and jawline, rather than the oily "T-zone" of the nose and forehead. The pimples themselves may be deeper and feel harder to the touch than adolescent zits. Finally, adult acne often comes and goes with menstrual cycles.

At the most basic level, these breakouts stem from the oil, or sebum, released by the sebaceous glands, which are found on the face, upper back and chest. We all produce sebum. ("Our faces would be incredibly dry without it," says Elizabeth Vierra, M.D., a dermatologist in Poway, California.) But too much sebum can cause problems. The pores get clogged with dead skin cells and extra oil, and bacteria begin to grow. Alarmed, your body rushes to fight off this tiny infection with white blood cells, and all of sudden, you've got a pimple that's red, swollen and sensitive to the touch.

But adult acne is often more than skin-deep, says Diane Berson, M.D., a dermatologist in New York City. These breakouts can be a symptom of hormones gone awry, thanks to your menstrual cycle, stress, or even medical problems.

Regardless of the source, though, the problem is generally too much of an influx of testosterone for us to handle. This androgen, or so-called male hormone, circulates through the body, combining with an enzyme known as 5-alpha reductase. This creates an even more powerful androgen known as dihydrotestosterone, or DHT. It's got a complicated name but a very simple impact on acne: DHT is the hormone that tells our sebaceous glands to make more oil, leading to the breakouts we hate.

Where is this extra testosterone coming from? It varies. In some women, acne may indicate polycystic ovary syndrome (PCOS), a condition in which growths on the ovaries produce the excess testosterone. (See chapter 9.)

In others, it comes from the adrenal glands, which sit on top of the liver. They may be releasing too much of a hormone called dehydroepiandrosterone sulphate (DHEAS). In the body, this androgen soon turns into testosterone, then the oil-causing DHT, and, finally, acne. But if the extra testosterone is coming from the adrenal glands, it's due to something more serious than a skin problem: adult-onset congenital adrenal hyperplasia, a blockage in the production of cortisol from the adrenals, leading instead to excess production of androgens, which requires a doctor's care.

Women with diabetes may also struggle with acne. Insulin resistance leads to lower-than-normal levels of a chemical (sex hormone-binding globulin) that binds with testosterone. As a result, women with diabetes may have more testosterone floating around in their bodies – and more pimples on their skin.

But remember that not all hormonally related acne springs from serious health problems.

You may simply be extra-sensitive to androgens at the skin level. That means that when free testosterone appears near your sebaceous glands, your overeager hormone receptors snatch it up and quickly convert it to DHT.

The blame could also lie with 5-alpha reductase, the enzyme that helps testosterone turn into DHT. Researchers suspect this enzyme is either more active or more abundant in women with acne.

Finally, you might just be too stressed-out. If you're balancing work, family, home and the care of elderly parents, your skin may show it, Dr. Berson says. When you're under pressure, your body responds by releasing stress hormones that prepare you for "fight or flight". The problem is, those adrenal glands don't just release a stress hormone, such as adrenaline – they also release its acne-inducing buddy, testosterone. In terms of the skin breakouts that result, "the stress reaction is similar to being premenstrual," Dr. Berson says. (For more information on premenstrual breakouts, see "Why Your Skin Breaks Out before Your Period" on page 329.)

## Over-the-Counter Acne War

When you've struggled with your skin since your teenage years, it's easy to lose faith in over-the-counter acne products.

Maybe you used the products wrongly dabbing a little medication here and there.

"Never spot treat," Dr. Fields says. "That may be fine if you only get one pimple a month, but if you're getting a nice colony of three to five pimples on a regular basis, you need a different programme. Treat your entire face every day."

Here's what she suggests.

**Benzoyl peroxide.** This familiar zit zapper is still tops when it comes to killing *Propionibacterium acnes*, the bacterium that infects our clogged pores, causing pimples. To clear your skin without irritation, look for a 2.5 per cent benzoyl peroxide product, Dr. Fields recommends. "More only burns your face."

**Salicylic acid.** Under the name "beta hydroxy acid", this treatment also fights wrinkles, but dermatologists know salicylic acid best for its pimple prevention. This oil-loving ingredient penetrates deep into our pores, keeping them clear of the plugs that turn into pimples. For maximum benefit and minimum skin irritation, look for an oil-free lotion or cream with 2 per cent beta hydroxy acid, Dr. Fields says.

Finally, skip alcohol-based astringents and toners. "All they do is strip the top layer of the skin," Dr. Fields explains. Failing to penetrate deep enough to unplug pores, "they only make things worse," as oil glands then overcompensate for the temporary dryness of just-toned skin.

## By Prescription Only

But over-the-counter products can do only so much for acne, especially if your blemishes and pimples stem from a hormonal problem such as polycystic ovary syndrome. "Without hormonal control, we're not going to help the acne," Dr. Fields says. The same applies to women whose blood tests for excess testosterone or DHEAS are normal but whose acne appears to be hormonally influenced.

To accomplish this, doctors rely on medications such as low-dose oral contraceptives and anti-androgen drugs. Here are some of the most common.

**Cyproterone acetate/ethinylestradiol.** The hormone treatment licensed for prescription use in the UK is Co-cyprindol, a combination of the anti-androgen hormone Cyproterone acetate and the oestrogen ethinylestradiol. Prescribed as Dianette, it is recommended for women with severe acne who also wish to have oral contraception.

**Norgestimate/ethinylestradiol (Cilest).** While some doctors say that any birth control pill helps acne by regulating hormones, dermatologists say that's not true. Women with androgen sensitivity and hormonally based blemishes need an oral contraceptive such as Cilest. Cilest uses a progestin called norgestimate; unlike progestins in many other pills, this synthetic hormone doesn't encourage the release of acne-causing androgens. "It helps decrease the hormonal output from the ovaries," Dr. Berson says of the therapy. "You also get the benefit of oestrogen, which decreases free testosterone."

**Desogestrel/ethinylestradiol (Marvelon).** While not approved explicitly for acne, this oral contraceptive also contains a low-androgenic progestin – desogestrel – which can clear up hormonal breakouts.

**Other anti-acne contraceptives.** Birth control pills Microgynon and Ovranette (levonorgestrel and ethinylestradiol) can also keep breakouts at bay with their low-dose formulations, Dr. Berson says.

**Spironolactone (Aldactone).** Usually reserved for women whose acne doesn't respond to oral contraceptives, this anti-androgen drug has fewer systemic and more specific effects than the Pill: it blocks testosterone at the hormone receptor level. "The hormone then can't interact with the skin to produce extra sebum," Dr. Berson explains. This makes it a good choice for women whose acne may stem not from extra testosterone from the ovaries or adrenal glands but from hormone receptor or enzyme problems that affect skin.

## Medical Approaches to Clearer Skin

Unfortunately, the Pill alone won't make pimples disappear. "While acne is hormonally driven, it also has lots to do with bacteria and plugged pores," Dr. Vierra says. To kill acne-causing bacteria and unplug clogged pores, doctors generally turn to a mix of retinoids (vitamin A derivatives that both treat and prevent pimples), antibiotics (both topical and oral), and other medications.

Here's what your dermatologist might prescribe for you. (Individual dosages will vary.)

**Tretinoin.** More familiar to us as Retin-A, Acticin or Aknemycin Plus, tretinoin is one of the most popular and effective topical acne medications. It encourages more rapid turnover of skin cells, unplugging pores and preventing them from becoming infected. But it also irritates many women's skin. To avoid that, your doctor will probably start you on a low-strength formulation, then gradually increase the potency. If Retin-A still proves too harsh for your skin, you might want to consider two other forms that promise less irritation: Retin-A Micro, which delivers the active (and skin-drying) tretinoin more slowly, or Avita, which doesn't penetrate as deeply into the skin. Whatever retinoid you choose, only apply it to your dry face; wet skin absorbs the medication too quickly, causing stinging, redness and other irritations.

**Adapalene (Differin).** This retinoid gel prevents skin breakouts, like tretinoin, as well as reducing the inflammation that creates painful pimples.

It also doesn't appear to cause the dryness or burning that tretinoin can.

**Tazarotene (Zorac).** Often prescribed for psoriasis, this retinoid (available in a gel) behaves like tretinoin or adapalene.

**Azalaic acid (Skinoren).** Long used for rosacea (an adult condition causing facial flushing), azalaic acid has been rediscovered as an acne treatment by dermatologists, who suspect it unclogs pores and perhaps acts as a mild antibiotic. Less irritating than a retinoid, it needs to be used with benzoyl peroxide.

**Erythromycin (Eryacne, Stiemycin or Zineryt).** This antibiotic, which can be taken orally or as a topical treatment, targets the bacteria responsible for skin breakouts. Combined with benzoyl peroxide, it becomes benzamycin.

**Tetracycline (Topicycline).** Taken orally or used topically, this antibiotic (with its relatives doxycycline and minocycline) reaches the pores to banish pimple-causing bacteria. But it's not the best choice for women taking oral contraceptives for hormonal reasons and birth control: the tetracycline drugs may interact with the Pill, reducing its contraceptive effectiveness.

**Clindamycin (Dalacin T or Zindaclin).** This antibiotic also kills bacteria.

**Isotretinoin (Isotrexin).** If your skin fails to respond to topicals or antibiotics, the next step is often isotretinoin, an oral medication that significantly decreases the skin's production of sebum. Make no mistake: it's strong medicine, with potential side effects like psychiatric problems and birth defects. Women of childbearing age who take Isotrexin must use two forms of birth control for at least 1 month before taking Isotrexin, during treatment, and for 1 month after treatment is stopped. In addition, a pregnancy blood test must be done within 1 week before beginning treatment and once monthly during treatment, and one must be done a month after completing Isotrexin.

## Fewer Drugs, More Patience

If you have patience, natural remedies may help correct the nutritional or hormonal imbalances contributing to skin breakouts.

It's a more holistic approach than many conventional doctors take, says Tori Hudson, N.D., a naturopathic physician and professor at the National College of Naturopathic Medicine in Portland, Oregon. "Sometimes when women go to dermatologists for acne, their doctors just treat the skin and ignore bodywide health," she says.

That's not the case with natural remedies, although they can be slower-acting and less dependable than traditional acne prescriptions. "In some people they work fine," Dr. Hudson says. "In others, nothing helps except tetracycline."

For women hesitant about taking the Pill or Isotrexin, though, they might be worth exploring. Here's what Dr. Hudson recommends.

**Vitamin A.** This vitamin moderates both skin cell turnover and the production of sebum, the fatty lubricant matter secreted by glands of the skin. Do not self-treat with vitamin A – an overdose (more than 10,000 IU a day) can cause serious health problems, including loss of vision. For a safe and effective dosage for you, talk with a naturopath or doctor.

**Zinc.** Often lacking in acne sufferers, this mineral helps vitamin A function properly. Dr. Hudson prescribes 30 to 45 milligrams daily, but check with your own doctor before exceeding 30 milligrams.

---

### THE HORMONE CONNECTION
# WHY YOUR SKIN BREAKS OUT BEFORE YOUR PERIOD

Women have long suspected that pimples – along with crabbiness and undeniable chocolate cravings – were a fact of premenstrual life.

We were right – at least about the pimples.

"Any hormonal fluctuation, if you're someone who's prone to acne, can exacerbate acne breakouts," says Diane Berson, M.D., a dermatologist in private practice in New York City. That includes having your period, going off the Pill, entering perimenopause, or carrying a pregnancy, all of which are hormonal events that may affect your skin in negative or positive ways. "While women are pregnant, they can have severe breakouts," she says. "On the other hand, other women with a history of acne may find that when they get pregnant, their acne improves."

The issue, Dr. Berson explains, is hormonal balance, which is influenced by the menstrual cycle. Just before your period begins, both your oestrogen and your progesterone levels drop, but then progesterone begins to rise and sebaceous gland activity may increase. "Some women, in the week before their period, say their scalp, hair, and skin all feel more oily," Dr. Berson says. Progesterone itself may also play a role, having androgenic effects similar to many of the man-made progestins used in older birth control pills.

What's the solution? If your skin is simply breaking out premenstrually, the answer is probably a low-dose oral contraceptive in addition to standard acne therapies, says Dr. Berson.

**Vitamin E.** Take 400 IU of this vitamin, which the body needs to use vitamin A, Dr. Hudson explains.

**Selenium.** Women with acne often have less of this trace mineral. To maximize your body's use of vitamin E and prevent inflammation, aim for up to 200 micrograms of selenium daily from diet and supplements combined, Dr. Hudson says.

**Vitamin B$_6$.** This seems to be particularly helpful for women with premenstrual acne, says Dr. Hudson, who recommends 100 milligrams daily of B$_6$ or a B-complex supplement.

**Saw palmetto.** Often recommended to men for prostate gland health, this herb checks your body's production of 5-alpha reductase, the enzyme that converts testosterone into oil-stimulating DHT. Dr. Hudson recommends taking 160 milligrams twice daily of standardized saw palmetto extract, with 85 to 95 per cent fatty acids.

**Tea tree oil.** If you suffer from mild acne, you may want to try this natural antiseptic. For acne emergencies, place a few drops on a cotton pad and dab it on the pimple before going to bed.

# Varicose Veins and Spider Veins

Dressed in her tennis outfit and looking trim and well-muscled for a woman in her fifties, Carole was aghast when her granddaughter lovingly ran a finger over her leg and said, "Grandma, you're so pretty! Your legs have designs!"

Those "designs" were spider veins, squiggly lines that may form a web-type pattern under the skin, each about the width of a hair. They may be red or purplish. Some doctors believe spider veins form in response to minor trauma – a run-in with a filing cabinet drawer, for instance. Others blame knee-high socks or stockings or the tight elastic bands at the base of girdles (in women who still wear them). The tendency to develop spider veins is somewhat inherited, and taking birth control pills, becoming pregnant, or taking hormone replacement therapy may make you more susceptible to them. Spider veins are a cosmetic problem, not a serious health problem.

Varicose veins are larger than spider veins, and more pronounced. These abnormally dilated veins may look like a hyperactive mole has been tunnelling under your skin, leaving behind a raised, purple-hued path. Symptoms may include a feeling of leg heaviness or tension, ankle swelling, aching, or itching.

To understand how varicose veins develop, think of your blood vessels as an irrigation system on a mountainside. When blood pumped by your heart flows through your arteries to your toes, it has gravity and muscles within the arterial walls to help. But when blood needs to return uphill, through veins, it needs help, and finds it in the pumping muscles of your calf while you walk and a series of valves that direct the flow in the proper, uphill direction. Varicose veins occur when weakened vein walls enlarge, pulling apart the "gates" of your valves. The veins overfill with blood so that the pumping system can no longer efficiently propel toward the heart. In extreme cases, the valves no longer work at all, and blood flows backwards. This complication, called reflux, may require surgery.

## Female Hormones at Work?

Although men, too, get varicose veins, women get them more often. What's more, in one study, nearly 30 per cent of women who had never suffered from varicose veins developed them during pregnancy, although in many cases the condition resolved itself after delivery. The next big rise in the incidence of varicose veins is around the time of the menopause, when levels of reproductive hormones are falling off.

Other clues pointing to a hormonal role in varicose veins: oestrogen and progesterone receptors are located in the saphenous veins, the major veins of the leg. Oestrogen receptors are more abundant in the varicose portion of a vein than in normal segments of the same vein, while the pregnancy hormone progesterone has more receptors in the normal segments. And many women complain that pain from their varicose veins is worse prior to their menstrual periods.

Researchers aren't certain what it is about pregnancy that seems to set the stage for varicose veins. But one thing is clear: the more babies a woman has, the more likely she is to develop varicose veins. Some experts believe enlargement of the uterus (and increased pressure within the abdomen) changes the careful pump-and-flow mechanism that allows blood to flow upward to the heart, putting pressure on the vein walls. Others believe women with a genetic predisposition to varicose veins develop them in the presence of altered hormones. Gabriel Goren, M.D., a surgeon at the Vein Disorder Center in Encino, California, believes hormones play a dominant role. He sees new varicose veins in women so early in pregnancy that the weight and pressure of the uterus are inconsequential. And he notes that when young women go on birth control pills, which simulate pregnancy, they often develop spider veins within 2 to 3 months. That said, in most women varicose veins that develop during pregnancy disappear with no treatment by several months after delivery.

Besides pregnancy, the use of birth control pills, or oestrogen therapy for menopause, other risk factors for varicose veins include advancing age, occupations, like hairdressing, that require standing for long periods of time, family history of varicose veins and obesity.

Spider veins, too, may have a hormonal link – albeit a weaker one. David Duffy, M.D., a phlebologist and associate clinical professor of dermatology at the University of Southern California and assistant clinical professor of dermatology at UCLA, suspects that the link may be a vascular endothelial growth factor (VEGF) that promotes vessel growth in the presence of hormones. This might very well be the switch that turns on vessel growth and may be a major player in the development of spider veins.

"Once a month, a woman develops new vessels to line the uterus and, in the corpus luteum, to nurse the egg," says Dr. Duffy. "VEGF appears to kick off this new vessel growth. Some women may simply have too big a dose of VEGF or lack the inhibitors that keep the process in check, so that when they run into an armrest on an aeroplane (or bump their legs in other ways), their bodies respond by creating spider veins." It doesn't happen so much in men – possibly because they lack the hormonal trigger that's programmed to create new blood vessels once monthly.

## Outsmarting Your Family History

You can't hide from your family tree, and your decision to have children certainly shouldn't hinge on whether you're going to develop varicose veins as a result. But there are steps that you can take to prevent varicose veins and to minimize their dysfunction once they've developed.

**Step right up.** Anything you can do to strengthen the muscles that pump blood towards your heart will help to preserve your veins. "Walking is absolutely great," says Dr. Goren. If you're in a situation where you can't move around, flex your foot repetitively, tapping your heel on the ground. This definitely applies to long airline flights, he stresses. Even in a person with normal veins, blood will stagnate in the superficial and deep veins on intercontinental journeys because of the lack of movement and the pressure.

**Stay trim.** Although no one knows exactly why, obesity is associated with varicose veins in women, but not in men. So keep your weight down.

**Wear compression stockings.** These specialized support stockings do just what they advertise: they compress spider or varicose veins, squeezing blood on its merry way. Compression stockings, once heavy and cumbersome, now come in sheer styles and fashionable colours and are available over the counter in pharmacies. If you're fighting spider veins, select stockings that state they have 15 to 20 mm Hg, a rating that describes the strength of their compression in millimetres of mercury. For varicose veins, look for stockings with a higher level of compression, 20 to 30 mm Hg. Choose a length that extends to the knee, upper thigh, groin, or waist, depending on the location of the veins you want to compress, says Dr. Goren.

**Keep your legs level with or above your chest as often as possible.** Once the force of gravity is equalized, blood can flow more easily back to the heart regardless of the condition of your veins or valves. You might want to put your legs on some pillows while you watch TV or read, and you should consider elevating the foot of your bed.

**Try horse chestnut.** Seven double-blind, placebo-controlled trials involving more than 500 patients provide some solid evidence to back up the enormous popularity of this herbal remedy for varicose veins. The standardized extract of horse chestnut seeds (*Aesculus hippocastanum*) works by strengthening blood vessel walls, says Varro E. Tyler, Ph.D., Sc.D., dean emeritus of the Purdue University School of Pharmacy and Pharmacal Sciences in West Lafayette, Indiana, and distinguished professor emeritus of pharmacognosy. In Germany, the approved dose of 250 to 312.5 milligrams of the extract, taken twice a day, is considered safe and effective for relieving symptoms. One study found that foot and ankle swelling was reduced in long-distance air travellers who took horse chestnut extract before they embarked on their flights.

**Sweep them away with butcher's broom.** Though less well-studied than horse chestnut, the rhizome, or underground stem, of *Ruscus aculeatus* – commonly known as butcher's broom – may also work. When used in connection with other measures, such as compression stockings and elevation, extract containing 7 to 11 milligrams of total ruscogenin, the active principal ingredient, taken daily may help to narrow blood vessels. You would receive this amount of ruscogenin in about 300 milligrams of butcher's broom products. Because such products vary, for best results follow the dosage recommendations on the label, says Dr. Tyler.

**Cover them up.** If all else fails, you can camouflage small spider veins and even moderate varicose veins with special cover-up makeup sold at pharmacies or department store makeup counters. One brand to try is Dermablend, recommends Dr. Duffy. An approach that works for women with light skin tones is to use a natural tanning product so the veins won't be so obvious.

## Your Doctor Can Help

One of the most effective treatments for varicose veins and spider veins is sclerotherapy: simply put, a doctor trained in the procedure injects an irritating solution into veins causing you trouble. The technique can be very quick, particularly for larger veins, involves only minor discomfort, and clears about 90 per cent of veins that are properly selected (those that are large enough to respond and that do not have reflux, the backup of blood through faulty valves). You may need several treatments. Sometimes small visible veins may crop up where larger veins were treated. Called matting, this complication is difficult to treat.

Several vein experts confess to having special leg vein laser units gathering dust in their surgeries. Early promises of a painless alternative to sclerotherapy for spider veins or surgery for varicose veins haven't quite lived up to their billing. Laser treatments are expensive and often ineffective, and may cause skin burns when they are used at settings powerful enough to reach their target, leg veins deep within the skin. (They do work for small spider veins on the face, however.) So, according to Dr. Goren, the best alternative for leg spider veins remains sclerotherapy.

If your doctor sees signs of reflux (a backup of blood that can lead to discolouration of the skin, bleeding, leg ulcers, and even more serious complications, like clots), he may carry out a more extensive evaluation to make sure the valves that keep your blood moving in one direction are functioning properly. Surgery, or new techniques that involve thermal closure of larger veins, may be used to remove or close the malfunctioning veins, redirecting bloodflow into functional alternative veins to relieve the symptoms of varicose veins (fatigue, discomfort, and swelling).

Once, your only option for getting rid of varicose veins was "vein stripping", a painful and cosmetically unsatisfactory procedure in which large incisions were made at the groin and/or behind the knees or along the course of the varicose vein (depending on which veins malfunctioned). This was a hospital procedure, performed in an operating room under general anaesthesia. However, today this is carried out as an outpatient surgical procedure. And, thanks to improved instruments, it can produce almost scarless results, says Dr. Duffy.

Other alternatives include:

**Ambulatory phlebectomy.** Done under local anaesthesia, this minimally invasive procedure originated in Europe. It basically involves making several 1.5- to 3-mm ($\frac{1}{16}$- to $\frac{1}{8}$-inch) openings in the skin through which the involved veins are removed in segments with a specially designed instrument that looks like a crochet hook. The long veins of the thigh or calf are gently peeled out, instead of stripped. The procedure is called "ambulatory" because patients walk out of the surgery afterwards, wearing special compression stockings. They can return to work or play almost immediately. The cosmetic and long-term results are excellent, says Dr. Goren.

**Closure.** This newer technique uses radiofrequency energy to shrink veins. A small incision is made behind the knee, and a catheter is threaded to the groin through the large saphenous vein, then heated. The collagen within the vein shrinks in response to heat. The procedure cannot be used on veins below the knee or on "twisted, tortuous" branches of the saphenous vein because nerve damage could result. Therefore, it is often done in combination with ambulatory phlebectomy, says Salvador Yunez, M.D., a specialist with Vein Care Specialists of Chicago.

# Upper Lip and Facial Hair

Most women take for granted the simple acts of shaving, waxing and plucking unwanted hair from their legs, underarms, bikini line, eyebrows and upper lip. But when hair growth is excessive, temporary methods can be time-consuming and tiresome. What's more, growing unwanted hair where it's most visible to others – on your upper lip and face – can be troubling to women worried about looking less feminine.

Technically speaking, hirsutism is excess facial and body hair in a male pattern, says Wilma F. Bergfeld, M.D., head of clinical research at the Cleveland Clinic. Heredity and hormones – or both – may be at play, prompting hair to grow in areas where men attract hair, like the face, including the moustache and sideburns, neck, chest, back, arms, legs, and inner thighs. Hirsute hair, also called terminal hair, is coarser and darker than the finer hair on other parts of the body.

Hirsutism isn't as rare as you might think – about 1 in 10 women experiences male-pattern hair growth. If excess hair growth doesn't bother you, you don't necessarily have to remove it or seek treatment – unless you also experience acne, abnormal menstrual cycles, obesity, scalp hair loss and clitoral enlargement. Though rare, undetected medical causes of hirsutism can potentially lead to infertility, heart disease, high levels of fat in the blood, high blood pressure, osteoporosis and endometrial cancer, and should be checked out.

More commonly, though, hirsutism is a cosmetic problem, rather than a medical problem. Either way, excess hair growth is treatable, says Stephen Schleicher, M.D., director of the Derm Dx Center for Dermatology in Philadelphia.

## Male Hormones at Work

Noticeably heavy hair growth in women is often inherited. Also, certain ethnic groups are predisposed to hair growth. But the most common causes include an excess production of androgens, male hormones, or increased sensitivity to these hormones, Dr. Schleicher says.

Small quantities of androgens circulate in every woman. Yet when those levels increase, or if hair follicles become more sensitive, then women may become hirsute.

"When this happens," Dr. Bergfeld says, "hair follicles are stimulated to grow terminal hair on the body, including the face." In other words, many women register a normal level of androgens but are simply more sensitive to those hormones.

"For example, with polycystic ovary syndrome (PCOS), one of the most common causes of hormonal imbalance, the ovaries secrete too much androgen," says Mary Jane Minkin, M.D., clinical professor of obstetrics and gynaecology at Yale University School of Medicine. Symptoms of PCOS – which occurs most often in premenopausal women – include irregular or no menstrual cycles, high blood pressure, baldness, acne, infertility, diabetes and weight gain. Treating PCOS normalizes hair growth. (For more details on the treatment of PCOS, see page 150.)

Hair growth may also become more noticeable – though still normal – during menopause, when ovaries decrease production of the female hormone oestrogen. Levels of testosterone (a "male" hormone present in both men and women in different amounts) may stay the same, creating an imbalance. "When that happens, the woman's body responds to the testosterone, and that could cause facial hair to grow," says Dr. Minkin.

Also, women who take postmenopausal hormone replacement therapy containing small amounts of testosterone could grow noticeably more hair on the upper lip, the face, or elsewhere.

More rarely, excess androgens can also be traced to ovarian or adrenal gland tumours, says Dr. Schleicher says. Surgery can remove the tumour, which will then stop the production of excess androgen.

# Plenty of Options

If excess hair growth is a problem for you, don't be embarrassed to seek medical attention. A family doctor, a dermatologist, or an endocrinologist can work with you to recommend the best treatment.

Commonly prescribed medications, often used in combination, include the following:

**Oral contraceptives.** Often prescribed for PCOS, birth control pills, especially those with low levels of progesterone, suppress the level of androgens produced by the ovaries.

**Glucocorticoids.** Drugs like prednisolone block excess amounts of male hormones.

**Antiandrogens.** Antiandrogens – like flutamide (Drogenil), and finasteride (Propecia or Proscar) – either decrease the production of androgens or block androgen uptake by the hair follicles, thus reducing unwanted hair growth. (Interestingly, they're also used for hair loss, as explained on the following page.)

**Topical medication.** The most recently developed treatment for excess hair growth, eflornithine (Vaniqa), blocks the enzyme that stimulates hair growth. It requires a twice-a-day application and may yield results in as little as 8 weeks, compared with 6 months for other medications. It is not yet available in the UK.

Regardless of what course your doctor may prescribe, give it time. To be effective, treatment must be administered regularly and should be considered long-term. Once treatment is stopped, the hair will return. But gradually, if treatment is successful, your hair will be finer and grow less, you'll have less need to cosmetically camouflage or remove hair, and your self-esteem will get a boost, Dr. Bergfeld notes.

# Other Hair-Removal Methods

How you deal with excess hair growth is up to you. If you're experiencing noticeably heavy growth and no other symptoms, if you don't tolerate drug treatment or decide against it for other reasons, simple hair-removal techniques may suffice. Or you may need to combine medical treatment with cosmetic hair removal, for best results. Unlike medical treatments, most cosmetic treatments get rid of hair currently on your face, rather than prevent future hair growth.

**Shaving.** Shaving takes seconds and is simple, provided it doesn't irritate your skin. Stick to unscented shaving cream and a clean double-edged razor blade. Do your upper lip and sideburns first, then your legs and underarms.

**Plucking.** Best for eyebrows only, says Vicki Morav, spa director at Minardi Salon in New York City. Otherwise, plucking facial hair is cumbersome and may cause skin irritation and ingrown hairs.

**Waxing.** Although you might experience temporary discomfort and skin irritation, this popular treatment is one of the best methods for removing unwanted facial hair. Results may last several weeks. For best results, find an experienced beauty consultant who can choose the right wax for your face. (Ask your hairstylist for a referral.) Also, check the cleanliness of the salon. "You don't want your face exposed to dirt and bacteria," Morav says.

**Depilatory creams.** Hair-removal creams dissolve hair but may cause allergic reactions or skin irritation, Dr. Schleicher says. Follow the manufacturer's instructions, which typically call for testing a coin-sized portion of the cream on an inconspicuous body part and waiting 24 hours before using it extensively.

**Electrolysis.** A needle and electric current destroy hair follicles one by one. Electrolysis is the only way to remove hair permanently, but it can be time-consuming and expensive and may cause skin irritation, pigment abnormalities, and in rare cases scarring, Dr. Bergfeld says. However, it's an effective option, especially for women who don't respond well to medication.

**Lasers.** Lasers treat larger areas with minimal discomfort and destroy hair follicles by heating hair. While lasers rarely remove hair permanently, results can last up to several months, making them a useful option for women who don't tolerate hormonal or drug treatments very well.

# Hair Loss and Thinning Hair

E very day the follicles in your scalp are working to produce slivers of hair so tiny it takes a month or two to grow just an inch.

Or *almost* every day. Those follicles get holidays after anywhere from 2 to 8 years. When the follicle takes a break, the hair shaft falls out. If you have workaholic follicles, your hair could grow as long as 2.5 metres (8 feet) – maybe even longer – without falling out. (Assuming you didn't cut it first, that is.)

The key to such Rapunzel-length hair is the hormone oestrogen, says Geoffrey Redmond, M.D., director of the Hormone Center of New York in New York City. When oestrogen levels are optimal, your hair keeps growing (2 to 4 years is also normal).

When oestrogen levels are low, follicles take more frequent holidays. The result is shorter hair. Men have lower oestrogen levels than women, so their hair never gets as long, even if they don't cut it.

Normally, about 100 follicles go on holiday each day. The result is hairs shedding onto your pillow or comb, or clogging your drain. And with about 100,000 follicles on your scalp, you can spare a few.

But if follicles go on holiday at a faster pace, or they fail to return to work, you will have a thinner head of hair.

By their fifties, about 40 per cent to 50 per cent of women have some hair loss, says Mary Sawaya, M.D., Ph.D., dermatologist and principal investigator of Clinical Research at Alopecia Research and Associated Technologies (ARATEC) in Ocala, Florida. Shedding may be sudden or gradual, depending on the cause.

A sudden drop in oestrogen due to childbirth can prompt masses of follicles to walk off the job. Gradual declines in oestrogen that herald the menopause lead to gradual thinning. So can androgenetic alopecia, a genetic predisposition to hormone-related hair loss.

If you seem to be losing your hair, don't panic. Talk to your doctor. She probably won't test your hormone levels unless you're experiencing other symptoms – such as irregular menstruation, excessive body hair growth, severe acne, or other signs of hormone imbalance.

## How Wide Is Your Parting?

Normally, we lose about 100 hairs a day, more or less. So collecting more hair in your hairbrush, sink, or pillow isn't necessarily a sign that you're losing hair any faster than normal. Instead, check out your parting.

With fewer hair follicles on the job, you will have a wider parting, especially on top of the head. A normal parting is just a thin line, like the edge of a ruler. If the parting is as wide as a pencil, you may be in the early stages of hair loss. If it is as wide as your comb, you have advanced hair loss.

Remember how thick your ponytail was when you were a teenager? A thinner ponytail is another sign of hair loss.

If your parting seems to be widening or your ponytail thinning, consult your doctor. To help diagnose hair loss, she may examine your hair more closely, with a magnifying glass, to see if some of your strands are turning into thinner, shorter vellus hairs, then treat you accordingly.

If you suspect you have alopecia areata (hair loss in sharply defined areas, usually the scalp or beard), your doctor may need to test for antithyroid antibodies and antimicrosomal antibodies, says Dr. Sawaya. Thyroid supplements and other medications are often effective, along with medications applied to the scalp. (See chapter 4.)

Your pattern of hair loss – where you're losing it, when it started, and so forth – will help pinpoint the cause. Your doctor will also need to rule out (or treat) non-hormonal conditions such as anaemia, intense stress, crash dieting, surgery and a high fever, which can all trigger shedding. With some trial and error – and patience – you can work with your doctor to find a treatment that works for you.

And don't delay. It's easier to keep those follicles on the job than to coax them out of retirement.

## The Testosterone Connection

The male hormone testosterone is to blame, at least indirectly, for what many experts believe is the most common form of hair loss in men and women: androgenetic alopecia (aptly called male-pattern baldness in men and female-pattern baldness in women). "Alopecia" is simply science-speak for hair loss.

Having androgenetic alopecia does not mean you have above-normal levels of testosterone; it just means your hair follicles are genetically predisposed to damage from a by-product of testosterone called dihydrotestosterone (DHT), an enzyme made within hair follicles.

"DHT packs a double whammy," says Angela M. Christiano, Ph.D., associate professor of dermatology and genetics and development at Columbia University College of Physicians and Surgeons in New York City. It both prompts hair follicles to go on more frequent holidays and causes some of the follicles to shrink a little each time they return to work.

The follicles are still working, but in rocking chair mode, producing an extremely thin shaft of colourless hair that might get only 5mm (¼ inch) long, called vellus hair. (It's the same "peach fuzz" that grows on your arms.) Androgenetic alopecia can cause hair thinning as early as your teens or twenties, though it may not be noticeable until decades later. Contrary to popular belief, androgenetic alopecia, male or female pattern, can be inherited from either side of the family.

If you're diagnosed with androgenetic alopecia, don't take the over-the-counter supplement DHEA, sold as an antiageing remedy. It can increase

*Escape from* **HORMONE HELL**

# HER HAIR IS FALLING OUT, AND SHE'S WORRIED

**Q:** I'm 32, feel great, exercise, and eat well. But I'm really worried about my hair. Over the past few months, I've been noticing more and more hair than usual in my shower drain and coming out in my comb. I see more scalp, especially when I part my hair.

When I asked my doctor about this, he said my hair looked great and seemed to think I was exaggerating and overreacting. It seemed to be getting worse, so I went to a dermatologist, who did a scalp biopsy. But the results were normal.

At this rate, I'm afraid I'll go bald. What should I do?

Geoffrey Redmond, M.D., director of the Hormone Center of New York in New York City and author of *The Good News about Women's Hormones*, replies: first, find a doctor who is interested and knowledgeable, and cares about your problem. Most doctors have little expertise in hair loss in women.

A key question is, How long have you been losing your hair? If it had occurred suddenly, it might have signalled a deeper medical problem. But since it has been progressing gradually, over a year or more, it sounds like you have androgenetic alopecia, a genetically caused form of hair loss, which can start as early as

the twenties and is common in women.

There is no medical test for androgenetic alopecia. A scalp biopsy, where a small piece of scalp is punched out and examined under a microscope, is of little value here.

The doctor should look through all areas of the scalp carefully. If the hair is thinner on the top, or "crown", and the "vertex", or point at the back of the head, and thicker on the sides and back, that is an indication of androgenetic alopecia.

The doctor should, however, rule out other possible causes, such as sudden crash dieting, recent surgery, or a high fever.

Prompt treatment for androgenetic alopecia is important because it is easier to prevent further hair loss than to get hair to grow back. Left alone, androgenetic alopecia tends to get worse.

Given your age and assuming no contraindications, I would prescribe spironolactone at a dose of 100 milligrams a day. If that didn't work, I'd recommend increasing the dose to 200 milligrams a day. If that didn't work, I would recommend trying minoxidil (Regaine).

With appropriate treatment, most women can prevent additional hair loss: hair may even grow back.

testosterone levels and speed up your hair loss, says Dr. Redmond.

While no drug will restore all your hair, three are worth a try. And, as with most drugs for non-life-threatening conditions, discontinue treatment if you're planning to become pregnant.

## First Choice: Minoxidil (Regaine)

This is the only drug approved by the US Food and Drug Administration for treating hair loss in women. And it seems to work.

"I've had a very good response treating women and men with minoxidil, even in women in their sixties and early seventies," says Dr. Sawaya.

How, exactly, minoxidil promotes hair growth is not clear. Dr. Sawaya believes it works by opening potassium channels and increasing hair follicle growth.

Still, minoxidil isn't perfect.

- *In a study of women aged 18 to 45, about 60 per cent had some hair regrowth after using Regaine 2 per cent solution for 8 months, but most of this was rated "minimal" growth.*
- *It may take a year to work. "It takes 4 months alone to wake up follicles and begin producing hair," says Dr. Sawaya.*
- *The directions call for applying it twice a day, and even though it can leave a residue, Dr. Sawaya says, it can enhance hairstyling.*

On the other hand, even if minoxidil doesn't fully restore your lost hair, it seems to prevent further hair loss (at least according to studies on men).

While you can buy over-the-counter versions of minoxidil and treat yourself, it's not a good idea. You need to talk to a doctor to get a realistic assessment of how effective minoxidil might be for your type of hair loss and to assess any underlying health problems, advises Dr. Sawaya.

If you decide to try minoxidil, here's some expert advice.

**Give it time.** Use it for 6 to 12 months to see if there are results.

**Let it work overnight.** Instead of applying it twice a day, Dr. Sawaya suggests using almost twice the amount in the evening. Leave it on overnight and shampoo it out in the morning. "It will still work very, very well," she says.

**Spray it on.** It takes less than a minute to apply minoxidil, by either a dropper or sprayer, to the scalp in the area where there is hair loss, says Dr. Sawaya. She recommends using a sprayer. "Rub it in and you're done," she says. If you accidentally spray the solution in your eyes, rinse with large amounts of cool tap water.

**If the 2 per cent version doesn't work, try 5 per cent.** Minoxidil is available over the counter in 2 and 5 per cent solutions, though the 5 per cent version has been tested and shown to be of added benefit only in men. Nevertheless, Dr. Sawaya recommends the stronger version for women.

If you have sudden or patchy hair loss, don't use minoxidil without first consulting a specialist. And don't use it if you have a red, inflamed, infected, irritated, or painful scalp. Stop using minoxidil and call your doctor if you develop chest pain, a rapid heartbeat, dizziness, or faintness. Stop using it and call your doctor if you experience a sudden, unexplained weight gain, swollen hands and feet, or scalp irritation that continues or worsens.

## Second Choice: Finasteride (Propecia)

If minoxidil doesn't work, ask your doctor about finasteride. Licensed for male pattern baldness in men, as Propecia, this drug blocks the conversion of testosterone into DHT (as Proscar it is licensed for benign prostate enlargement). The European Medicines Commission does not approve the use of finasteride by women – mainly because it causes underdeveloped genitals in *male* lab animals. So it could cause birth defects if women take the drug during pregnancy. But if you are postmenopausal, have had a tubal ligation, or are otherwise not planning to have a baby, it's safe, effective and legal. So doctors in Europe may prescribe finasteride for women.

Finasteride is taken as a pill. It will probably take from 6 months to a year to see results. A study found finasteride to be ineffective in women over the age of 60. This may be because by then androgen levels fall to insignificant levels, Dr. Redmond says.

If you do plan to get pregnant and want to try finasteride:
- *Stop taking finasteride 3 weeks before you start having unprotected sex, so that your body has plenty of time to excrete the drug, Dr. Sawaya says.*
- *Use oral contraceptives, condom plus spermicide, or other form of pregnancy protection while using finasteride.*
- *If you no longer plan to get pregnant, consider a tubal ligation, or a vasectomy for your husband.*
- *One side effect that may occur when taking this medication is a loss of sexual desire. If it continues or is bothersome, call your doctor. If you develop a skin rash or a swelling of the lips, call your doctor immediately. These are the signs of a toxic reaction. If you're pregnant and have handled broken or crushed tablets, call your doctor right away.*

## Third Choice: Spironolactone

The drug that Dr. Redmond most often recommends for premenopausal women with hair loss is spironolactone, a prescription medication that decreases production of testosterone. And less testosterone means less of the follicle-zapping DHT.

Nevertheless, there are side effects to consider. Spironolactone appears to have a potential for birth defects similar to finasteride. And it may cause periods to come closer together, as frequently as every 14 days, which is probably safe for a few months but not over several years, cautions Dr. Redmond. Still, he finds spironolactone to be generally safe.

---

### THE HORMONE CONNECTION
# PREMATURELY GREY HAIR: ENDOCRINE GLANDS UNDER ATTACK?

If more than 50 per cent of your hair gradually turns grey before you reach 40, most likely you have nothing to worry about. If everyone in your family tends to turn grey early, and you have no health problems, prematurely grey hair is no doubt simply genetic, like blue eyes or high cheekbones.

But if you're under 40 and your hair suddenly turns grey over a couple of months, your doctor may look for Hashimoto's disease, an autoimmune disorder in which the thyroid gland is underactive.

"Sometimes premature grey hair can be an obvious feature of the disease," says Raphael Kellman, M.D., director of the Kellman Center for Progressive Medicine in New York City. But hair that is going grey is not by itself a sign of disease. Other autoimmune disorders associated with an overactive thyroid – namely Graves' disease – can indirectly cause grey hair by attacking the endocrine glands. With Graves' disease, antibodies sometimes attack the melanin cells that give your hair and skin their pigment. The hair may turn grey, or even white.

Sometimes people who have decreased adrenal function also get prematurely grey hair, says Diana Bihova, M.D., a dermatologist in private practice in New York City. The adrenal glands in particular play a critical role in producing melanin. Also, premature ovarian failure may occasionally cause prematurely grey hair. Should your doctor find an underlying autoimmune disorder or related endocrine problem, treatment may reverse the loss of pigment.

Some medications or medical conditions contraindicate the use of spironolactone. Inform your doctor or pharmacist of all medications that you are taking. Do not take this medicine if you are taking supplemental potassium. If you're taking ACE inhibitors or other medicine for heart conditions, your doctor may need to monitor how much you're taking and how well it's working. If you're taking spironolactone, don't use salt substitutes.

Spironolactone (Aldactone) is mainly used for heart failure as a diuretic in the UK. This use by Dr. Redmond is not widely known in the UK.

## A Herbal Alternative: Saw Palmetto

Herbalist James A. Duke, Ph.D., believes saw palmetto might help treat hair loss, citing the herb's similar benefits to finasteride in treating enlarged prostate glands in men, where the enzyme DHT also is the main culprit.

The tropical berry has been used for centuries and appears to be safe in women, says Dr. Duke, a retired ethnobotanist with the United States Department of Agriculture and author of *The Green Pharmacy*. However, he does not know of any scientific studies showing that saw palmetto works for hair loss.

Dr. Christiano is conducting experiments at Columbia University to see whether saw palmetto affects hair growth. Based on previous studies, saw palmetto has been shown to work by a mechanism similiar to that of Propecia.

"I know quite a few women using it successfully," says Dr. Christiano, adding that some have seen improvement in their androgenetic alopecia in just 2 months from using saw palmetto.

If you decide to try saw palmetto:

**Take the right form.** Dr. Duke recommends 320 milligrams a day of saw palmetto extract in a capsule concentrated to 80 per cent fatty acids and sterols.

**Try synergy.** Dr. Duke suggests using saw palmetto in combination with other treatments, such as minoxidil or finasteride.

# Birth Control Pills: Newer, Hair-Saving Prescriptions

If you are on the Pill, the problem might be in your prescription.

Taking birth control pills can trigger hair loss because the progestin in some birth control pills acts a little like male hormones. For many women this is no problem. But if you have the genes for androgenetic alopecia, the extra DHT produced could put many of your follicles out of commission, says Dr. Sawaya.

If that happens, and you either begin to lose hair or you lose hair faster, you have a few options.

**Talk to your doctor about switching to a low-androgen prescription.** If you're taking high-androgen pills – such as those that contain 1.5 mg norethisterone (such as Loestrin 30) your doctor may instead prescribe one that contains less (such as Loestrin 20, that contains 1 mg norethisterone) or that gives a three-phase dose of progestin over the whole cycle (such as Tri-Minulet, Triadene or TriNovum).

**Consider non-hormonal methods of birth control available.** Depending on whether you're temporarily or permanently delaying getting pregnant, tubal ligation or other means of birth control may solve your hair-loss problem.

In some instances, discontinuing birth control pills could cause a drop in oestrogen that might trigger temporary shedding. But hair growth should return to normal after 4 months or so.

## Childbirth: Be Patient

Once you decide to become pregnant, your belly won't be the only part of your body getting fuller. Your head of hair probably will, too. That's because the higher oestrogen levels during pregnancy keep more hair follicles on the job, Dr. Redmond says.

But when oestrogen levels fall after delivery, you may experience some shedding.

"It's definitely noticeable but, for most women, not severe," says Dr. Redmond.

And it's temporary. Shedding usually occurs about 2 to 4 months after birth and lasts about a month, though it can continue a bit longer if you breastfeed. The welfare of your baby should come ahead of your hair, says Dr. Redmond. So don't curtail breastfeeding for the sake of your tresses.

Once your period returns, oestrogen levels should be back to normal and the shedding should stop. But it will typically take another 4 months for your hair to be noticeably fuller.

If your hair is not back to normal 6 to 8 months after childbirth, see a doctor. It may signal a more fundamental hormonal imbalance or other health problem, says Dr. Redmond.

## Hair Loss with Menopause: Not Inevitable

Since any decline in oestrogen production seems to initiate hair loss, and menopause (like the period after giving birth) is marked by a decline in oestrogen production, it's no surprise that many women experience accelerated hair loss at the menopause. In extreme cases, women can lose close to 80 per cent of their hair by their seventies. On the other hand, some don't lose any.

Hair loss isn't inevitable. Here's what to do if your hair loss is related to the menopause.

**Consider hormone replacement therapy.** If losing oestrogen causes hair loss, replacing oestrogen prevents hair loss. Sounds simple. But the dose of oestrogen needed to help hair is usually 1.5 to 2 times higher than that used for general symptoms. "It is still within the accepted range, just at the higher end of it," says Dr. Redmond.

Dr. Redmond finds a dose of 1.25 milligrams daily of conjugated oestrogens (Prempak) is more likely to be effective than the usual dose of 0.625 milligrams.

**Talk to the right doctor.** While postmenopausal hair loss is common, not all doctors are aware of – or agree with – the oestrogen connection, cautions Dr. Redmond. So if your gynaecologist doesn't go along with the idea, you may need to consult a dermatologist or an endocrinologist with expertise in hair loss, he says.

**Work with your hairstylist.** If you've lost some of your hair and can't take hormone replacement therapy, or prefer not to, or can't tolerate higher doses, enlist the help of your hairstylist. The right cut – plus hair colour, teasing, perms, sprays, gels, spritzes and blow-drying techniques – can help make the most of the hair you do have. Or, if you've lost a considerable amount of hair, a natural-looking hairpiece or even a wig can help you look your best.

# Allergies

Imagine the cells of your immune system as an army at the ready, waiting for dangerous organisms to invade. Normally your ally, this militia can turn from friend to foe fast if you suffer from allergies.

Allergic reactions are the by-products of an immune system so anxious to do its job that it forms antibodies called immunoglobulin E (IgE) against harmless substances. Those antibodies attach themselves to mast cells – which, it just so happens, most densely populate your nose, eyes, lungs and gastrointestinal tract. When you come in contact with an allergen, the mast cells release histamines (the chemical responsible for unpleasant allergic reactions) and an assortment of other chemicals, and you end up with a stuffed-up nose, watery eyes, and a scratchy throat or other hallmarks of allergy.

Scientists aren't sure why some people react to things like animal dander, dust mites, and pollen, but 20 per cent of the population suffer from some type of allergy. If you count yourself among them, keeping allergic reactions at bay will be a priority. That's where hormones come in.

Cortisol and epinephrine – and, some experts believe, even oestrogen – can influence your body's response to allergens. What's more, allergist Russell Roby, M.D., director of the Texas Allergy Center in Austin, suggests that some women can actually develop allergies to their own hormones, including progesterone, oestrogen, or thyroid hormones.

## Oestrogen – For Better or Worse

Your neighbour told you her allergies disappeared after menopause. You discovered during perimenopause that your hay fever actually got worse. This confounding situation is one example of how female sex hormones may be linked to allergies. Exactly what the connection is, however, isn't clear. One theory holds that high oestrogen levels may elevate your body's response to allergens and could even increase your likelihood of developing allergies. Another holds that low oestrogen levels may create a hormonal imbalance that minimizes your ability to fight off allergies.

"We're at a very early stage in understanding the association between hormones and allergies," says Baizhuang Xu, Ph.D., epidemiologist at the Imperial College School of Medicine in London. "We still have a long way to go before we can have a better knowledge of the mechanism of allergy development linked with hormones."

Dr. Xu theorizes that elevated levels of oestrogen could be a factor in the development of allergies. "It is commonly observed that women at reproductive age have more allergic disorders. This could be linked with sex hormones," he says.

Dr. Xu conducted a study that sought to determine whether the age at which a woman begins menstruating influences the development of allergies in her children. Interestingly, of the 5188 people (half were men and half were women, all from Finland) tested, 35 per cent of those whose mothers had begun menstruating at the age of 12 or younger had allergies. By contrast, allergies affected only 26.4 per cent of those whose mothers hadn't started their periods until the age of 16 or later. Since women who begin menstruating early are believed to have higher oestrogen levels in adulthood, Dr. Xu says his study could point to a connection between oestrogen and allergy development.

In an earlier study, women were found to be more reactive to histamines during skin-prick tests that were conducted on days 12 to 16 of their menstrual cycles, when oestrogen levels peak. So that, too, would seem to indicate a correlation between high oestrogen and allergies. The correlation is bolstered by the observation that postmenopausal women in general are far less likely to develop allergies, says Dr. Xu.

But Dr. Roby says he sees many women who experience a worsening of allergies in both perimenopause and postmenopause. He blames low oestrogen levels. Dr. Roby theorizes that women low on oestrogen have a hormonal imbalance that impacts all the other hormones in their bodies. It happens, he says, because your body prioritizes hormone production. Because oestrogen is responsible for reproduction, it is given a top priority – second only to adrenaline, which you need for survival. To compensate for low oestrogen levels experienced during perimenopause – and, for some women, premenstrually – the body's DHEA (the basic building block of hormones) is diverted from the production of other hormones. The consequence is diminished levels of testosterone (causing a lower sex drive) and greatly diminished levels of cortisol – resulting in more allergies, less energy and less ability to deal with stress.

## THE HORMONE CONNECTION
## ARE YOU ALLERGIC TO YOUR OWN HORMONES?

Occasionally, people with chronic hives are found to have developed immunoglobulin E (IgE) antibodies to their thyroid hormones, says Ira Finegold, M.D., chief of allergy and clinical immunology at St. Luke's–Roosevelt Hospital in New York. Progesterone and oestrogen sensitivities have also been discovered in women whose hives and rashes reoccur premenstrually.

Progesterone and oestrogen allergies are rare, but not unusual. In fact hormone sensitivity could be responsible for cyclical changes in hay fever and asthma symptoms, says Marianne Frieri, M.D., Ph.D., associate professor of medicine and pathology at the State University of New York, Stony Brook, and director of allergy and immunology at Nassau University Medical Center on Long Island, New York. Oral contraceptives can help since they diminish hormonal fluctuations, but they can also trigger a runny nose, so you should discuss their use with your doctor.

Unfortunately for allergy sufferers, the hormone with the lowest priority is cortisol, Dr. Roby says. With less cortisol being produced, women may experience worsening of allergies, due to greater inflammation and heightened response of the immune system.

*Escape from* **HORMONE HELL**

## HER ALLERGIES GET WORSE BEFORE HER PERIOD

**Q: I'm 41 years old, and I've had allergies since I was at college. After I turned 35, I've noticed that every year my allergies have become a bit more severe. This year was the absolute worst! And right before I get my period – it never fails – my allergies go out of whack. My nose is so stuffed, and my eyes are so itchy, I find it hard to concentrate on anything. During allergy season, I've come to dread my period. Yet when I told my doctor, he said there is absolutely no reason why my allergies should flare up premenstrually. Am I imagining a connection?**

Russell Roby, M.D., an allergist and director of the Texas Allergy Center in Austin, replies: what you describe sounds to me like a progesterone sensitivity. And you're not alone: progesterone sensitivity may be responsible for a number of premenstrual symptoms, including an exacerbation of hay fever right before you get your period. Invariably, symptoms get worse each month when the oestrogen level drops about a week before your period begins. You may even have seen your hay fever disappear during pregnancy, when all your hormone levels would have been high, especially oestrogen. Some other common disorders associated with hormone reactions are dry or oily skin, thinning scalp hair, PMS, increased body hair, asthma, migraines and weight gain. Each may be treated by a different specialist, but I believe the first step towards treatment is to correct the imbalance. This usually means boosting oestrogen.

Birth control pills help some women, but for others they make symptoms worse, especially if given the wrong dose. So instead, I recommend you try to improve the imbalance by improving your overall health. This means maintaining your ideal weight and getting at least a half-hour of exercise every day, and avoiding carbohydrates and caffeine, both of which can aggravate a hormonal imbalance.

Dr. Roby acknowledges that some women see their allergies improve after menopause. That may be because an imbalance of the hormones progesterone and oestrogen during perimenopause can stimulate swelling. Once hormones balance out at menopause, swelling subsides and allergic reactions abate, he says.

If your allergies are worse premenstrually or if they seem to be getting worse as you get older, here's what to try.

**Fight it with phyto-oestrogens.** Some women improve with supplements of isoflavones and other plant forms of oestrogens (collectively known as phyto-oestrogens), available online (www.healthstore.co.uk). (However, before you try supplements, you should try to get as much of your isoflavones as possible by eating one to two servings a day of foods containing soya.) Dr. Roby suggests experimenting with taking a dose right before you get your period. The recommended dose for isoflavone supplements is usually 30 to 50 milligrams a day. You may need to adjust the dose several times before you see an improvement. Ask your doctor to help determine whether oestrogen is safe for you or if it poses a risk.

**Go for a walk.** Thirty minutes to an hour a day of gentle exercise could keep your allergist away, says Dr. Roby. Walking is the best exercise because it's not overly strenuous, and it will help reduce weight gain, another factor in optimal hormone balance, he adds.

**Cut back on carbohydrates.** According to Dr. Roby, carbohydrates encourage fat production. He says that women whose diets are high in carbohydrates may suffer more from allergic reactions because they have more soft tissue (i.e., fat). While eating more in general, and more carbohydrates in particular, leads to overweight – especially without enough exercise – people who crave carbohydrates are especially prone to overeating and gaining weight. He claims that reducing the amount of simple sugars that you eat, or even eliminating them altogether, could make you feel better during allergy season. (For more details on following a reduced-carbohydrate diet, see "Protein, Fat and Carbohydrates: The Key Is Balance" on page 114.)

## Hormone-Based Drugs That Help Allergies

Corticosteroids are hormones produced naturally by the adrenal cortex (the outer layer of your adrenal gland). Synthetic corticosteroids are often prescribed for allergies and asthma because they suppress tissue inflammation and quell the immune response. In the case of allergies, they tell your immune system to stop overreacting to foreign substances.

If you have seasonal allergic rhinitis (hay fever), your doctor may prescribe a corticosteroid nasal spray. These drugs are considered safe because although the medicine comes in direct contact with the nasal passages, at normal (small) doses, very little is absorbed into your system; therefore, they don't suppress the adrenal hormones you naturally produce. Oral corticosteroids may be prescribed for severe allergies associated with asthma or hives.

Long-term use of oral corticosteroids can wreak havoc on your adrenal hormones, says Ira Finegold, M.D., chief of allergy and clinical immunology at St. Luke's–Roosevelt Hospital in New York City. "It shuts off your natural steroid. If you shut it off for a long enough time – usually several years – your body doesn't make it naturally even when you go off the medication," he explains. So oral corticosteroids can be taken safely when they are used only for several days at a time or, with long-term usage, on alternating days.

While nasal sprays are far safer, they can create similar problems if you exceed the recommended dose, usually two spurts per day, says Dr. Finegold. Nevertheless, both oral and inhaled corticosteroids have been demonstrated to decrease bone density in people who use high doses for long periods of time.

Yet another adrenal hormone, epinephrine, is produced by the adrenal medulla (the inner layer of the gland). A natural mechanism that keeps you ready for action, epinephrine shores up your blood pressure, constricts your blood vessels, and increases your heart rate. Once stimulated, epinephrine can help your body fend off an allergic reaction, even in minor cases.

In severe cases, a food or drug allergy can cause anaphylaxis, a life-threatening reaction that includes shortness of breath, a drop in blood pressure, and even loss of consciousness or shock. This creates the need for emergency treatment – normally an injection of synthetic epinephrine, which reverses the allergic reaction.

A number of other medications are used to treat allergy symptoms. These include antihistamines, which block histamines and therefore reduce annoying symptoms, and over-the-counter decongestants, like pseudoephedrine (brand name Sudafed), which help relieve congestion caused by allergies and have the advantage of not being as likely to make you drowsy. Over-the-counter antihistamines come with side effects, most notably drowsiness, but nonsedative antihistamines are available by prescription.

**Beware of ephedra.** Also known as ma huang, this Chinese herb is sometimes used for treating allergies, says Marianne Frieri, M.D., Ph.D., associate professor of medicine and pathology at the State University of New York, Stony Brook, and director of allergy and immunology at Nassau University

## THE HORMONE ZONE

# FOODS THAT FIGHT – OR FOSTER – ALLERGIES

Your allergies are acting up and you're miserable. So you cuddle up with a nice, hot cup of camomile tea. Sound good? Not if you're allergic to ragwort, says Marianne Frieri, M.D., Ph.D., associate professor of medicine and pathology at the State University of New York, Stony Brook, and director of allergy and immunology at Nassau University Medical Center on Long Island, New York. Camomile can cross-react with ragwort, aggravating your allergies. Likewise, people who suffer from birch tree allergies should avoid apples and kiwifruit when birch trees are pollinating, since these fruits may be related to the birch pollen protein.

It's not always easy to link allergy symptoms – asthma, sneezing, diarrhoea, and so on – to food allergies, says James Balch, M.D., of Rancho Santa Fe, California, co-author of *Prescription for Natural Healing*. Proteins found in cow's milk, for example, are common but often unrecognized allergens.

Refined sugars, caffeine, and most processed foods can also work against your immune system, prompting it to overreact to allergens, says Dr. Balch. Better to set your table with immune-supportive foods full of bioflavonoids, vitamins and friendly bacteria. Yoghurt, for example, contains lactobacilli – bacteria essential to immune function.

If you have allergies, Dr. Balch suggests making the following changes to your diet.

### FOODS TO ADD
- Bananas (magnesium) and other fruits (vitamin C, quercetin, and other nutrients)
- Yoghurt (lactobacilli)
- Vegetables, raw grains, and seeds

### FOODS TO SUBTRACT
- Milk and milk products, peanuts and nuts that grow on trees, wheat, soya, fish and shellfish, and eggs (these foods are responsible for 90 per cent of all food allergies)
- Refined sugars
- Chocolate, coffee and other caffeinated beverages
- Foods containing Azo dyes

Medical Center on Long Island, New York. Though natural, ephedra contains ephedrine, the same ingredient found in pseudoephedrine (such as Sudafed) and can cause insomnia or other, potentially dangerous side effects such as elevated blood pressure. So ephedra should be used only under the care of a knowledgeable health care practitioner, and then used with great caution.

And, as with Sudafed, if you are taking thyroid or high blood pressure medication, you should definitely avoid this herb, says Dr. Frieri, since it can cause heart palpitations when used with those drugs.

**Quiet symptoms with quercetin.** A supplement derived from bioflavonoids naturally found in citrus fruits and buckwheat, quercetin can stifle your body's reaction to allergens because it stabilizes mast cells so they don't release so many histamines, says James Balch, M.D., of Rancho Santa Fe, California, co-author of *Prescription for Nutritional Healing*. Dr. Balch recommends taking 500 milligrams twice a day. For best results, combine it with 100 milligrams of bromelain, a natural enzyme.

## Stress Hormones Worsen Allergies

Given the role of stress hormones in allergic reactions, one way to feel better during allergy season is to reduce stress, says Chris Meletis, N.D., naturopathic doctor and dean of clinical education and chief clinical officer at the National College of Naturopathic Medicine in Portland, Oregon. Stress causes your adrenal gland to secrete cortisol, a natural corticosteroid that is also essential for managing allergic reactions.

Too much stress can cause your body to exhaust its limited daily supply of cortisol, says Dr. Roby, causing a lot of adrenaline (its backup hormone) to be released into your system.

The problem is that adrenaline, which is supposed to be an emergency hormone, gives you "superhuman energy," according to Dr. Roby, and this is exhausting. If you are pumped up with adrenaline at bedtime, you won't be able to get the restful, REM (rapid eye movement) sleep you need. So, the next morning, until your body can replenish its daily cortisol supply, you'll still be running on adrenaline, causing a cycle of increasing tiredness that makes your body less resistant to allergy attacks.

There are a few things you can do to keep your adrenal hormones in balance.

**Take time out for yourself.** If you notice your allergies acting up after a stressful day, try to eliminate any additional stress. "Stress is usually a culmination of a number of stressors. Every straw you keep off your back helps," Dr. Meletis says. He recommends that you carve out a 20-minute block of time each day for some peaceful, stress-relieving activity, such as prayer or meditation. For other stress-reducing strategies, see Phase 2 of the Hormone-Balancing Programme, starting on page 275.

**Seek help from supplements.** Vitamin C and pantothenic acid are important antistress vitamins because they support the adrenal system, says Dr. Balch. "They are used together in the body in order to produce adrenal hormones," he says. If you're deficient in either of these vitamins, your system won't be able to manufacture enough cortisol to quell allergic reactions. Dr. Balch recommends taking between 100 and 300 milligrams of pantothenic acid a day, along with 100 milligrams of a B-complex supplement. He also recommends taking between 2000 and 5000 milligrams of vitamin C, in divided doses to obtain maximum benefit.

**Get to bed on time.** The US National Sleep Foundation has found that most women aged 30 to 60 sleep only a little more than 6 hours a night during the working week and that more women than men are likely to report they have insomnia. If you don't get enough sleep, you're not allowing your body the rest it needs to replenish those adrenal hormones that might have been used up the day before. Try to get an optimal 8 hours of shut-eye every night.

# Asthma

For some mysterious reason, more people have asthma now than they did a generation ago. And doctors are noticing nearly twice as many new cases of asthma in women as in men. So while it's not a female-only disease, women are clearly experiencing more than their fair share of wheezing, coughing and shortness of breath – the hallmarks of asthma.

The emerging mini-epidemic of asthma has been blamed on air pollution, obesity and demographic changes. But the prevalence of asthma in women points to another, recently discovered link: female hormones.

"Hormones need to be emphasized as a cofactor in asthma, along with other factors," says James Myers, M.D., clinical associate professor of medicine in the department of pulmonary medicine at Brown University in Providence, Rhode Island.

Part of the evidence is circumstantial: in children, it's boys, not girls, who seem most prone to asthma. In fact, boys are admitted twice as often to hospitals for asthma. Curiously, that trend begins to reverse itself around puberty – until, by the age of 20, an adult woman is nearly three times likelier to suffer from asthma than a male of the same age. Women are also more apt to be admitted to casualty for acute attacks. What's more, women may find symptoms affected by their menstrual cycles, pregnancy, or hormone replacement therapy.

# Premenstrual Asthma: The New "PMS"?

During an asthma attack, the lungs respond to some allergen or irritant in a way that makes it more difficult to breathe. The airway becomes inflamed, the muscles stiffen and the cells of the bronchial tubes produce mucus. Hence the tightness in your chest, wheezing, or coughing.

Asthma can be provoked by a number of things – allergens (like pollen, dust, or cat dander), irritants (like tobacco smoke or perfume) or even a change in the weather or exercise. Only recently, however, have researchers discovered that many women also find that their menstrual cycles aggravate asthma.

In fact, if you find yourself grabbing for your inhaler more frequently whenever you have your period, you're in good company. Studies have shown that as many as 40 per cent of women report significant asthma flare-ups during the perimenstrual phase (that is, 3 premenstrual days and 4 menstruating days).

Why, no one knows. "The mechanism underlying perimenstrual asthma is not well-understood," says Molly Zhongxin Gong, M.D., a senior research associate at the University of Michigan in Ann Arbor, who is conducting an intervention study on health education for women with asthma. Progesterone levels could be to blame. Several days before your period begins, the amount of progesterone in your body drops, explains Dr. Gong. "A lot of researchers think perimenstrual asthma is related to the decrease in progesterone because progesterone can relax the smooth muscle and decrease contractions, kind of like a bronchodilating drug often prescribed to relieve asthma symptoms." With a lower amount of progesterone available, your airway muscles are more inclined to tense up, stimulating or aggravating an asthma attack, Dr. Gong speculates. Progesterone may also have an anti-inflammatory effect, so a decrease in progesterone could increase asthma inflammation.

Fluctuating levels of oestrogen, the other reproductive hormone involved in menstrual cycling, could also be a factor, says Emil Skobeloff, M.D., clinical associate professor of emergency medicine at MCP-Hahnemann Medical College in Philadelphia and president of Consortium Clinical Research in Upland, Pennsylvania. Dr. Skobeloff conducted a study that found a fourfold increase in the number of asthmatic women going to casualty during the perimenstrual phase of their cycles. So he has reason to believe it's the sudden drop in oestrogen, rather than progesterone, that may make perimenstrual asthma flare-ups likelier.

"When the serum oestradiol levels fall sharply after being elevated during the third week, there are changes in the way the body and the lung respond to asthmatic challenges," he explains. "Stimuli that might not cause a problem during the rest of the month do [perimenstrually] because the receptors on and in the cells of the lung change and the internal environment of a woman's body is changing."

Though the pattern is less clear, hormones may also be responsible for pregnancy-related asthma changes. During pregnancy, asthma symptoms improve in about one-third of women, worsen in one-third and remain unchanged in one-third. That probably has to do with some very complex differences in the body's makeup. "Some people have oestrogen receptors where oestrogen will bind in the lung. It's a variable thing. Some people have more receptors than others," Dr. Myers says.

If you have asthma and you're still menstruating:

**Talk to your doctor.** "All women should remind their doctors that they have asthma," says Dr. Gong. "And let your asthma and allergy nurse know if it changes during your cycle." She can help you decide whether or not you need to step up treatment during the perimenstrual phase.

**Pay attention to where you are in your cycle.** "Women need to become more aware that the likelihood of a significant flare-up is very real during the perimenstrual interval," says Dr. Skobeloff. That means letting your doctor know that you're susceptible to hormonal influences, and possibly that asthma attacks should be treated aggressively on the days before and during your period. Consult your doctor to develop a treatment plan that will be appropriate for you. If you see no improvement after an hour, go to casualty where you can be treated effectively.

**You should avoid overusing bronchodilators.** If you are going through more than one canister per month, let your doctor know. She may need to change your treatment plan.

**Know your peak flow.** Because asthma by its very nature tends to come and go, you, too, may be unsure of whether or not you suffer from perimenstrual asthma. In a pilot study, Dr. Gong interviewed 22 women with asthma and found that the symptoms of one-third were exacerbated by their menstrual cycles. But many of the women interviewed had never before considered the possibility of a connection between asthma and their periods.

Dr. Gong recommends that all women gauge their peak flow rate twice daily for 1 month, using a peak flow meter. Your doctor will instruct you in the proper use of the meter, which measures the amount of air you can exhale with your strongest effort. By keeping a daily record, you will notice whether fluctuations occur around your period.

**Consider the Pill.** If asthma symptoms are severe, oral contraceptives can sometimes alleviate perimenstrual asthma. "With oral contraceptives, the hormonal fluctuation gets reduced and the symptom fluctuations get reduced, too," explains Dr. Gong.

## Corticosteroids: Breath Savers, Bone Breakers

If you take oral corticosteroids – that is, prednisone (Sterapred) or similar drugs in pill form – your doctor has probably already cautioned you that long-term use puts you at risk for osteoporosis. So doctors typically try to keep their use to a minimum.

A new study has revealed that high doses of *inhaled* corticosteroids, long considered safe for bones, also can pose a risk if used long term. The study, conducted by researchers at the University of Nottingham, tested 196 people (119 of whom were women) who had been taking inhaled corticosteroids. They found a definite correlation between the use of inhaled corticosteroids and a decrease in bone mineral density. The researchers warned that people taking high doses (over 800 milligrams a day) would enter their "fifth and sixth decades with lower bone mineral densities" than people on low doses.

For that reason, people taking more than 1000 milligrams per day of an inhaled corticosteroid should be monitored for bone density, says Gary Gross, M.D., of the Dallas Allergy and Asthma Center. "Just like any other medication, they should be used at the lowest-possible effective dose," he said. If a bone scan shows significant loss, your doctor may prescribe a biphosphonate drug to help rebuild bones. "That is the most effective treatment in steroid-induced osteoporosis," says Dr. Gross.

Dr. Gross notes that even high doses of inhaled steroids are better than oral corticosteroids, which are more directly absorbed into your system and, therefore, have a greater impact on bone formation. But, with both inhaled and oral medications, the risk of osteoporosis becomes amplified when other factors, such as chronic alcohol abuse and smoking, come into play. If you must use inhaled corticosteroids, at least take measures to minimize bone depletion from other causes by not drinking to excess or smoking.

**Another reason to get sufficient calcium.** "If you're not taking in enough calcium and you're on corticosteroids, you have two strikes against you," observes Dr. Gross. He recommends taking each day between 1000 and 1500 milligrams of calcium in a supplement to keep bones healthy.

**Include 800 IU of vitamin D every day.** It's essential for optimal absorption of calcium.

**Get up and go.** "Bone density is somewhat regulated by how much pressure you put on your bones," says P. Brock Williams, Ph.D., director of research at the IBT (ImmunoBioTech) Lab, a testing centre for allergies and other immunologic diseases, and clinical associate professor at the University of Missouri Medical School, both in Kansas City. Weight-bearing exercises – like walking, jogging and aerobics – can help ensure that your bones remain healthy as you age. Dr. Williams suggests exercising at least a half-hour each day to ensure that bone loss from corticosteroids is not compounded by inadequate activity.

## Live Right, Breathe Easy

Asthma can be controlled, but it can't be cured: once you have it, you can't get rid of it. Drugs like corticosteroids and bronchodilators can help. So always use them as directed. But there are plenty of ways to help manage your asthma and prevent it from getting worse.

**Get your quota of magnesium.** "Magnesium is a marvellous mineral," says Ann Louise Gittleman, C.N.S. (certified nutrition specialist), N.D., a clinical nutritionist and naturopathic doctor in Bozeman, Montana, and author of *The Living Beauty Detox Program*. It's an antispasmodic, so it may help to relax the bronchial tubes – and that improves the quality of your breathing and allows the severity of an asthma attack to be reduced, according to naturopathic practice. About three out of four women (and men) are magnesium deficient, however. To make sure you're covered, eat lots of leafy green vegetables, pulses and almonds – plus enough supplemental magnesium in divided doses throughout the day to be sure you're getting 350 milligrams each day.

**Fortify your adrenals.** Your adrenal glands are responsible for producing natural corticosteroids, anti-inflammatory hormones that keep down the swelling of your lungs and bronchial tubes. Vitamin C is essential to proper adrenal functioning, says Dr. Gittleman. In addition, alternative health researchers have shown that it can reduce histamine levels in the blood – important if your asthma is brought on by allergies. To realize these benefits, take up to 1,000 milligrams of vitamin C a day if you have asthma, suggests Dr. Gittleman.

**Fight it with fatty acids.** Omega-3 fatty acids are the precursors to the production of anti-inflammatory prostaglandins, says Dr. Gittleman. So they may control swelling of the bronchial tubes and better your breathing. Omega-3s are found in fatty fish – like salmon, mackerel and sardines – and also in flaxseeds, walnuts and pumpkin seeds. Dining on fatty fish three times a week can provide you with a good supply. Or take a fish oil supplement containing essential fatty acids. You'll benefit most from a dose of 1000 to 2000 milligrams a day, says Dr. Gittleman.

**Shed excess pounds.** Here's one more reason to lose weight if you carry extra pounds. The Nurses' Health Study – an ongoing study of 85,911 registered nurses – found that women who were overweight were more likely to develop asthma, particularly women who had put on weight since the age of 18. Another study, done at Helsinki University Central Hospital in Finland, found that symptoms and lung function significantly improved in obese people with asthma who lost weight.

"A couple of factors work against you when you're overweight," says Dr. Gross. For one thing, you have extra weight on your chest wall, and that exerts additional pressure on your lungs. In addition, the stomach and abdomen push up on the diaphragm, so breathing can be impaired by extra abdominal weight. How much weight must you lose? The Helsinki study found improvements in patients who cast off between 5 and 10 per cent of their original weight.

**Get your exercise.** Make every effort to get regular, purposeful exercise, says Dr. Williams. "It really helps those with asthma to breathe," he explains. The kind of heavy breathing you do with exercise conditions the muscles of your airways and rib cage, strengthening your ability to fight off asthma attacks. If, like many, your asthma is triggered by exercise, you may need to start out slowly, pace yourself, and possibly use your inhaler as directed before physical effort. "A lot of people can get by just by slowing down for a few minutes," says Dr. Williams. "Work within your limitations."

**Step up your stress control.** A high-stress lifestyle takes its toll on asthmatics. "When your body is under stress, it uses up vitamins and minerals you need to keep your body in balance," says Dr. Gittleman. Magnesium, for example, is eliminated through urine when you get stressed-out. Stress also influences how well you respond to inflammation, according to naturopathic medicine. That's because in order to handle stress, your body relies on cortisol, a natural corticosteroid that provides the same anti-inflammatory benefits of synthetic corticosteroids. When you use up all your natural cortisol battling stress, you'll have little left to quell inflammation in your airways.

While you might not be able to eliminate stress from your life, you can relieve tension through relaxation techniques like meditation and deep breathing. (See Phases 1 and 2 of the Hormone-Balancing Programme.) This may be especially important if you find yourself becoming stressed-out premenstrually. Women who suffer from PMS are likelier to suffer from other menstrual-related problems, like perimenstrual asthma, says Dr. Gong.

---

### THE HORMONE CONNECTION
## CAN HRT HELP ASTHMA?

Women who suffer from perimenstrual asthma may see symptoms improve after menopause, according to Molly Zhongxin Gong, M.D., a senior research associate at the University of Michigan in Ann Arbor. That's because the hormonal fluctuations that triggered asthma are gone. However, if you are undergoing hormone replacement therapy (HRT), your hormonal fluctuations may return, and your asthma symptoms may change again.

Women with severe asthma sometimes realize dramatic improvements from HRT. On the other hand, women who use oestrogen replacement at menopause may experience an increase in symptoms.

"Women vary greatly in how they react to oestrogen," says James Myers, M.D., clinical associate professor of medicine in the department of pulmonary medicine at Brown University in Providence, Rhode Island. "So HRT can help or hurt."

Dr. Myers has seen patients who require high doses of corticosteroids to manage their asthma. Putting them on oestrogen to protect them from bone loss proved so beneficial to their asthma that they were able to eliminate high-dose steroid treatments.

For that reason, only women with severe cases of asthma should consider undergoing hormone treatments to improve symptoms.

"It's still okay to give asthmatic women oestrogen," says Dr. Myers. "You and your doctors just need to be aware that you may get better, or you may get worse."

# Migraines

S ome women don't even have to look at the calendar or notice spotting on their underwear to know their period has arrived: they can
count on a headache to herald the start of their menstrual period.
Fluctuations in levels of oestrogen – especially a plummet of oestrogen just
prior to menstruation – affect not only the ovaries and uterus but the whole
body, including the brain, triggering migraines in sensitive women.

"Only 7 or 8 per cent of women have true menstrual migraines – that is,
migraines that occur only with menstruation," says Merle L. Diamond,
M.D., associate director of the Diamond Headache Clinic in Chicago.

Hormonal fluctuations at midcycle or just after your period can also
produce a migraine. Since migraines are often (but not always) associated
with changing oestrogen levels, many women experience migraines during
the first 3 months of pregnancy, when oestrogen is usually higher. For
others, migraines go on holiday during pregnancy – a good thing because
taking painkillers (and even herbal remedies) isn't safe during pregnancy,
especially during the first trimester, when the foetus is at a vulnerable stage
of development.

"In women with migraines, one-third get better when they're pregnant,
one-third get worse and one-third stay the same," says Dr. Diamond.

Taking – or stopping – oral contraceptives or hormone replacement therapy (HRT) may bring on migraines.

"Older, high-dose contraceptives worsened headaches in women," says Dr.
Diamond. "Newer, low-dose contraceptives are better tolerated. But you
should track your headaches in a headache journal to make sure their frequency doesn't change." Migraines may get worse (or disappear) during the
hormonal chaos we know as perimenopause, 7 to 10 years before your periods are gone for good. Migraines that occur more often in the middle of the
night may be associated with hot flushes. Some women feel a migraine
coming on when they're sexually aroused during lovemaking, while others
can enjoy foreplay only to find that orgasm induces a migraine, taking all the
fun out of sex, says Dr. Diamond.

## Temples of Doom

"Not all headaches are migraines, nor are they hormonal, and they need to
be treated accordingly," says Dr. Diamond.

If you come home from work feeling like someone has clamped a vice around your head and is pulling it tighter and tighter, you may have a tension-type headache.

If your stomach is doing flip-flops, blinking lights are dancing in front of your eyes, you have a severe, pounding pain (often on one side of the head), you're sensitive to light and sound, you don't want to move an inch, and all you want to do is stagger into bed, you have a migraine. If your headache lasts for most of the day or up to 3 days, you definitely have a migraine.

Doctors once believed that tension-type headaches and migraines were two entirely different entities. Now, this distinction isn't so clear-cut. Both types of headaches seem to be aspects of the same disorder, which may be caused by an abnormality – both electrical and chemical – deep in an area of the brain called the brain stem.

Many experts blame migraines on a disruption in the level of serotonin, a hormone-like pain-regulating chemical that conveys messages along nerve cells in your brain. If this chemical change in the brain is not corrected, the migraine triggers in the brain stem become activated. This in turn generates in the back of the brain a wave of electrical activity that moves slowly forwards. In some people this electrical activity excites nerve cells, creating an aura, most commonly experienced as flashing lights or tingling in the face or hands, says Roger Cady, M.D., medical director of the Headache Care Center in Springfield, Missouri. Other common warning symptoms are fatigue, mood changes, food cravings (chocolate, for example) and muscle pain in the head and neck.

If the migraine proceeds, nerves begin to lose control of blood vessels in the covering of the brain, called the meninges. As a result, these blood vessels begin to dilate, or swell. "The nerves at some point in this process can release peptides, and inflammation follows," says Dr. Cady. "If head movements or heartbeats stretch these inflamed vessels, you feel the throbbing pain of a full-blown migraine attack."

It was only in the past decade, in a breakthrough some have called "revolutionary", that K. M. A. Welch, M.D., vice chancellor for research at the University of Kansas Medical Center in Kansas City, discovered that migraines aren't caused by blood vessel abnormalities at all but may be caused by an electrical disorder in the brain. This discovery may lead to treatments for headaches that resist the best that modern and herbal medicine has to offer.

## Hormones Aren't the Only Trigger

"If you could keep your oestrogen levels high all the time, you probably would not get menstrual migraines," quips Kathleen Farmer, Psy.D., administrator of the Headache Care Center in Springfield, Missouri. According to the serotonin theory, stable levels of oestrogen may protect against migraines by assisting serotonin, says Dr. Cady.

In both men and women, oestrogen stabilizes serotonin, a chemical in the brain that allows nerve cells to communicate with one another. During a migraine, serotonin levels drop and the nervous system loses its ability to regulate some of its activities. Women prone to migraines become more vulnerable to an attack during their period, when the levels of oestrogen decrease, says Dr. Cady.

---

**THE HORMONE ZONE**

# HORMONAL HEADACHE?
## AVOID YOUR TRIGGER FOODS

Certain foods are associated with migraines.

Tyramine, a type of compound commonly found in food, seems to cause an immediate increase in serotonin, a brain chemical that triggers or contributes to migraine attacks. "A tyramine-free diet alleviated migraine symptoms in about 30 to 35 per cent of my patients," says Seymour Diamond, M.D., executive chairman of the National Headache Foundation in Chicago.

A diet rich in soya and other plant-derived oestrogens can help even out fluctuating hormone levels.

That wonderful caffeine lift you get from beverages containing caffeine is due to vasoconstriction or narrowing of the walls of blood vessels – blood moves through narrow veins faster, delivering oxygen and sugars to the brain more efficiently. Caffeine stimulates the adrenal glands to produce extra noradrenaline, the hormone that instructs your liver to convert its stored glycogen into blood sugar. Unfortunately, your head may ache after the effects of the caffeine have worn off, as veins dilate and your blood sugar level drops.

Caffeine is also a diuretic and washes magnesium out of the system. Low magnesium levels have been associated with migraines. It also overstresses the liver – the organ that breaks down reproductive hormones such as oestrogen. A dysfunctional liver causes extra hormone fluctuations that trigger migraines.

Between 40 and 60 per cent of migraine sufferers report that having beer, wine, or a cocktail precipitates a migraine, says Dr. Diamond.

Women's lives are punctuated by hormonal ups and downs during the menstrual cycle, pregnancy and menopause (which may partially explain why migraines afflict 23 million American women, yet only 8 million American men).

All these changes are registered by the supersensitive systems of those with migraines, says Seymour Diamond, M.D., executive chairman of the National Headache Foundation in Chicago. Women (and men) with migraines react to non-hormonal factors – say, weather, noise, or food – that might not affect others. When non-hormonal triggers converge with

**Refined sugar is quickly absorbed and burned, according to Connie Catellani, M.D., medical director and facilitator of family and internal medicine at the Miro Center for Integrative Medicine in Evanston, Illinois. After the sugar is used up, you'll start to feel tired, an energy deficit precipitated by low blood sugar. This will follow the initial energy rush (a condition called *reactive hypoglycaemia*). The up-and-down fluctuation in blood sugar levels can trigger migraines. Reactive hypoglycaemia also overtaxes the liver, which must work overtime to convert stored glycogen into usable sugar. Headache is often a symptom of hypoglycaemia and makes a migraine more likely, says Dr. Catellani.**

### FOODS AND ADDITIVES TO SUBTRACT

- Red wine, beer, mature cheese, yeast extracts and sauerkraut (some common foods that contain the amino acid tyramine*)

- Chocolate (contains phenylethylamine, related to tyramine)

- Processed and cured meats (like hot dogs and salami) and smoked fish, such as smoked salmon (contain the preservatives nitrites)

- Asian cooking, soya sauce, hydrolysed vegetable or plant protein, glutavene kombu extract and calcium caseinate (contain monosodium glutamate, MSG, a widely used flavour enhancer)

- Diet cola (contains aspartame, an artificial sweetener associated with headaches in many people, including those with migraine)

- Coffee, tea, caffeineated fizzy drinks

- Alcoholic beverages

- Refined sugar

*The tyramine content in foods will vary depending on processing and storage methods.

hormonal changes, you reach what experts call your "headache threshold" and you get a migraine, says Dr. Seymour Diamond.

Eliminating known migraine triggers, especially during times of hormonal flux, such as premenstrually or perimenopausally, is the first step towards managing migraines, says Dr. Farmer.

**If you smoke, quit.** One study found that women with menstrual-related migraines were more likely to be regular smokers, to smoke heavily and to have smoked longer than those free of migraines. If you have migraines with an aura, there is a minimally increased risk of having a stroke. But if you smoke and have migraines with aura, your chances of having a stroke increase dramatically, says Alan Rapoport, M.D., founder and co-director of the New England Center for Headache in Stamford, Connecticut.

**Get some exercise.** As explained in Phase 2 of the Hormone-Balancing Programme, exercise helps balance insulin and other critical hormones such as cortisol, in myriad ways. If you have migraines, regular aerobic exercise can cut down on the frequency and intensity of your headaches: it counterbalances the effects of stress, releases endorphins (painkilling neurotransmitters in the brain) and improves blood circulation everywhere, including the brain. "I recommend 20 to 30 minutes of exercise, four to five times a week," says Alexander Mauskop, M.D., director of the New York Headache Center in New York City.

**Follow a routine.** Women with migraines are especially sensitive to disruptions of *chronobiology*, or the internal rhythmic body clock. Irregular eating or sleeping habits can be devastating. Don't skip meals, and resist the urge to sleep late during weekends. "It's better to get up at the usual time and nap later in the day than to allow yourself to sleep in," says Dr. Farmer.

**Destress.** Scientists no longer believe that having migraines is a sign of psychological disturbance. Yet they do acknowledge that under stress the body increases production of adrenal hormones. These hormones constrict blood vessels, which expand once the adrenaline rush passes, triggering off a migraine. (For details on how to reduce stress, see Phase 2 of the Hormone-Balancing Programme starting on page 275.) Dr. Mauskop also recommends yoga, meditation and prayer.

**Try biofeedback.** Dr. Farmer specifically recommends thermal biofeedback, which she says is especially effective for migraines. During a session, you're hooked up to a special thermometer, which measures the temperature in your finger. The goal is to consciously warm your finger. You'll be taught how to do this through relaxation techniques.

Finger temperature is a measure of the overall amount of stress your body is carrying. In women with migraine, finger temperature is in the 20s°C (70s°F), compared with 29.5°C (85°F) for others. To benefit from biofeedback, migraine sufferers learn to voluntarily increase finger temperature to 36°C (96°F) – the first step in the process of relaxation and pain management, says Dr. Farmer.

**Consider acupuncture.** This ancient Chinese technique is helpful in treatment and prevention of migraines. A single session may bring relief, although some people may need more than six sessions before experiencing results. A few people may need monthly treatments to control the headaches.

According to traditional Chinese teaching, headaches are caused by blockages in the flow of energy. Evidence supports use of acupuncture in treating headaches of various causes. Acupuncture can help relieve headache pain because it rebalances a person's whole system, allowing blocked energy to flow again, says Joseph Blustein, M.D., a practising acupuncturist in Madison, Wisconsin.

## Start Simple

If avoiding the usual headache triggers doesn't work, dozens of medications, both over-the-counter and prescription, plus some herbs, are available. Finding what works for you might take some trial and error, especially if your headaches are hormonally related. As discouraging as this can be, don't give up – chances are, you'll find something that works for you.

"If one product doesn't work, try another," says Dr. Merle Diamond.

### THE HORMONE CONNECTION
## DON'T LET HEADACHES RUIN YOUR SEX LIFE

If your headaches heat up during a hot session of lovemaking, the cause is most likely changing levels of cortisol and oxytocin, hormones that rise during arousal, peak at orgasm, then fall afterwards. If this is a problem for you, Alexander Mauskop, M.D., director of the New York Headache Center in New York City, recommends taking NSAIDs (nonsteroidal anti-inflammatory drugs) an hour before intercourse. Whether you should use prescription or nonprescription medication depends on the severity of your headaches. Check with your doctor first.

"I always tell people to try the simple things first," says Dr. Seymour Diamond.

**Supplement with magnesium.** About 50 per cent of people with migraines have low magnesium levels, says Dr. Mauskop. He recommends 400 milligrams of supplementary magnesium daily, taken once a day with a meal.

**Give feverfew a try.** Evidence suggests that this herb (*Tanacetum parthenium*) may prevent as well as relieve migraines, says Dr. Mauskop. He recommends 100 milligrams a day, taken with meals, if you are migraine-prone.

Be aware that a few people – one out of 10 – who regularly use feverfew experience rebound symptoms (anxiety, sleep problems and muscle and joint aches) after stopping use. These may be signs of withdrawal from melatonin, a light-sensitive hormone present in feverfew.

**Look for butterburr.** Dr. Mauskop often recommends this herb (*Petasites hybridus*), first studied in Germany and now available in the United States. Dr. Mauskop recommends using a preparation of butterburr called Petadolex, which is available in 50-milligram capsules. Take one capsule of Petadolex twice a day. (Petadolex is not available in the UK but many US Web sites will ship it.)

**Make a cup of ginger tea.** Some people report less pain and frequency of migraines while drinking ginger tea. It's available in tea bags, or you may use the fresh root. Make a tea from ½ to 2 teaspoons of fresh, grated ginger and pour into a thermos. You'll have enough to sip all day. Drink this to prevent a migraine or to ease the pain if you already have one, says Connie Catellani, M.D., medical director and facilitator of family and internal medicine at the Miro Center for Integrative Medicine in Evanston, Illinois.

## The Right Way to Use Pain Pills

If you've been popping aspirin, paracetamol and ibuprofen like sweets, stop. They may be making your headaches worse, called the rebound effect.

Used correctly, though, over-the-counter medication can help. Some women with mild migraines respond well to over-the-counter medications, particularly if they're taken at the first sign of an impending attack. Look for combinations of aspirin and/or paracetamol with caffeine and/or codeine.

You should always consult your doctor after your first serious headache, whatever time of month it occurs. You should also consult your doctor if you're suffering from chronic headaches, to rule out (or treat) any serious illnesses.

Let your doctor know what you've already tried and how the headaches are

*Escape from* **HORMONE HELL**

# SHE WANTS TO FEEL HUMAN AGAIN

**Q:** Every month without fail, a few days before my period, I get racking headaches that last a day into my period. My head feels like it's going to explode. I see flashing lights and large black blotches. My arms and legs are numb, and sometimes they get very cold. I feel queasy, and often I throw up. I can't work, I can't cook, I can't make love or take care of my kids. Painkillers seem to make things worse. For 23 days a month, I'm a wife, mother, employee, and human being. But for the other 5, I'm a whimpering wreck. I've got to find an answer!

Alexander Mauskop, M.D., director of the New York Headache Center in New York City, replies: Start by making an appointment with your doctor. While hormonal changes associated with your cycle seem to be the main trigger, they may not be the only trigger. Various irritants may be assaulting your sensitive system. Falling oestrogen levels right before your period may merely be the proverbial straw that breaks the camel's back.

Do you like smoked foods? Do you order Chinese takeaways? Are you fond of diet cola? Are you a chocoholic? Do you crave your morning coffee? All have been associated with migraines. Eliminate them from your diet, especially during your migraine-prone days.

You should also eat at regular hours and avoid skipping meals. Your body is unusually sensitive to changes in routine at this time of month. Make sure you go to sleep and get up at roughly the same time each day.

Next, try some holistic remedies, such as magnesium and a B-complex supplement, along with herbs (such as feverfew or valerian), and aerobic exercise. If the headaches persist, find a practitioner who uses acupuncture or biofeedback.

Nondrug treatments usually take some time to kick in. It may take two or three cycles to see improvement. If you're desperate and want rapid and dramatic changes, try NSAIDs such as naproxen (Naprosyn or Synflex) or prescription drugs in the family of triptans. Taken preventively for a few days before your usual migraine is expected, one of these may bring fast relief. Be sure to follow label directions with the over-the-counter forms. If not, you can take a prescription medication (such as sumatriptan) if you develop symptoms.

Medication can give you time for the dietary changes and other lifestyle improvements to correct whatever system imbalance has been causing your headaches in the first place.

affecting your life, and whether or not they seem to be related to hormonal fluctuations. That way, you can tailor the treatment to your particular needs.

Your doctor may suggest certain prescription drugs that abort migraines in progress (although they, too, can create a rebound effect if overused).

**Triptans.** Available in self-injectable or oral form, a newer family of drugs – such as sumatriptan (Imigran), naratriptan (Naramig), rizatriptan (Maxalt) and zolmitriptan (Zomig) – seem to imitate some of the beneficial actions of serotonin and also block inflammation. These drugs start working in less than an hour and may stop the pain in 2 to 4 hours. Triptans have "revolutionized the treatment of migraine headaches," says Dr. Rapoport.

**Prescription nonsteroidal anti-inflammatory drugs (NSAIDs).** NSAIDs such as naproxen sodium (Naprosyn, Synflex) and rofecoxib (Vioxx) reduce inflammation, raise the pain threshold and seem to prevent blood vessels from dilating.

## Heading Off Migraines Before They Start

Sounds like an oxymoron, but taking certain prescription medications before you have pain can reduce the frequency, duration, or intensity of headaches with no rebound effect. If your migraine attacks are frequent (three times a week or more), your migraines don't respond to triptans, or you are unable to take triptans because of heart disease, your doctor may put you on a daily, preventive medication, says Dr. Rapoport. Options include:

**Beta-blockers.** Originally developed for control of blood pressure, these medications work on the blood vessels and the nervous system to decrease migraines. They do so by regulating serotonin and noradrenaline production, which keeps the blood vessels in the head from dilating. Some of the most commonly used beta-blockers are Inderal, Corgard, Tenormin and Lopresor.

**Calcium channel blockers.** The three main calcium channel blockers are diltiazem (Tildiem, Istin), nifedipine (Adalet) and verapamil (Cordilox). These drugs stabilize blood vessels in the brain, but they aren't as effective as the beta-blockers for migraine.

**Antidepressants.** These include so-called tricyclic antidepressants (such as Anatramil, Prothiaden, Sinequan, Gamanil, Allegion and Tofranil), MAO inhibitors (such as Nardil), and selective serotonin reuptake inhibitors, or SSRIs (such as Prozac, Lustral and Seroxat). All three may be useful, especially if your headaches are accompanied by depression or sleep disturbance. With the advent of triptans, they're prescribed less frequently for headache alone.

**Anti-epileptics.** Many anti-epileptic drugs – such as valproate (Epilim), gabapentin (Neurontin) and topiramate (Topamax) – are used for migraine prevention.

**Asthma drugs.** The newest category of medications being used for migraine prevention includes asthma drugs such as montelukast (Singulair) and zafirlukast (Accolate). They treat asthma by decreasing inflammation in the lungs and probably treat migraines by decreasing inflammation in the brain.

All medications have side effects. Some interact poorly with other drugs or should be avoided by women with particular conditions. Your doctor can help you choose a drug that's most suited to your unique profile, including your hormone status.

## Premenstrual and Menstrual Headache Relief

Most experts recommend treating these headaches without drugs when possible. Start by eliminating triggers, as well as trying aerobic exercise, biofeedback, acupuncture, herbs and vitamin/mineral supplementation. If these measures don't work, or if you need immediate relief, you may need pharmaceuticals or hormone therapy – at least for a while.

"I prescribe a large dose of a powerful NSAID such as Naprelan (Naprosyn) to be taken preventively for 3 to 4 days before the period, and stopped just before the period ends," says Dr. Rapoport.

If NSAIDs aren't effective, Dr. Rapoport adds oestrogen replacement to the regime just prior to the start of menstruation to boost and stabilize falling oestrogen levels.

Dr. Catellani recommends trying natural progesterone for premenstrual headaches. Progesterone counterbalances the impact of falling oestrogen levels, which can lower the headache threshold in many women.

## Safe Solutions during Pregnancy

"Avoiding medication during pregnancy begins *before* you become pregnant," says Dr. Cady. "Adopting a healthy lifestyle and modifying your diet is your best chance at a pain-free pregnancy."

"Learn biofeedback before you become pregnant," suggests Dr. Farmer. "Then if you do develop a migraine, you're already versed in a drug-free way to relieve the pain."

Vitamin and mineral supplementation is safe during pregnancy, notes Dr.

Rapoport, who recommends magnesium and riboflavin to pregnant women prone to migraines. While pregnant, discuss the proper supplement dosage with your doctor before you start taking them. Magnesium comes in different types, and some may cause diarrhoea. If this happens, try other types of magnesium until you find the right one for you.

If natural measures don't work, drugs may be necessary because repeated bouts of nausea, vomiting and loss of appetite can lead to dehydration, which can be harmful to both mother and foetus. Check with your doctor before taking any prescription or nonprescription medication, says Dr. Cady.

Acupuncture is drug-free and safe – with an important caveat. Certain acupuncture points that bring relief to nonpregnant women might be of concern during pregnancy. "Acupuncture can be used effectively for headaches associated with pregnancy, as long as the practitioner knows what he or she is doing," says Dr. Blustein. So if you're considering acupuncture, be absolutely certain your acupuncturist has experience working with pregnant women.

"Some pregnancy-induced headaches are caused not by hormones but by the shift in gait and the stress on the back caused by the growing baby," says Dr. Catellani. "Often, these structural changes place pressure on the base of the skull and can lead to headaches." In that case, Dr. Catellani recommends chiropractic or massage therapy. If you decide to give one of these a try, make sure your practitioner has experience working with pregnant women.

## Migraines from Birth Control Pills

Some studies have suggested a link between oral contraceptives and strokes in people with migraines. These studies generally refer to older oral contraceptives, released during the 1960s and 1970s, which contained higher levels of oestrogen. If you're migraine-prone, check with your doctor to be sure you're taking low-dose oestrogen oral contraceptives.

"Unless their migraines are extremely complicated – that is, accompanied by confusion, partial paralysis, or vision loss – women who already suffer from migraines can probably start taking today's new low-oestrogen pills," says Dr. Seymour Diamond. But if you've developed migraines only *after* beginning oral contraceptives, you should find another form of birth control, he advises. Barrier methods, such as diaphragms and condoms, provide protection without introducing hormones into your system.

"Also, if you smoke and take the Pill and have migraines, quit," says Dr. Merle Diamond. (Smoking significantly contributes to your risk for stroke.)

Some women experience migraines while taking oral contraceptives for the same reason that they experience migraines during the menstrual cycle. The usual contraceptive regime involves taking oestrogen for 21 days, followed by a 7-day break, followed by another 21 days of oestrogen. Menstruation takes place during the break.

Eliminating that break can prevent migraines, says Dr. Rapoport. Women who are taking oestrogen consistently without pause should take additional progesterone if it's not in their birth control pills, he adds, because this will reduce their risk of endometrial cancer. All of this should be done only under a doctor's supervision.

## Help for Menopausal Migraines

If you have migraines in your twenties, thirties, or forties, you could get lucky: migraines often abate after menopause because cyclical fluctuations are no more. If they don't, diet, exercise, biofeedback and acupuncture may relieve menopausal headaches. NSAIDs taken preventively might help but should be used cautiously. Antidepressants might be a better choice, especially if

### ON THE WEB & Other Resources

The best organization for migraine in Britain is the City of London Migraine Clinic, run by an excellent doctor, Dr. Anne McGregor.
**City of London Migraine Clinic**
22 Charterhouse Square
London ECIM 6DX
Tel: 0207 251 3322
*www.colmc.org.uk*

**Migraine Trust**
45 Great Ormond Street
London WCIN 3HZ
Tel: 0207 831 4818

**Migraine Action Association**
Unit 6
Oakley Hay Lodge Business Park
Great Folds Road

Great Oakley
Northants NN18 9AS
Tel: 01536 461333
E-mail: *info@migraine.org.uk*

**The International Headache Society**
Oakwood
9 Willowmead Drive
Prestbury
Cheshire SK10 4BU
Tel: 01625 828663
E-mail: *rosemary@ihs.u-net.com*
*www.@w-h-a.org*
(the IHS is linked to the World Headache Association, hence w-h-a)

**The World Cluster Headache Support Group**
*www.clusterheadaches.com*

you're experiencing mood swings as well as headaches, says Dr. Merle Diamond.

Hormone replacement therapy can help some women but doesn't work for everyone. Replacing oestrogen may have little or no effect on menopausal migraines. And when it helps, it's not because the oestrogen has been replaced but because the oestrogen levels have been stabilized. "When a perimenopausal woman with migraines comes to see me, sometimes I try HRT – always in the form of a patch because that provides a steady intake of oestrogen without fluctuations," says Dr. Mauskop.

Exercisers, take note: "Wearing the patch during exercise can increase absorption of oestrogen and cause headaches. The solution may be to switch to an oral form of instead of the patch," says Dr. Merle Diamond.

If your migraines started after you began HRT, you should discontinue it, says Dr. Rapoport. Try the alternatives in chapter 11 and in the chapters Hot Flushes on page 298, Night Sweats on page 304 and Vaginal Dryness and Irritation on page 305.

# Fibromyalgia

Think back to the last time you had flu – not just a cold, but real influenza, the kind where you ache all over and getting out of bed is as daunting as climbing Mount Everest.

This is what fibromyalgia can feel like – only there is no chance of you getting better after a week.

With fibromyalgia, muscles are achy and hurt more when used or when any kind of pressure is applied. It is as though the slightest sensations were amplified in an echo chamber until they are unbearable, says David Nye, M.D., who has specialized in treating fibromyalgia for more than 10 years in the department of neurology at Luther Midelfort–Mayo Health System in Eau Claire, Wisconsin.

When you have fibromyalgia, this hypersensitivity can last a lifetime; there is no cure. But there are plenty of things you can do to break fibromyalgia's vicious cycle of pain, poor sleep, exhaustion and stress and return to a productive life.

Many of the recommendations for ME also apply to fibromyalgia. (See page 383.) "There is a great deal of overlap in the symptoms," says Dr. Nye. About two-thirds of people with ME also have fibromyalgia, and vice versa.

## Not a Bunch of Whiners

To those who do not have fibromyalgia, the complaints of constant pain may sound suspiciously like hypochondria. After all, the condition has no outward symptoms. Even if you have it, you look healthy. So for a long time, many doctors did not take these complaints seriously, often dispensing bad advice, says Devin J. Starlanyl, M.D., who lives with fibromyalgia and myofascial pain and has written two books on the subject, including *Fibromyalgia and Chronic Myofascial Pain Syndrome: A Survival Manual.*

"I spent years being told to work out the pain," says Dr. Starlanyl. "My doctors suggested I get involved in sports, so I was playing ice hockey several times a week. It didn't work.

"Or doctors often prescribe pain pills for fibromyalgia and tell people to go back to work, saying 'There is nothing wrong with you; it's all in your mind,'" says Dr. Starlanyl. But extreme exercise and pain pills are not the answer.

## A Real Test for Real Pain

Though they don't know exactly what causes it, researchers have built up a growing body of evidence that fibromyalgia is very real. No one can feel or see your pain, but they can see abnormalities in brain functioning, and changes in body chemistry, that are associated with it. And there is a simple test that a doctor can perform by using a single finger.

People with fibromyalgia don't just ache all over; they hurt when you press on specific spots on their bodies. This is the key to diagnosing fibromyalgia.

The doctor simply pushes on 18 of these "tender points" with about 1 kilogram (2 pounds) of pressure (enough to whiten the base of the fingernail) – and, provided you also have had widespread pain for at least 3 months – if you experience pain, not just tenderness, in at least 11 of these spots, you have fibromyalgia.

Actually, the tender point test was originally intended as a tool for research, to decide who qualifies for inclusion in fibromyalgia studies, rather than who qualifies for treatment, says Dr. Starlanyl. So even if you have pain in fewer than 11 tender points, you may still have the symptoms of fibromyalgia – widespread pain and hypersensitivity – and you may well benefit from the treatments for fibromyalgia.

## Why You Wake Up Tired and Sore

Another factor that distinguishes women with fibromyalgia from others is their levels of substance P (for "pain"), the key chemical neurotransmitter for sending pain signals to the brain. In those with fibromyalgia, substance P levels in the spinal fluid are three to four times normal, which provides strong evidence the pain is not imaginary. (This is the key difference between fibromyalgia and ME; typically in people with ME, substance P levels are normal.)

These high substance P levels appear to be a key cause of the pain amplification characteristic of fibromyalgia. In technical terms, doctors classify pain as either "allodynia" (nonpainful sensations are transformed into pain sensations) or "hyperalgesia" (pain sensations are amplified).

If you have fibromyalgia and could watch your brain waves while you sleep, you'd notice that you get a less-than-normal amount of slow, delta-wave sleep, the deep sleep essential for the repair of the body. As a result, you probably wake up frequently throughout the night and are still tired when morning comes.

This lack of deep sleep has broader implications.

"It's during delta sleep that growth hormone is produced and that most muscle repair takes place," says Laurence Bradley, Ph.D., professor of medicine at the University of Alabama at Birmingham who specializes in fibromyalgia research. "Growth hormone apparently facilitates muscle tissue repair."

The theory is that the disruptions in delta sleep result in lower levels of growth hormone, says Dr. Bradley, which might explain the muscle damage and pain in people with fibromyalgia.

In those without fibromyalgia, vigorous exercise not only builds muscles; it also triggers an increase in growth hormone levels. But in those with fibromyalgia, it does not. This may be due to abnormally high levels of other hormones that inhibit growth hormone production.

## What Hormone Tests Don't Tell

Doctors can't diagnose fibromyalgia by measuring blood hormone levels. Hormone levels in those with fibromyalgia aren't normal, yet they are not abnormal either.

"There is no diagnostic hormone that's consistently high or low," says R. Paul St. Amand, M.D., an endocrinologist and assistant clinical professor at UCLA School of Medicine in Marina Del Rey. They sometimes tend to be near the upper or lower limits for what is considered normal. What researchers have focused on instead is the production of one hormone in response to the level of another hormone and the timing of this response. As with so many other hormone-related conditions, scientists cite this as an abnormality in the hypothalamic–pituitary–adrenal axis.

"Fibromyalgia is more a syndrome – a group of symptoms – than a specific disease," says Robert McMurray, M.D., associate professor of medicine at the University of Mississippi at Jackson, who is studying hormonal and neuroendocrine therapies for fibromyalgia.

Fibromyalgia may not even be a single syndrome, says Dr. Starlanyl. "There arc so many different hormonal axes that can be out of balance in each fibromyalgia patient. Hormonal levels can be different in different patients." But overall, the patterns of hormones and neurotransmitters appear to be different from those of people without fibromyalgia.

While disabling fatigue is the primary problem for those with ME, pain and tenderness are the overriding concern for those with fibromyalgia, says Harvey Moldofsky, M.D., professor emeritus of psychiatry and medicine at the University of Toronto, who has been a leading researcher into fibromyalgia since 1975.

Or as Dr. Starlanyl puts it: "People with CFS (ME) tend to sleep an awful lot, while people with fibromyalgia can't sleep much."

Until scientists find a cure, a good diet, moderate exercise, stress reduction and improved sleep can all work together to help those with fibromyalgia.

## The Stress–Diet–Pain Connection

As discussed in Phase 2 of the Hormone-Balancing Programme, stress has a huge effect on hormones. It triggers the fight-or-flight response, causing your glands to produce epinephrine (adrenaline) and norepinephrine, hormones that normally speed up your system, giving you more energy. But with fibromyalgia, the body is struggling because it has a limited capacity to generate energy, and the added burden of stress makes it much worse.

"Whether it's physical stress or mental stress, you are calling on reserves you don't have," says Dr. St. Amand.

To get at the cause of any chronic pain condition, you have to identify the factors that are contributing to it. Excess sugar and other refined carbohydrates, and stimulants such as caffeine, can cause your body to produce excess adrenaline, and generally throw your hormones out of whack, says Dr. Starlanyl. "So one of the best ways to restore hormonal balance is to eat a good diet." She's found that a diet with 30 per cent of total calories from protein and 40 per cent from carbohydrates is helpful in balancing hormones, whether or not you have fibromyalgia. (For details on following this type of diet, see "Protein, Fat and Carbohydrates: The Key Is Balance" on page 114.)

*Escape from* **HORMONE HELL**

# DRUGS MAKE HER CHRONIC PAIN WORSE

**Q:** I've had fibromyalgia-type pain for 5 years. It started when the car I was driving was rear-ended by another vehicle. It was bearable until I fell hard on a slippery floor at work 2 years ago and twisted my neck.

Before then I never had the severity of pain I have now. Sometimes I ache all over, and it just won't go away. I get up in the morning feeling like I never got any sleep, and I can't hold down a job. The doctors seemed sceptical and told me I just had to work through it. I had a full-time job for years and brought up a daughter; I am not faking it.

Recently I've been seeing a rheumatologist, who diagnosed me with fibromyalgia. She put me on venlafaxine (Efexor), an antidepressant and pain reliever, but my blood pressure went sky-high, and I had to stop after a few days. I tried other medications, and they didn't help either. What can I do for the pain? I'll try anything!

David Nye, M.D., who has specialized in treating fibromyalgia for more than 10 years in the department of neurology at Luther Midelfort–Mayo Health System in Eau Claire, Wisconsin, responds: painkillers won't solve your problem. Anti-inflammatory medications – such as Vioxx, Celebrex and other NSAIDs – do nothing for fibromyalgia because there is no inflammation. And they interfere slightly with deep sleep.

Though they may help for a while, you should also avoid narcotics and other prescription painkillers because the pain actually increases as they wear off. And they block the deep sleep you vitally need.

With fibromyalgia, it doesn't work very well to treat the individual symptoms, such as pain. You need to treat the underlying fibromyalgia problems, and then all the symptoms will improve. In at least half of cases, we can get patients free of pain most of the time.

Start with exercise. Through the right amount of aerobic exercise, you can trigger the production of endorphins. These are the body's own hormones that relieve pain, help you sleep better, and trigger other benefits.

Daily exercise will help you sleep better, and deep sleep helps restore your hormonal balance. Make sure you go to sleep at the same time each night to reset your hormonal rhythms. There are prescription antidepressants that may help you sleep, such as Trazodone, so talk to your doctor.

# Exercise: Easy Does It, Please

If you have fibromyalgia, it's easy to fall into a cycle of inactivity, poor fitness, negative attitudes, despondency and increasingly poor sleep, says Dr. Moldofsky. After all, you hurt. And when you exercise too much, you can hurt for days.

There may be a hormonal reason for this. Researchers at Oregon Health Sciences University in Portland put people with fibromyalgia on a treadmill until they were exhausted, and then checked their growth hormone levels. Unlike in other people, in those with fibromyalgia, growth hormone levels did not increase. Because growth hormone seems to play a key role in repairing muscles, this could explain why strenuous, muscle-building exercise does not work for those with fibromyalgia.

**Walk around the block.** Dr. Moldofsky recommends walking for his out-of-shape patients, and he starts by asking them how far they can walk without being tired.

"One woman told me she could walk one block, so I told her to start by walking a block every day. 'But doctor,' she said, 'how do I get back home?' So she had to start by walking a half-block a day," says Dr. Moldofsky with a laugh.

The point is you have to start somewhere and then gradually increase the amount of exercise at a comfortable pace.

"We're not talking about muscle building or weight lifting," says Dr. Moldofsky. "You don't want to tear up muscle. It should be aerobic exercise. This improves oxygen circulation and your general metabolism." Housework and running up and down stairs are more likely to wear you out and are not a substitute for an aerobic workout, says Dr. Nye. The key is to trigger your body's production of endorphins, the body's own hormonal pain relievers, but not overdo it.

In addition to brisk walking, try swimming or other water exercises, bicycling or stationary bikes, a treadmill, or gentle aerobic dance, says Dr. Nye. Jogging, vigorous aerobic dance and weight lifting are too strenuous for most patients.

**Midday is best.** For people with fibromyalgia, the best time to exercise is the middle of the day – between 10 a.m. and 3 p.m. – when they have the least fatigue and pain, recommends Dr. Moldofsky.

**Check your pulse.** Dr. Nye recommends starting with 3 to 5 minutes of gentle aerobic exercise a day, and gradually increasing this to 20 to 30 minutes a day. Take a few minutes to first stretch your muscles, and start out slowly. Then get your heart rate up above your normal resting rate and into the lower aerobic exercise range. If you don't exercise hard enough, you're wasting your time, but if you exercise too much, you're hurting yourself.

Check your pulse, using a watch or a heart rate monitor, available at sports shops. Find your resting heart rate, and then calculate your aerobic heart rate target, using the following formula:

*(220 − age − resting heart rate) × 0.6 + resting heart rate*

For example, for a 50-year-old woman with a resting heart rate of 70:

*(220 − 50 − 70) = 100 × 0.6 + 70 = 130*

So for this woman, the goal of aerobic exercise is to get her heart rate up to 130 beats per minute. As you get into shape and your resting heart rate changes, recalculate the formula.

A treadmill that automatically adjusts its pace by monitoring your heart rate is ideal, says Dr. Nye. But with practice, you can learn to sense your limits without a heart monitor.

**Exercise every day.** An aerobic workout apparently triggers a cascade of good hormonal responses. If you find that aerobic exercise gives you more energy and reduces your pain, try exercising more often during the day. And best of all, it helps you sleep more soundly, which is vital to getting back to normal. (You may need to do a lighter workout on days you are feeling worse.)

## Sleep Well

Anyone who has spent a night tossing and turning knows she's not going to wake up feeling refreshed. With fibromyalgia, this is a chronic problem that seems to play a central role in the cycle of pain.

When Dr. Moldofsky first observed the brain waves of fibromyalgia patients during sleep, he found that when they entered deep sleep – characterized by slow, delta brain waves – faster, alpha brain waves appeared on top of the delta waves, apparently disrupting patients' deep sleep. Later, he performed a classic experiment, disrupting the sleep of healthy but sedentary test subjects with noise whenever they entered deep sleep. After several days of that, they were aching all over, as if they had fibromyalgia. When he tried this experiment on long-distance runners, however, they still got a good night's sleep.

When you don't get that good "delta" sleep, you don't produce the growth hormones needed to repair your aching muscles, says Dr. Moldofsky. Another consequence of disrupted sleep is that your immune system becomes overactive, says Dr. Nye, causing your body to make excess cytokines, chemical messengers that trigger aching, fatigue and weakness, making you feel like you had the flu. And that aching does not make getting to sleep any easier. Somehow you have to break that cycle.

Sleeping pills generally don't help people with fibromyalgia, says Dr. Moldofsky. Sure, they will put you to sleep, but some (including benzodiazepines, like Nitrazepam, Dalmane and Rohypnol) actually reduce delta-wave sleep. What counts is not the quantity of sleep but the quality.

**Ask your doctor about medication to improve deep sleep.** Some antidepressants may help you get a good, sound sleep, says Dr. Nye. He often prescribes Trazodone for those he treats for fibromyalgia, typically starting with 50 milligrams, then gradually increasing the dose until the person is sleeping well. Amitriptyline (Triptafen) also works but is less popular because of side effects. He sometimes also prescribes muscle relaxants like dantrolene (Dantrium). The medications all help by fostering deep sleep, says Dr. Nye.

**Go to bed at the same time every night.** "Keeping to a regular schedule helps restore the body's hormonal rhythms," says Dr. Nye.

**Eliminate stimulants.** That means nicotine and caffeine.

**Don't overdo it during the day.** Learn your limits, says Dr. Nye.

**Get checked for other sleep disorders.** People with fibromyalgia may also have other sleep disorders that require medical treatment, such as sleep apnoea or periodic leg movements. So if you snore, your legs twitch, or you are excessively sleepy during the day despite getting enough sleep at night, see your doctor.

**Avoid troublesome foods.** Many individuals with fibromyalgia seem to do better on a simple, low-fat diet, minimizing fatty meats and dairy fat, fried foods, spicy foods and sauces, and simple sugars. Experiment by eliminating suspect foods from your diet. This may help you sleep better, especially if you have irritable bowel syndrome (which seems to occur in up to 50 per cent of patients). For those sensitive to lactose, eliminating milk products might help relieve disturbances in bowel functions.

When you add it all together, chances are you will sleep better, says Dr. Nye. And then your hormonal balance will improve, resulting in less pain and more energy during the day.

## Break the Stress Cycle with Meditation

With fibromyalgia, your nervous system does not quieten down as quickly as normal when you go to sleep, says Dr. Moldofsky. Meditation – or any activity that turns your mind away from your pain – may help you break your stressful response to your pain.

Dr. Starlanyl agrees: "Fibromyalgia is like an amplified sensory system, and there's nothing better for turning it down than meditation."

Brain wave biofeedback and other relaxation techniques also may help reduce stress.

The slow, meditative exercises of tai chi and chi gung (qi gong) can both help you relax and provide gentle exercise. But to avoid hurting your muscles, you need to be careful not to do too many repetitions of the same move, advises Dr. Starlanyl.

Other options Dr. Starlanyl recommends trying are acupuncture and myofascial trigger point massage.

Dr. Nye reports that many individuals with fibromyalgia find that weekly massages are great for reducing pain and stiffness. Massage therapists will often provide a discount for a package of 5 or 10 visits.

## Staying Well

There's no cure for fibromyalgia, so you should be prepared for occasional flare-ups, warns Dr. Nye. Relapses can be caused by increased stress, skipping exercise for a day, staying up as little as 1 hour late, a disruption in your daily routine – or for no apparent reason.

Don't fight it; try to get some extra rest. Take a warm bath, and perhaps get a massage. But don't miss your daily aerobic exercise, even if you have to ease up a bit. And continue stretching.

Once you are feeling better, try to figure out what caused the relapse, and correct the problem.

"With a little effort, most patients can eventually make it to the point where they feel significantly better most of the time," says Dr. Nye.

But don't just depend on your doctor.

Says Dr. Nye: "Patients who learn as much as they can about fibromyalgia generally fare better than those who don't."

## Still Troubled? Consider Counselling

Naturally, being in pain can be pretty stressful. But not knowing what's wrong with you can really frazzle your nerves. One of the benefits of getting accurately diagnosed with fibromyalgia, even if there is no cure for it, is knowing you don't have some more frightening and fatal disease.

Still, fibromyalgia can be pretty depressing, and sometimes people need

## ON THE WEB & Other Resources

The Arthritis Research Campaign (ARC) produce free booklets on aspects of arthritis, one of which is on fibromyalgia:
**The Arthritis Research Campaign**
 PO Box 177
Chesterfield
Derbyshire S41 7TQ
*www.arc.org.uk*

The Fibromyalgia Association is a pressure and self-help group:
**The Fibromyalgia Association**
PO Box 206
Stourbridge
West Midlands DY9 8YL
Tel: 0870 220 1232
*www.fibromyalgia-associationuk.org*

Arthritis Care offers self-help support and leaflets on various subjects including fibromyalgia:
**Arthritis Care**
18 Stephenson Way
London NW1 2HD
Freephone: 0808 800 4050
Tel: 0207 380 6555
*www.arthritiscare.org.uk*

STIFF is a small national charity which provides information and support for fibromyalgia sufferers:
**STIFF**
PO Box 1484
Newcastle-under-Lyme
Staffs ST5 7UZ
Callback service at: 01782 562366
*www.stiffuk.org*

cognitive therapy to help them overcome the negative attitudes they have accumulated about themselves and their capabilities.

"They will often say 'I can't do anything.' Counselling helps them deal with their life in a much more constructive way," says Dr. Moldofsky.

A psychologist, a psychiatrist, or someone who is skilled in psychotherapy may be able to help.

# ME (Myalgic Encephalomyelitis)

D enise Sasiain wants her life back.

Before she came down with ME (Myalgic Encephalomyelitis), also known as chronic fatigue syndrome, Denise thrived at her job as a certified public accountant, proud of her ability to analyse reams of numbers for 60 hours a week or more.

Out of the office, she loved to run – 25 miles a week. And she played tournament volleyball.

Then, 3 years ago, Denise herniated some disks in her neck while lifting heavy boxes. For a couple of weeks, she was bedridden with severe pain. And her life hasn't been the same since.

"As the months passed, I couldn't concentrate at work," Denise recalls. "A month after my accident, I'd try to run, but I hurt all over. I just couldn't do it."

At 35, Denise desperately wanted the energy to have children and bring up a family. "And I wanted to be able to enjoy life again," she says.

## What Goes Wrong?

Denise is typical of women diagnosed with ME: once whirlwinds of energy, they now struggle just to get out of bed or walk around the block, says Charles W. Lapp, M.D., a physician in Charlotte, North Carolina, who specializes in CFS and is a medical adviser to the CFIDS Association of America.

But when someone like Denise goes to the doctor, the usual battery of tests generally show nothing wrong, apart from the initial illness that may have triggered the condition. There is no infection, no hormonal abnormalities like hypothyroidism or diabetes that typically cause fatigue – in short, nothing that can be cured by a pill or an injection.

And so it is tempting to assume that depression – or perhaps hypochondria – is to blame.

"A lot of doctors treat ME as a form of depression or anxiety, rather than a physical illness," says Nancy Klimas, M.D., professor of medicine at the University of Miami and founding editor of the *Journal of Chronic Fatigue Syndrome*. "Yet putting ME patients on antidepressants and anti-anxiety drugs without addressing what's really going on just further saps their energy."

Strictly speaking, ME is defined as severe fatigue lasting at least 6 months, along with at least four of eight other symptoms: impaired short-term memory or concentration; sore throat; tender lymph nodes; muscle pain; multijoint pain (but no swelling or redness); headaches of a new type, pattern, or severity; unrefreshing sleep; and feeling bad for more than 24 hours after exercise.

## The *Real* Hormone Connection

There is a physical basis for ME. And while it's not all in your mind, it can be traced, in part, to your brain. Specifically, researchers theorize that a trio of hormone-producing glands – the hypothalamus, pituitary and adrenal – may be out of whack in those with ME. This creates a domino effect that saps your energy, fogs your brain, and interferes with your ability to handle stress.

Researchers call this "dysregulation of the hypothalamic–pituitary–adrenal (HPA) axis." Basically, three things happen.

The hypothalamus doesn't produce enough corticotropin-releasing hormone (CRH). CRH is the final common element directing the body's response to all forms of stress. And the pituitary gland is not producing enough adrenocorticotropic hormone (ACTH) because it is not being triggered by the CRH. ACTH is needed to tell the adrenal gland to make more cortisol. Cortisol plays a key role in the body's response to stress and infection, and helps regulate blood sugar levels.

Low cortisol levels may explain a lot. Normal levels are key to reducing inflammation and keeping the immune system on standby. When cortisol levels fall, the immune system revs up, producing inflammation and widespread aches and pains.

Yet because hormone levels vary widely during the day, and overall hormonal levels in ME patients fall within "normal" boundaries, measuring hormone levels provides little help in diagnosis.

## You *Can* Recover

What throws the trio of energy-regulating glands out of whack?

Typically, some form of physical stress – such as a severe flulike illness.

"Most women with ME remember the date and circumstances that marked the beginning of their illness," says Dr. Klimas.

Some experts believe an emotionally stressful event may trigger ME. And sometimes it begins gradually, with no identifiable trigger. And ME may disappear as mysteriously as it starts. The US Centers for Disease Control and Prevention found that about one-third of people with ME recover within 5

### ON THE WEB & Other Resources

ME is a controversial subject, not least because we don't know nearly enough about it. So you need to be particularly careful where you go for information and advice. In the UK the best resources are the Arthritis Research Campaign and Arthritis Care listed in the Fibromyalgia box on page 383 (the illnesses are linked).

In Britain various ME charities seem to have come together under one banner:

**The ME Association**
4 Top Angel
Buckingham Industrial Park
Buckingham MK18 1TH
Tel: 08707 443011
Information line: 01280 816115
E-mail: *enquiries@meassociation.org.uk*
*www.meassociation.org.uk*

years, and about one half of all sufferers recover within 10 years.

As Dr. Lapp puts it: "Nature does heal most."

But that's a long time to wait.

By breaking ME into its components and tackling these step-by-step, many of those affected can climb back to health sooner. "The secret is to take the energy and willpower you have left and apply it to a structured programme," says Dr. Lapp.

First, make certain that what you have is ME and not some other disease. For that, you need to find a doctor who takes ME seriously. ME is relatively new – it wasn't officially recognized until the late 1980s. To find the right doctor, talk to people in a local ME support group, or check with your local hospital. (See "On the Web & Other Resources" on page 385.)

With step-by-step treatment, some people start feeling better in a little as a week or two. Improvement sometimes comes quickly, but usually it is gradual, says Dr. Lapp. Sometimes it leads to a full recovery and a return to work; others have fewer and less frequent symptoms.

"People start to get better and better, and finally, if they have been symptom-free for a year, the ME often never returns," says Dr. Lapp.

## Get Help ASAP

Dr. Lapp recommends a broad programme focusing on education, activity and exercise, nutrition and symptom-by-symptom treatment of fatigue, sleeplessness, headaches and pain. Options include a battery of supplements or drugs. Where to start – and what might work for you – will depend on the type and severity of your symptoms, he says.

The sooner you seek treatment, the better. Dr. Lapp found that about 80 per cent of patients are helped by his step-by-step therapy. The ones who came in early, with milder symptoms, had the greatest recovery.

"I've seen hundreds of women make full recoveries from ME," says Dr. Lapp.

Don't try to change everything all at once. Doing that not only takes more energy than you have but also makes it difficult to assess what is working and should be continued, and what is not. Generally, you should add another step every month or so, suggests Dr. Lapp.

## Stretch, Breathe, Walk

One difference between simple exhaustion and chronic fatigue syndrome is that with ME, getting more rest won't help. In fact, staying in bed will just make you more run-down as you lose muscle tone. But if you overdo it on a good day, you will end up sick in bed for several days.

The key is to begin with light, consistent activity alternated with rest, Dr. Lapp advises. And start slowly. His advice:

**Stand up straight – shoulders back, head held upright.** People with ME tend to slump forward because of tightness in their chest, which then tightens muscles in the neck and upper shoulders, causing neck pain and headaches. Make an effort throughout the day to stand tall.

**Take a deep breath.** Most people, including those with ME, breathe from the chest in "tiny baby breaths," leading to shortness of breath and an almost asthmatic feeling when you, say, walk up the stairs. Learn to breathe from your abdomen, and you will get more air with less strain. Practise deep breathing several times a day. (For details, see "Other Personal Cooling Tactics" on page 302.)

**Reach for the sky.** Pretend you are picking cherries off a branch hanging from your ceiling. Hold your hand up for 6 seconds. Then reach with the other hand, breathing while you stretch. Also use exercises to stretch your neck and shoulders. Tai chi (a traditional Chinese martial art distinguished by graceful, flowing movements) is an excellent alternative. To reap the benefits of tai chi, check with health clubs, martial arts schools, hospitals, or colleges for classes in your area.

**Take regular breaks.** You may have been able to run a 6-minute mile before, but for now you should be content with walking 2 to 5 minutes at a stretch. Then rest for at least 5 minutes. Repeat three to four times a day. One preliminary study found that even people with the most severe cases of ME were able to do that much and not relapse, Dr. Lapp says.

You can use a treadmill, stationary bike, or even weights or circuit training. Just stick with a level you are comfortable with, and don't push your heart rate too fast – in most cases no more than 60 per cent of the maximum heart rate for your age. In practical terms, that means you should be able to talk while you exercise. If you can't, back off.

## Nondrug Strategies for Aches and Pains

Thanks in part to hormonal disruptions at work, muscle aches and arthritis-like joint pains are typical of ME. There's plenty you can do for that allover-achy feeling.

**Massage those muscles.** It's great for reducing muscle aches. Dr. Lapp recommends craniosacral therapy, which stretches muscles along the spine and neck, to reduce headache and back pain. (For more on massage, see page 281.)

**Try acupuncture instead of aspirin.** Acupuncture can be a great pain reliever. It also can promote relaxation and increase energy, provided you find a skilled acupuncturist. Ask your doctor about local facilities and practitioners. Dr. Lapp recommends trying it for five or six sessions to see if it will help. (See "On the Web & Other Resources" on page 385.)

---

## THE HORMONE ZONE
# FOODS THAT RESTORE ENERGY – AND PREVENT LETHARGY

With chronic fatigue syndrome (ME), diet can make a big difference in restoring your energy, says Charles W. Lapp, M.D., a physician in Charlotte, North Carolina, who specializes in ME and is a medical adviser to the Chronic Fatigue and Immune Deficiency Syndrome Association of America. Aim for a diet that maximizes foods high in vitamins, minerals and other nutrients and minimizes fat and other substances that sap your energy.

"Anybody knows that if you go out to a steak house and have the typical big, heavy steak-and-potato meal, you're going to come home and feel lethargic," says Dr. Lapp. "If you have ME, you don't need that.

"Essentially, you want to eat a lot of complex carbohydrates and only light meats," says Dr. Lapp. "It's a good, prudent diet, and it's not hard."

As for what Dr. Lapp calls "verboten" items – sugar, caffeine, alcohol, the artificial sweetener aspartame and tobacco – he recommends eliminating them.

If following this plan doesn't help sufficiently, try giving up dairy products for 1 week, then wheat, especially if you have bloating or diarrhoea, common in those with ME.

**FOODS TO ADD**
- Fruit
- Vegetables
- Whole grain bread and cereal
- Rice
- Pasta
- Chicken
- Turkey
- Fish

**FOODS TO SUBTRACT**
- Red meat
- Greasy or fried food
- Sugar and sweets
- Aspartame
- Caffeine and caffeinated beverages
- Alcohol

**Try hot and cold packs.** Start with ice in a sealed plastic bag covered with a towel and place it on your shoulders and neck until they feel nice and cool. Then change to a comfortably hot, moist towel. This switch from cold to hot gets the blood flowing in those muscles and feels great, Dr. Lapp says.

**Warm is good; hot is bad.** Getting overheated can rev up your already turbo-charged immune system, making you feel sick and achy. So avoid hot showers or soaking in a hot bath. But 15 to 30 minutes soaking in a swimming pool heated to 30°C (85°F), or a bath at 35°C (95°F), will lower production of cytokines, immune substances that cause the flulike symptoms. Spending time in a bath two or three times a week also improves blood circulation. Use a pool or hot tub thermometer to get the bath temperature right.

## If You Still Hurt

If nondrug strategies don't do the job, aches and pains can be treated with over-the-counter or prescription nonsteroidal anti-inflammatory drugs (NSAIDs), such as ibuprofen and naproxen (Naprosyn), says Dr. Lapp.

But don't mix different types of NSAIDs with each other. NSAIDs can have dangerous side effects, particularly stomach bleeding, if you exceed the recommended dose or take them longer than recommended. Newer prescription NSAIDs – COX-2 inhibitors, such as Vioxx and Celebrex – are safer because they have fewer side effects, says Dr. Lapp. Ask your doctor or pharmacist about proper dosage.

## Maybe You Need More Salt

Cutting down on dietary sodium is standard for some people with high blood pressure. But nearly all people with ME have a form of low blood pressure called neurally mediated hypotension, where the brain sometimes signals the adrenal glands to produce too much adrenaline, causing blood pressure to fall instead of rise.

Standing suddenly or for a long time, or being out in hot weather, can trigger this. "The blood is going to their feet instead of their brains," says Dr. Klimas. The brain drain can make you feel light-headed and fatigued, and even produce rapid heartbeat (tachycardia). Doctors sometimes misinterpret this as a panic attack, and inappropriately prescribe anti-anxiety drugs, says Dr. Klimas.

Both Dr. Klimas and Dr. Lapp usually advise those diagnosed with ME and low blood pressure to consume more salt and water to bring the pressure up.

However, they caution, don't do this without a green light from your doctor. Even then, check your blood pressure before pouring on the salt, and keep checking it to make sure it does not get too high.

If increasing salt intake is not enough, Dr. Lapp prescribes fludrocortisone (Florinef) which tells the kidneys to retain more salt and water. Fludrocortisone is a synthetic adrenocortical steroid similar to a hormone produced by the adrenal glands.

## Supplements Can Help

A number of supplements may help ME, but don't go broke trying every supplement in the health food shop. Some work some of the time for some people, but no single supplement helps everyone. And some could be dangerous and should be avoided.

Here's what Dr. Lapp prescribes for those he treats for ME.

**A multivitamin with minerals.** These can help correct the minor deficiencies common in ME.

**Check out coenzyme $Q_{10}$.** Also known as $CoQ_{10}$, this may actually increase energy production at the cellular level. About half of Dr. Lapp's patients find modest improvement with doses of about 100 milligrams a day: "With this supplement, everything seems to get just a little bit better," he says.

**Fight inflammation with fatty acids.** Omega-3 fatty acids (found in evening primrose oil) and omega-6 fatty acids (found in fish oil) can reduce muscle pain and arthritic pain. Flaxseed oil and borage oil are also good sources of both. These fatty acids block the production of hormone-like compounds that trigger inflammation. Taking capsules containing up to 1000 milligrams of omega-3s per day has never been shown to be harmful, though you should tell your doctor what you're doing. (For more on fish oils, see "Foods That Fight Or Fan Inflammation" on page 33.)

## Get Quality Sleep

With ME, merely getting to sleep isn't enough. The key to waking up refreshed is deep, restorative sleep. Don't take all three of the following. Rather, see which one works best for you.

**Night-time sleep aids.** Dr. Lapp reports great success using preparations that combine the pain reliever paracetamol with the antihistamine diphenhydramine (such as Panadol Night). However, these preparations are not sold for long-term use. Talk with your doctor before straying from the label directions.

**Valerian root.** The active ingredients of this herb – one of the most widely used natural sleep aids in the world – include a group of compounds called valepotriates. Research indicates that components in valerian attach to the same brain receptors as tranquilizers like diazepam (Valium), but without causing dependency. Most people prefer taking the tincture or tablets, instead of the tea. Herbalists usually recommend one or two dropperfuls (½ to 1 teaspoon) of the tincture in a little water, or one or two capsules, 30 minutes before bedtime.

**Melatonin supplements.** A natural hormone that helps regulate the timing of sleep, melatonin will not knock you out, but it may help you sleep more soundly and wake up refreshed.

If you are falling asleep at 1 or 2 in the morning, melatonin may help you shift your sleep cycle back to a 10 or 11 p.m. bedtime. Combine this with light therapy in the morning to get your circadian rhythm in sync: open the blinds and turn on all your lights for 4 hours when you get up.

For people with ME, Dr. Lapp prescribes 3 milligrams of melatonin at bedtime if you are younger than 50; 3 to 6 milligrams if you're older. However, melatonin should be taken only under a doctor's advice. Children and a dolescents should not take melatonin. Melatonin is not available in the UK but it is widely available by mail order online; check with your doctor before taking it.

## Wake Up Your Brain

If you're finally getting quality sleep at night, but you feel sleepy during the day, unusually low levels of serotonin and dopamine – key brain chemicals called neurotransmitters – may be to blame.

"Increasing those two neurotransmitters can increase your energy and motivation levels," says Dr. Lapp.

To increase serotonin levels, doctors can prescribe SSRIs – selective serotonin reuptake inhibitors – such as fluoxetine (Prozac). Alternatives include sertraline (Lustral), paroxetine (Seroxat), venlafaxine (Efexor) and fluvoxamine (Faverin), all of which help keep more serotonin circulating in the brain.

When SSRIs don't deliver, Dr. Lapp looks for ways to increase dopamine levels through medications such as bupropion (Zyban).

Some of the symptoms of ME closely resemble those of attention deficit disorder (ADD): poor concentration, forgetfulness, using words incorrectly and reversing words and letters. And Ritalin (methylphenidate), a mild amphetamine-like drug typically used to treat children, works wonders in some adults with ME.

"It takes a sleeping brain and wakes it up. It gives you your old energy back," Dr. Lapp says.

It takes only a little Ritalin. Dr. Lapp prescribes doses about one-third that for ADD – 5 to 10 milligrams twice daily – and finds it very safe and non-habit-forming.

Alternatives are dexamphetamine (Dexedrine) and modafinil (Provigil).

However, very few doctors in the UK will prescribe Ritalin, Dexedrine, or Provigil without consultation with a psychiatrist.

## Symptom-by-Symptom Housecleaning

Women with ME can have problems from any and all zones of their bodies that compound the fatigue and pain of ME, says Dr. Lapp. Among them:

**Headaches.** Headaches associated with ME typically come in two types: pressure headaches and migraine-like headaches. For help, see page 362.

**Allergies and asthma.** Common in ME, both can sap your energy. See pages 347 and 355.

**Yeast infections.** Whether in the mouth, in the vagina, or under the arms, yeast infections also drain energy and need to be treated with oral medications like fluconazole (Diflucan) or ketoconazole (Nizoral).

---

### THE HORMONE CONNECTION
## THE OXYTOCIN HIGH

The hormone oxytocin helps explain the mystery of why women with ME can feel so much better when they are pregnant – a good thing since there are so few drugs they can take safely.

Oxytocin levels normally rise during pregnancy, and it is sometimes given to induce labour and stimulate lactation. Charles W. Lapp, M.D., a physician in Charlotte, North Carolina, who specializes in ME and is a medical advisor to the CFIDS Association of America, has seen dramatic improvement in nonpregnant women with ME when they got a shot of oxytocin. The hormone quickly increases bloodflow, especially to the eyes, muscles and brain. The result can be less pain and a clearer mind.

While the observation is intriguing, don't expect your doctor to prescribe it routinely. Providing supplemental hormones can have unexpected consequences, and the use of oxytocin is still controversial.

**Chemical sensitivity.** In people with ME, tobacco smoke, car exhaust and chemicals (like fragrances or household cleaning products) can aggravate symptoms. Do your best to avoid them.

**Stress.** Fighting at home and financial pressures don't help ME. Work them out, or find a counsellor to provide advice. For more stress-reducing strategies, see Phases 1 and 2 of the Hormone-Balancing Programme on pages 258 and 275.

**Restless leg syndrome.** Also common in ME, restless leg syndrome is characterized by cramps and twitching that interfere with sleep. Talk to your doctor about clonazepam (Rivotril) or doxepin (Sinequan) to help ease these symptoms.

**Cavities.** People with ME are prone to cavities because they tend to have dry, acidic mouths. Drinks lots of water, avoid sugar, and use a toothpaste with baking soda because it is more alkaline and tends to protect the teeth. And have regular dental checkups.

# Leaky Bladder

For many women, menopause is a mixed blessing: they rejoice at not having to deal with menstrual periods, and being able to enjoy sex without worrying about getting pregnant. But they also notice urinary leakage when they laugh, cough, or play tennis.

Menopausal women aren't alone. Women of all ages experience incontinence, or involuntary leakage of urine. Some have problems when they first stop having their periods. Other, much younger women find after having a baby that they can't hold their urine.

Most bladder control problems happen when muscles are either too weak or too active. Problems may also happen when nerve signals from the bladder to the brain are interrupted or don't work properly. The two most common types of urinary incontinence are stress incontinence and urge incontinence.

With stress incontinence, the muscles that keep your bladder closed are weak, and you have accidents when you sneeze, laugh, or lift a heavy object. Stress incontinence often occurs during pregnancy or after childbirth because the pelvic floor muscles stretch and weaken at this time. After a woman stops menstruating and becomes menopausal, the same muscles become weak because of the cumulative effects of ageing, gravity, childbearing and lower levels of female hormones.

With urge incontinence, just the opposite happens. The bladder becomes *too* active. You may feel strong, sudden urges to urinate, even if your bladder has little urine. A bladder infection, nerve damage (sometimes from childbirth), drinking alcohol and certain medications can overactivate your bladder.

Aside from gender, a number of other factors determine who will experience bladder control problems and who won't.

**Genetics.** If your mother or grandmother had bladder problems, chances are you might, too.

**Culture.** According to one study, 37 per cent of Americans have urinary incontinence, 26 per cent in continental Europe, 29 per cent in the United Kingdom and 20 per cent in Japan.

**Childbearing.** The incidence of urinary incontinence rises with the number of children women have given birth to.

**Bowel troubles.** Bowel problems, such as constipation and irritable bowel syndrome, can increase your risk.

**Diet.** Caffeine and alcohol have been shown to contribute to urinary incontinence.

**Medications.** Certain drugs can increase your risk, such as ACE inhibitors, beta-adrenergic agonists and antagonists, calcium channel blockers, diuretics and sedatives.

**Infection.** A history of urinary tract infections, such as cystitis, can increase your risk.

## How Your Bladder Works

Most of the bladder control system lies inside the bowl-shaped pelvis. If you stand with your hands on your hips, the bones under your hands are the pelvic bones.

At the bottom of this "bowl" are the pelvic floor muscles. These muscles should be strong and tight to hold up the bladder in its proper place. The bladder is a muscular, balloon-shaped organ located inside the pelvis, just below the belly button. When the bladder is full, it stays relaxed. When you urinate, the bladder muscles tighten, squeezing urine out of the bladder.

The urethra – the tube that carries urine out of the body – is surrounded by two sphincter muscles, which keep the urethra closed by squeezing like tight rubber bands. The pelvic floor muscles also help keep the urethra closed. When the pelvic floor and sphincter muscles are tight, and the bladder is relaxed, urine stays put and does not leak out.

When the bladder is full, nerves in your bladder signal the brain, prompting you to head for the toilet. Once you're seated, your brain sends a message down to the sphincter and pelvic floor muscles telling them to relax. The brain signal also tells the bladder muscles to tighten up, to squeeze urine out of the bladder.

Understandably, women with bladder control problems are embarrassed. But it's a medical problem and nothing to be ashamed of. Nor is urine leakage a normal, expected part of the ageing process, as some believe. Most of the time, it can be improved.

---

**THE HORMONE ZONE**

# IDENTIFY THE USUAL SUSPECTS

If you find yourself running to the lavatory frequently, pay attention to what you've been eating and drinking. Common bladder irritants include coffee, tea, alcohol, carbonated beverages, acidic fruits and juices (such as cranberry, orange, grapefruit and lemon), tomatoes and tomato-based foods, chocolate, artificial sweeteners and spicy foods. "If the carbonation isn't bothersome, some women find relief just by switching from colas to uncaffeinated soft drinks, such as Sprite or 7UP," says Nina S. Davis, M.D., assistant professor of urology at Oregon Health Sciences University in Portland. However, avoiding carbonation is best.

**FOODS TO ADD**

- Non-cola drinks
- Noncarbonated beverages
- Herb tea
- Water

**FOODS TO SUBTRACT**

- Coffee
- Tea
- Colas
- Alcohol (such as beer and wine)
- Carbonated beverages (including sparkling water)
- Acidic fruits and juices (such as cranberry, orange, grapefruit and lemon)
- Tomatoes and tomato-based foods
- Chocolate
- Artificial sweeteners
- Spicy foods

## Where Hormones Come into Play

With the approach of menopause, lower oestrogen levels reduce the muscular pressure around the urethra, permitting urine to leak. Menopausal women also have reduced sphincter strength from the decreased levels of oestrogen. Low hormone levels also make the urethra thinner, impairing its ability to hold urine.

"As hormonal levels wane – especially when oestrogen levels drop – there are changes in the bladder wall which cause problems like frequency of urination and urinary incontinence," says Nina S. Davis, M.D., assistant professor of urology at Oregon Health Sciences University in Portland. "The normally elastic tissue in the bladder changes into less elastic, stiffer tissue that does not allow the bladder to contract or store urine as effectively as it used to."

Like nearly every other part of your body, the urethra and bladder have oestrogen receptors, making them dependent upon oestrogen to function properly. You might expect that replacing the lost oestrogen – as part of hormone replacement therapy (HRT) for menopause – would ease symptoms. So far, studies haven't shown a consistent benefit. Some studies showed that HRT did improve symptoms of urinary incontinence, yet others showed it had no effect. In one study, for example, 33 postmenopausal women were given oestrogen, and 34 were given a placebo (dummy pill) over a 6-month period. The group that received the oestrogen did not experience any improvement of their symptoms.

## Bladder-Friendly Measures

Luckily, there are plenty of ways to regain control. Start with self-care strategies. If they don't work, explore your medical options.

**Drink plenty of water.** This may sound counterintuitive, but getting more liquid, not less, helps by diluting the urine. "Urine that's concentrated is more irritating to the bladder," says Dr. Davis. "The bladder becomes more sensitive as you get older, so keeping the urine diluted will result in less irritation." Aim for eight glasses of water a day. If you work in a hot environment or do strenuous exercise, you may need to drink even more water to keep your urine dilute.

**Crush that cigarette.** A chronic cough not only causes leakage but also can contribute to weakening the pelvic muscles. Also, nicotine constricts blood vessels, reducing bloodflow to the pelvic region.

**Give yourself time to go.** "Women are especially busy. With jobs, families, a home to take care of, they tend to put themselves last, and don't take time for themselves to go to the lavatory when they feel the urge," says Dr. Davis. "But the longer you wait, the more concentrated the urine becomes, irritating the bladder." Try to go every 3 to 4 hours.

**Plan ahead.** It's obvious, but it makes sense: "Empty your bladder before you start a trip of an hour or more," advises Dr. Davis. "And if you're out and about and you feel the urge to urinate, don't try to wait until you get home or until it is more convenient."

**Use a public toilet when needed.** "Women are concerned that they will get a disease, even though the actual risk is minimal," says Dr. Davis. "So they don't use it, or when they do, they squat instead of sitting down. That's not an anatomically correct way to urinate fully. When you squat, the urethra can't open properly, and you don't completely void." If you're still uneasy about sitting on community toilets at work, request toilet seat covers. Or do what your mother told you to do when you were a girl – place toilet tissue on the seat. Or carry antibacterial towelettes (sold with hygiene products everywhere) and wipe the seat down before use. Afterwards, dispose of them in the rubbish, not the toilet, as with tampons or sanitary towels.

**Retrain your bladder.** "Done properly, bladder retraining can increase your

---

## Herbs to Try

Connie Catellani, M.D., medical director of the Miro Center for Integrative Medicine in Evanston, Illinois, finds that three herbs – horsetail, marshmallow root and kava (currently under investigation in the UK and not available in Europe – or barley tea can promote healing and toning of the bladder and urethra tissues and the pelvic muscles.

For best results, says Dr. Catellani, purchase the herbs in tincture form and, using a dropper with demarcations, dissolve 1 to 4 cc in a glass of water. Try them one at a time to see which works best. "When taking horsetail, take a multivitamin that contains B vitamins because this herb accelerates the breakdown of these important vitamins," adds Dr. Catellani.

"To make barley tea, cook barley in a large pot of water," she says. "Save the leftover water and drink it as a tea. For an extra dose, eat the cooked barley as a side dish."

As usual, tell your doctor of any herbs you're taking, especially if you're taking medication of any kind for bladder control or other health conditions.

bladder capacity and cut down on how many times you urinate," says Dr. Davis. To retrain your bladder, when you get the urge to urinate, try to hold it for 5 extra minutes before going to the toilet. Each week, add 5 to 10 minutes to the length of time you hold the urine beyond the desire to go. The goal here is to hold your urine for at least 2 hours, at most up to 4 hours. If within 4 to 6 weeks you don't see improvement in how long you can hold your urine, says Dr. Davis, consult your doctor. You may be referred to a specialist for further evaluation. Inability to train the bladder may be a sign of a nerve problem. So further instruction may be beneficial.

**Exercise your pelvic muscles.** "Pelvic muscle exercises, or Kegel exercises, increase the strength of the muscles which support the bladder and urethra," says Dr. Davis. "Strong pelvic muscles give women better control in their ability to hold their urine." Pelvic floor muscles are just like other muscles. Exercise can make them stronger. Two pelvic muscles that stretch across the pelvic floor do most of the work. The biggest one stretches like a hammock. The other is shaped like a triangle. These muscles prevent leaking of urine and stools.

Start by finding the right muscles. Your doctor, nurse, or physiotherapist will help make sure you are doing the exercises the right way. Your goal is to tighten the "hammock" muscle and the "triangle" muscle. Here are three methods experts recommend to check for the correct muscles.

1. *Try to stop the flow of urine when you are sitting on the toilet. If you can do it, you are using the right muscles. Imagine that you are trying to stop passing wind. Squeeze the muscles you would use. If you sense a "pulling" feeling, those are the right muscles for pelvic exercises.*
2. *Lie down and put your finger inside your vagina. Squeeze as if you were trying to stop urine from coming out. If you feel tightness on your finger, you are squeezing the right pelvic muscles.*
3. *Don't squeeze other muscles at the same time. Be careful not to tighten your stomach, legs, or other muscles. Squeezing the wrong muscles can put more pressure on your bladder control muscles. Just squeeze the pelvic muscle. Don't hold your breath. Repeat, but don't overdo it. At first, find a quiet spot to practise – your bathroom or bedroom – so you can concentrate.*

After you've found the right muscles, follow these steps to exercise your pelvic muscles.

1. *Lie on the floor. Pull in the pelvic muscles and hold for a count of three. Then relax for a count of three. Work up to 10 to 15 repeats each time you exercise. Do your pelvic exercises at least three times a day.*
2. *Every day, use three positions: lying, sitting and standing. You can exercise while lying on the floor, sitting at a desk, sitting in your car, or standing in the kitchen. Using all three positions makes the muscles strongest.*
3. *Be patient. Don't give up. It's just 5 minutes, three times a day. You may not feel your bladder control improve until after 3 to 6 weeks. Still, most women do notice an improvement after a few weeks.*

---

*Escape from* **HORMONE HELL**

## HER BLADDER GIVES OUT ON THE FRONT PORCH

**Q:** I'm 53 and hit menopause 3 years ago. Lately I've been leaking urine at inopportune times. The situation is getting critical: one day this week, I was out shopping, and on the drive home, I really had to go. I made it as far as my front door, then the floodgates opened, and I was soaked, standing on my front porch.

Car trips, too, are a problem. Recently, my husband and I were stuck in traffic on holiday, with no way to pull off the road to find a lavatory, and I thought my bladder was going to burst. I had to climb into the backseat and use an empty bottle to urinate. My husband was disgusted. Am I going to have to wear incontinence pads for the rest of my life?

Nina S. Davis, M.D., assistant professor of urology at Oregon Health Sciences University in Portland, responds: rest assured, incontinence pads aren't in your immediate future. You can be helped easily. This is a classic scenario for many women your age. Your doctor should take a complete medical history to make sure there's nothing seriously incorrect with your pelvic anatomy, or to rule out nerve damage. Then you should look into behavioural interventions, such as biofeedback with a focus on urge inhibition techniques. You can learn how to hold your urine long enough to make it to the lavatory.

You also sound like an ideal candidate for any of the anticholinergic drugs.

**Squeeze before you sneeze.** You can protect your pelvic muscles from more damage by bracing yourself. Think ahead, just before sneezing, lifting, or jumping. Sudden pressure from such actions can hurt those pelvic muscles. Squeeze your pelvic muscles tightly and hold on until after you sneeze, lift, or jump. After you train yourself to tighten the pelvic muscles for these moments, you will have fewer accidents.

**Keep a bladder control diary.** Buy a small notebook and keep track of how often you do Kegels, just as you would keep a fitness log. Devote each page to a day of the week, and note how many times a day you exercised your pelvic muscles, how many minutes you spent exercising them and how many times you squeezed your pelvic muscles at each exercise session. This helps to continue doing the exercises and monitor your progress.

## High- and Low-Tech Bladder Control

If you've tried every bladder control trick in the book and you're still having accidents, don't despair. You've got plenty of other options, says Dr. Davis.

**Biofeedback.** This procedure, currently only available in the US, helps women find their pelvic muscles. A certified therapist places a patch over the muscles. A wire connects the patch to a TV screen. You watch the screen to see if you are exercising the right muscles. With the aid of the therapist, you learn to control these muscles without the patch or the screen.

**Pessaries.** A support device that's inserted in the vagina by a family doctor or gynaecologist – often to push a dropped bladder or uterus back into place – can help to mechanically control urine leakage.

**Urethral insert.** An elongated tube filled with mineral oil, this comes in various sizes that are fitted to a woman's urethra. Your doctor will give you the device that conforms to the inside of the urethra and closes it off so that urine can't leak out. It's like a plug. You remove the device when it's time to go to the lavatory, and reinsert a fresh device until it's time to go again.

**Magnetic stimulation.** The patient sits on a chair with a magnet below the seat. Magnetic forces of increasing intensity are delivered to the pelvic floor muscles to stimulate and strengthen them. The patient can feel muscle contractions induced by the magnetic stimulation. It usually requires 16 or so 20-minute sessions with a urologist or urogynaecologist to see results.

**Transvaginal electrical stimulation.** A vaginal electrode delivers a gentle electrical current to the pelvic floor to stimulate muscle contraction, to reduce bladder muscle overactivity and to strengthen pelvic floor muscles. This procedure must be authorized by a doctor, but the actual treatment and instruction may be given by a certified biofeedback therapist or a physio-therapist.

**Bladder control medication.** The most common medications, oxybu-tynin (Ditropan) and tolterodine (Detrusitol), work by interrupting the signals to the bladder that make it contract inappropriately, resulting in leakage. These medications work best for women with urge incontinence. Another medication – flavoxate (Urispas) – works very well for women with urinary frequency. Still other medications work by tightening the blad-der outlet and increasing resistance to urine flow.

If you don't respond to any of these medications, see a pelvic floor spe-cialist – preferably a urologist or a urogynaecologist, advises Dr. Davis. "These doctors have had advanced training in the evaluation and treatment of urinary disorders."

## Surgical Repair

There are several different types of surgery to improve bladder control. Which one your doctor may recommend for you depends on what is causing the problem. The goal of surgery is to restore normal anatomy, to provide necessary pelvic floor sup-port, to prevent urine leakage and to repair or replace a severely malfunctioning bladder. Most surgery of this type is extensive and requires a hospital stay.

**Periurethral bulking.** Either collagen, a natural protein, or Durasphere,

---

### ON THE WEB & Other Resources

For more information on bladder control problems, contact the following:
**The International Continence Society (UK section)** *www.icsuk.org.uk*

**The British Medical Association is also, as so often, an excellent source of information:**
**The British Medical Association**
Tavistock Square
London WC1H 9JP
Tel: 020 7387 4499
*www.bma.org.uk*

Alternatively, write, enclosing a large sae for leaflets, to:
**The Continence Foundation**
The Helpline Nurse
307 Hatton Square
London EC1N 7RJ
Tel: 0845 345 0165
E-mail: *continence-help@dial.pipex.com*
(giving your postal address so you can be sent relevant leaflets)
*www.continence-foundation.org.uk*

a string of tiny carbon-coated beads, is injected into the tissues of the bladder neck and urethra. This recreates the normal closure of the walls of the bladder neck and urethra to resist urinary leakage. The injection is usually performed in the operating theatre under anaesthesia.

**Sacral nerve root stimulation.** Electric wires are inserted next to the spinal cord to interrupt the overactive signals to the bladder. The wires (electrodes) are connected to a pacemaker-like device beneath the skin. The insertion procedure is done in the operating theatre under anaesthesia.

# Hysterectomy

For women who undergo a natural menopause, hormonal changes usually occur gradually over a period of 10 or so years, allowing time to adjust physically and emotionally. When a woman has a hysterectomy, however, she may undergo "instant menopause", with abrupt and often severe hormonal changes.

If her ovaries are removed along with her uterus, a procedure called "hysterectomy with bilateral salpingo-oophorectomy", done in about half of cases, a woman will have a precipitous drop in oestrogen, progesterone and androgens, male hormones, such as testosterone, made by the ovaries. Within 48 hours, she'll begin to have hot flushes, often severe, more than 20 times a day. The hot flushes will also cause sleep disturbances, which can lead to depression.

"The lack of oestrogen may also cause a change in bloodflow and vascular spasms that induce chest pain, headache, or shortness of breath, which makes some women think they've having a heart attack or a stroke," says Philip Sarrel, M.D., professor of obstetrics, gynaecology and psychiatry at Yale University School of Medicine. "Many women also are plagued by an exhausting kind of fatigue and muscle weakness following ovary removal," he says. That's due to a 50 per cent to 60 per cent drop in androgens. Many also experience a drop in sex drive, for the same reason.

Even when women undergoing a hysterectomy know what to expect – and often they don't – "they are frightened, in pain and going through a pretty unpleasant experience," Dr. Sarrel says.

That's why, whenever it's feasible, most doctors consider it good medical practice to start a woman on oestrogen as soon as possible after her ovaries are removed. Dr. Sarrel recommends putting a patch on a woman in the operating room, prior to removing her ovaries, so there is no "crash." Or he'll start a woman on Estratest, a combination of oestrogen and the androgen testosterone: "In my opinion, the androgen is just as important as the oestrogen," he says.

Studies show that women who have their ovaries removed and don't take oestrogen afterwards have twice the rate of bone loss as those who experience a natural menopause. That's because, even after menopause, normal ovaries produce a spectrum of hormonal substances for a number of years, says Herbert Goldfarb, M.D., assistant professor of clinical obstetrics and gynaecology at the New York University School of Medicine in New York City, director at the Montclair Reproductive Center in New Jersey and author of *The No-Hysterectomy Option*. Even when the ovaries aren't removed, women who have had hysterectomies have significantly lower bone density than women with intact reproductive organs and, so, are more likely to develop osteoporosis, says Dr. Goldfarb.

And the risk for having a heart attack for women who undergo complete hysterectomies and oophorectomies (removal of one or both ovaries) is more than twice that of women who go through menopause naturally. That's due to a drop in oestrogen and can be alleviated somewhat with oestrogen replacement therapy, Dr. Goldfarb says. "But it's due, in part, to removal of the uterus, he says. "The uterus produces substances called prostacyclins, which are critical to blood circulation because some of them inhibit clotting and dilate blood vessels," he says. "Once the uterus is no longer present, prostacyclin levels drop. Coronary artery disease may develop more easily in the presence of thicker blood within a narrower vessel."

## Keeping Ovaries No Guarantee against Problems

Insisting that your ovaries are not removed isn't always a guarantee that they will continue to produce hormones, Dr. Goldfarb says. "In about 15 to 20 per cent of women who have a simple hysterectomy, where only the uterus is removed, the ovaries start to fail, as a result of a disruption in their blood supply during surgery," he says. And that can happen no matter what type of hysterectomy you have, he says. "There currently is no good surgical technique to avoid this possibility." Ovarian failure may happen soon after the surgery, but more often the ovaries take a few years to completely peter out.

There's also increasing evidence that, whether the ovaries remain functional or not, hysterectomy reduces some women's sexual responsiveness and ability to achieve orgasm, says Irwin Goldstein, M.D., professor of urology at Boston University Medical Center. "We see scores of women who've had a marked decline in the ability to respond sexually and achieve orgasm after they'd had a hysterectomy," he says. He attributes that, in part, to damage to nerves of the vagina, clitoris and labia, particularly autonomic nerves, during surgery. "These nerves are very small – the size of hairs – but they're what allow your sex organs and brain to communicate. So they're indispensable for arousal and orgasm," Dr. Goldstein says. Doctors found this happened in men who underwent prostate surgery, which now is designed to preserve these nerves so men can retain normal sexual function.

At this writing, Dr. Goldstein and his colleagues have started to map these nerves and their major anatomical "landmarks" so that doctors can perform nerve-sparing surgery when they do a hysterectomy. In the meantime, he says, the best way to avoid having your autonomic nerves cut is to have a supracervical hysterectomy, one that leaves the cervix in place. This isn't an option for every woman, but it is for many. It can be done only via an abdominal incision, not by a vaginal incision. "There is no question that this type of surgery spares some of the autonomic nerves," Dr. Goldstein says.

Leaving the cervix in place also helps prevent other problems associated with hysterectomy. It avoids shortening of the vagina; it is less likely to result in prolapse (falling) of the upper vagina or in granulation – painful, hard, grainy changes in the tissue in the upper vagina. And it may help you avoid urinary incontinence as a result of a drop in the neck of the bladder. However, it does require that you continue to have Pap smears throughout your life.

## Know Your Options

Except when it's done for bona fide invasive cancer of the uterus or ovaries, almost every hysterectomy is elective surgery, done for a benign condition. "That means it's your choice, your decision, even if your doctor doesn't put it that way," says Michael S. Broder, M.D., assistant professor of obstetrics and gynaecology at the UCLA School of Medicine. According to the Public Health Service of the US Department of Health and Human Services, some 90 per cent of hysterectomies in the US are done for conditions other than cancer, and in nonemergency situations. Most often, the surgery is done for uterine fibroids, endometriosis and uterine prolapse. "You almost always have a chance to get a second opinion, to think about it, to get your questions answered, and to explore other options," Dr. Broder says. Unfortunately, he's found that many doctors are still performing hysterectomies without exploring other options first with women they treat.

In a study conducted at UCLA of nearly 500 hysterectomies, a panel of experts who reviewed medical records and talked to patients after surgery found that 14 per cent of the surgeries probably weren't warranted. "In other words, there just didn't seem to be any symptoms or indications to justify the procedure," Dr. Broder says. "It was hard to imagine anything that would have made these hysterectomies indicated."

And in another 56 per cent of cases, before recommending a hysterectomy, doctors hadn't done an adequate diagnostic evaluation or hadn't tried all of the alternative treatments suggested by American College of Obstetricians and Gynecologists (ACOG) guidelines.

The study's researchers concluded that altogether, about 70 per cent of these cases had significant quality problems in the way the preoperative evaluation was handled. On 77 per cent of the women with pelvic pain, neither a laparoscopy nor a laparotomy had been done before the hysterectomy. (The panel believed such an evaluation was necessary in most cases to exclude other causes of pain before hysterectomy.) Some 45 per cent of women with abnormal bleeding had not had endometrial sampling before hysterectomy, which might have uncovered a problem treatable by hormones. Some 21 per cent with pain or bleeding had not received (or had not been offered) a trial of medical treatment for pain or bleeding. "Rates of inappropriateness do appear to be higher for hysterectomy than for other types of surgery," Dr. Broder says.

**Get as much information as possible before you make a decision.** And

## ON THE WEB & Other Resources

**The HERS (Hysterectomy Educational Resources and Services) Foundation** provides free information on alternative treatments for hysterectomy as well as on coping with hysterectomy. The foundation publishes a newsletter, sponsors conferences and offers telephone counselling (by appointment only). You can also write to request a free package of information. Contact HERS at:
**The HERS (Hysterectomy Educational Resources and Services) Foundation**

422 Bryn Mawr Avenue
Bala Cynwyd, PA 19004
*www.hersfoundation.org*

For a good account of what to expect in Britain check out the BUPA factsheets:
*www.bupa.co.uk*

**Hysterectomy Association**
8 Newby Close
Burton upon Trent
Staffordshire DE15 9GG

don't let anyone rush you. Ask your doctor about other treatment options, including the benefits and risks of both surgical and nonsurgical alternatives, such as medication. Ask your doctor if he is following the Royal College of Obstetricians and Gynaecologists (RCOG) guidelines, which evaluate the appropriateness of hysterectomy for a variety of conditions, such as abnormal bleeding, chronic pelvic pain and endometriosis. If he's not following the guidelines, find out why. He may have a good reason.

"Patients who are involved in their care tend to get better care," says Dr. Broder. "If your doctor is dismissive of your questions, it's time to find a new doctor."

Get an independent second opinion. A second opinion is always warranted in the case of hysterectomy, but it can be hard to find a doctor who doesn't think along exactly the same lines as your usual doctor, says William Parker, M.D., clinical professor of obstetrics and gynaecology at UCLA–Santa Monica. The *worst* way to get a second opinion: asking your doctor for a referral, because he (or she) will send you to someone he knows will agree with him. Ask around as much as you can.

Although there is a feeling in America that all doctors may be out to get your money, in Britain, in the NHS, where most hysterectomies are performed, there is no incentive for surgeons to operate. They are paid a salary regardless of how many operations they perform. There could even be said to be an incentive the other way – *not* to operate – as unnecessary surgery means extra costs.

## Coping With the Aftermath

Even when you feel you're better off after a hysterectomy, there are some aspects you just can't compensate for. You can take hormones, but they can't make up for the loss of structural support, changes in placement of the bladder or colon that can lead to urinary incontinence or chronic constipation, or damage to nerves and loss of feeling in the sex organs. "These problems can be prevented, but they can't always be fixed," Dr. Goldstein says. Here's what you *can* do.

**Give yourself plenty of time to recover.** "Gynaecologists tell women that they will feel better after 6 weeks, and that often is not the case," Dr. Broder says. "Studies show that even 6 months after the surgery, women are having problems." The most common ones – pain, weakness, fatigue, general malaise. These problems may go away by themselves, given time, but they're slow in going. "You may need 6 months to a year to really feel better," he says.

**Use a stool softener, and take in plenty of fibre.** You don't want to have to strain to attain normal bowel function. Pain medications can cause constipation, Dr. Goldfarb says. He suggests that you eat plenty of whole grains, fruits and vegetables for fibre. If necessary, use a stool softener until you can evacuate normally. Follow the manufacturer's recommendations for dosage, and take it once a day with a meal. Drink at least two large glasses of water with each dose, Dr. Goldfarb says. Use this combo for painless evacuations.

**Wear wraparound abdominal support.** Women who have had a hysterectomy say a support garment provides needed abdominal support, and helps reduce fatigue and lower-back pain. But instead of struggling to pull on a girdle, you can get a wraparound abdominal binder that fastens with Velcro-type hook-and-loop fasteners. These are available without a prescription at surgical supply stores, but be sure to check with your doctor first that this is right for you, says Dr. Goldfarb. Better yet, ask your doctor for a prescription.

---

### THE HORMONE CONNECTION

## US FINDINGS – TESTOSTERONE MAY HELP EASE EFFECTS OF OVARY REMOVAL

In both men and women, testosterone helps maintain strong bones and muscles as well as their sex drives and improves general mood and energy. Doctors may continue to debate its use in women who go through menopause naturally. But more and more agree – and studies support the stance – that women who have had their ovaries removed benefit from its use, says Glenn Braunstein, M.D., chairman of the department of medicine at Cedars-Sinai Medical Center in Los Angeles.

A testosterone patch for women is currently under development, and some doctors believe that this patch is the way to go.

In the meantime, doctors in the US have their own ways of providing synthetic testosterone to women who need it. It is available in combination with oestrogen in prescription drugs such as Estratest. It can be made up at a compounding pharmacy and used as a vaginal or topical cream. And some doctors adapt the products used for men – skin patches or a gel – to women's use, although this needs to be done very carefully.

"Doctors are developing common knowledge protocols for 'off-label' use of these products in women," Dr. Braunstein says.

**Insist on oestrogen.** If you've had your ovaries removed, the sooner you start on oestrogen after your surgery, the better you'll feel, Dr. Sarrel says. (You may heal faster, sleep better, and feel less depressed.) He also suggests that you ask your doctor to consider adding androgen treatment as well since most of the cells producing androgens are removed along with the ovaries. Oestrogen replacement therapy (HRT) will also help to reduce your risk of urinary incontinence later in life. If your ovaries haven't been removed, and you are technically "premenopausal", you may still need HRT at some point after your surgery. You won't have an end to menstrual cycles to mark this point. So, if hot flushes begin to make your life miserable, make sure your doctor tests your hormone levels and starts HRT even if you're younger than the typical age for menopause, Dr. Goldstein says. (For more details on hormone replacement therapy, see chapter 11.)

If you can't or won't take HRT, you still have many alternatives to make your life easier and your health better.

**Do Kegel exercises.** After hysterectomy, there is often some displacement and loss of structural support from pelvic floor muscles, the sling of muscles that goes from your tailbone to the front of your pubic bone. So you'll want to maintain as much muscle tone in that area as you can. Kegel exercises contract this muscle group, helping to keep it strong and making it easier to contract your vagina and the muscles that stop the flow of urine. Better yet, insist on preserving your cervix unless abnormalities call for surgical removal, says Dr. Goldfarb. (For details on doing Kegels, see page 398.)

# Breast Lumps and Tenderness

Finding a breast lump can be one of the most worrisome symptoms a woman can experience. Perhaps it's happened to you. As you step out of the shower to call your doctor, one question races through your mind: is it cancer?

Over a lifetime, half of all women become concerned enough about a breast change to see a physician. However, most breast lumps and other changes turn out not to be cancer. Among breast conditions for which biopsies are often done, the results show that some 80 per cent are not cancer.

Should you find a lump, don't panic – but don't ignore it, either. Only a doctor can tell for sure whether a lump is malignant (cancer) or not.

## Some Breast Changes Are Normal

To understand how and why breasts sometimes become lumpy or tender, it helps to know what lies beneath the surface. Each breast has 15 to 20 sections, called lobes, each with many smaller lobules. The lobules end in dozens of tiny bulbs that can produce milk. Thin tubes called ducts link all lobes, lobules and bulbs. These ducts lead to the nipple, which is centred in a dark area of skin called the areola. The spaces between the lobules and ducts are filled with fat. There are no muscles in the breast, but muscles lie

---

### Escape from **HORMONE HELL**
# HORMONE TREATMENT SOLVED ONE PROBLEM, TRIGGERED ANOTHER

**Q: A couple of years ago, I developed abnormal uterine bleeding due to a hormone imbalance, and my doctor prescribed conjugated oestrogens. The bleeding is under control, but ever since, my breasts are constantly tender and swollen. I can't stand to be touched, and it's even painful to do a breast self-examination. The thought of a mammogram makes me cringe. Now my fingers, hands, and ankles are swelling, too. I feel like I'm filling up with fluid. Is there anything I can do?**

Blake Cady, M.D., director of the Breast Health Center at Women and Infants Hospital in Providence, Rhode Island, replies: it sounds like you're taking too much oestrogen, and you've been taking it for too long. The high amount of oestrogen is causing fluid to build up, and that's what's causing the symptoms, especially the breast sensitivity. You need to get off the oestrogen pills and return your body back to a normal state. Try staying off the oestrogen for 6 months and see if the symptoms clear up.

And by all means, let your doctor know what's going on. Patients also need to be proactive and contact their doctor immediately to tell them they're experiencing these other changes with their bodies. Too many women are put on oestrogen, and then the doctor doesn't follow up and touch base periodically with the patient to see if they prescribed the correct dose. The same amount and type of oestrogen won't work for all women. (*Editor's note*: It's always a good idea to inform your doctor of any side effects from medication and get approval before discontinuing medication of any kind.)

under each breast and cover the ribs.

These normal features can sometimes make the breasts feel lumpy, especially in women who are thin or who have small breasts. And from the time a woman begins menstruation, her breasts undergo regular changes each month. Many women experience swelling, tenderness and pain before and sometimes during their periods. At the same time, one or more lumps or a feeling of increased lumpiness may develop because of extra fluid collecting in the breast tissue. These lumps normally go away by the end of a woman's period.

"Eventually, about half of all women will experience symptoms such as lumps, discomfort, pain, or nipple discharge, but these symptoms generally quieten down after they reach menopause," says Blake Cady, M.D., director of the Breast Health Center at Women and Infants Hospital in Providence, Rhode Island.

Benign (noncancerous) breast lumps are usually found in the glandular tissue of the breast and are common in all women of childbearing age.

## Not All Lumps Are Alike

The most common types of benign breast lumps are cysts, fibroadenomas and fatty necrotic lumps. All these lumps can appear at any time, in one or both breasts, may be large or small, soft or rubbery, fluid-filled or solid.

**Cysts.** These fluid-filled sacs occur most often in women aged 35 to 50, and they often enlarge and become tender and painful just before the menstrual period. They are usually found in both breasts. Some cysts are so small they cannot be felt; rarely, cysts may be several centimetres across. Cysts show up clearly on ultrasound, a test that uses sound waves to produce a picture of tissues inside the breast. The diagnosis of cysts is usually handled by observation or by the withdrawal of fluid with a needle, called fine-needle aspiration.

**Fibroadenomas.** Solid, round benign growths made up of both structural (fibro) and glandular (adenoma) tissues, these lumps are usually painless and found by the woman herself. They feel rubbery and can easily be moved around. Fibroadenomas are the most common type of growths in women in their late teens and early twenties, and they occur twice as often in women of African origin as in other women. Although fibroadenomas do not become malignant, they can enlarge with pregnancy and breastfeeding. Most surgeons believe removing fibroadenomas is a good idea, to make sure they are benign.

**Fat necrosis.** Painless, round, firm lumps formed by damaged and disintegrating fatty tissues, this condition typically occurs in obese women with very large breasts. It often develops in response to a bruise or blow to the breast, even though the woman may not remember the specific injury. Sometimes the skin around the lumps looks red or bruised. Fat necrosis can easily be mistaken for cancer, so such lumps are removed surgically and tested.

## Cyclical Tenderness

No one knows exactly why some women develop benign breast lumps, but breast care specialists blame a woman's menstrual cycle for the appearance and disappearance of breast lumps. "Throughout the menstrual cycle, the levels of oestrogen and progesterone fluctuate, which causes the breast tissue cells to respond," says Ellen Yankauskas, M.D., director of the Women's Center for Family Health in Atascadero, California. "Breast tissue is on 'standby' for breastfeeding and at times will thicken and retain fluid. These premenstrual changes trigger the development of tiny, fluid-filled cysts in the breasts' milk-producing glands, which then may reduce in size after your period," she adds. The cysts and the thickening can be felt as lumps. The medical term is fibrocystic breast disease. (*Fibro* means "thickening", and *cystic* means "sacs of fluid".) "But I don't like to think of it as a disease – these tiny fluid-filled sacs are actually quite normal; I just attribute the condition to the normal variation among women," says Dr. Yankauskas.

"Most women will experience cycles of increasing lumpiness and tenderness," says Dr. Cady. "Women seem to go through broad periods of 2, 3, up to 6 months at a time, then they disappear, and she won't feel any more lumps," explains Dr. Cady. "Then, years later, there will be another time period where she'll feel lumps or tenderness for several weeks or months."

According to Dr. Cady, breast tenderness is caused by this buildup of fluid in the breast tissue. "Some women actually put on 1 to 1.5 kilograms (2 to 3 pounds) prior to the onset of their periods. They notice an engorgement of their breasts, and their bras feel tighter. Their breasts become painful and difficult to touch."

Generalized lumpiness sometimes feels "ropy" or "granular" and can often be felt in the area around the nipple and areola and in the upper, outer part of the breast. During pregnancy, the milk-producing glands become swollen, and the breasts may feel lumpier than usual. This new lumpiness can make it difficult for a woman to examine her breasts while she is pregnant. However, if you are pregnant, don't stop performing breast self-examination. Although very uncommon, breast cancer has been diagnosed during pregnancy. Lumpiness may become more obvious as you approach middle age and the milk-producing glandular tissue of the breasts increasingly gives way to soft, fatty tissue. Unless you are taking hormone replacement therapy, this type of lumpiness generally disappears after menopause.

Rest assured, most benign breast changes do not increase a woman's chances for getting cancer. Recent studies show that only certain very spe-

---

### THE HORMONE ZONE
# A DIET PLAN THAT'S KIND TO YOUR BREASTS

Studies have shown that women who live in countries where a low-fat diet is eaten have fewer breast complaints. "Leading health authorities say to follow a diet consisting of less than 30 per cent fat," says Ellen Yankauskas, M.D., director of the Women's Center for Family Health in Atascadero, California.

Blake Cady, M.D., director of the Breast Health Center at the Women and Infants Hospital in Providence, Rhode Island, agrees. "This is not only good for general breast health, but it's also recommended for overall health. Westerners eat too many fatty foods and calories. Instead of a plant-based diet, we have a cholesterol-based diet, which stimulates the endocrine system to produce more hormones. Each generation of Western women is getting heavier and taller, and they're menstruating earlier and having menopause later than their ancestors. The body converts animal-based foods into hormone-like compounds."

A breast-friendly diet, say these two experts, contains less meat, salt and caffeine and more soya.

"Most US beef today contains growth hormones, either from injections or from the feed they eat," notes Dr. Yankauskas. "Although we're not completely certain yet of the possible connection between growth-stimulating hormones and breast problems, why add more hormones to your diet, since most breast lumps are hormone-related.

"In cultures that consume a large amount of soya in the diet, women have fewer breast problems," notes Dr. Yankauskas. Soya beans, and foods made from soya, contain isoflavones, naturally occurring substances that are converted to hormone-like substances that may be beneficial in decreasing the overall oestrogen level in the body, thereby cutting breast discomfort. "Aim for at least two servings of soya a day," says Dr. Yankauskas.

"Salt, and foods that are high in sodium, cause the body to retain fluid, which adds to breast discomfort," says Dr. Yankauskas. Switch your table salt to low-sodium products and cut back on tinned and processed foods. Fast-food

cific types of microscopic changes, featuring excessive cell growth, or hyperplasia, put a woman at higher risk. According to the National Cancer Institute, about 25 per cent of benign breast biopsies show signs of hyperplasia.

restaurants also dish up many high-sodium meals.

According to Dr. Yankauskas, many women feel the difference in breast comfort very quickly when they cut back on coffee. "Some women are very sensitive to caffeine and have to eliminate it completely from their diets. But when they do, their breast discomfort improves."

Caffeine is found in coffee, tea, soft drinks, chocolate, and some over-the-counter pain medications.

"Switching from coffee to herbal tea can help many women with breast problems because some herbal teas act as a diuretic, removing extra fluid from breast tissues," says Dr. Yankauskas. "The extra fluid causes swelling and discomfort."

Dr. Yankauskas also recommends drinking purified water. "I believe there are many pesticides in the environment and water systems today, which the body turns into hormonal substances." Recent animal studies have shown that pesticides can be converted into hormonal substances. This association justifies further investigation into the link between pesticides and breast and prostate cancers, she adds.

You can purchase a tap water purifier at many large DIY shops or speciality water suppliers. Take a bottle of purified water to work with you so you can have it anytime. It's also a good idea to take along your own purified water when you travel.

**FOODS TO ADD**

- Nuts and seeds (for vitamin E)
- Soya milk (on breakfast cereal) and other soya products
- Tofu burgers
- Purified water
- Herbal tea

**FOODS TO SUBTRACT**

- Meat that is not hormone-free
- Tinned or processed foods (unless low-sodium)
- Coffee and fizzy drinks (unless decaffeinated)
- Fast-food meals

## What Does It Feel Like, Exactly?

If you find a breast lump, do not try to diagnose it yourself. While most breast lumps are benign, it's still important to consult a doctor to confirm that the lump is nothing serious. If you find a lump, follow these tips from Dr. Yankauskas, so you can describe it accurately to your doctor:

**Is the lump becoming larger, or harder?** Be sure to tell your doctor the date you found the lump or change, and the time in your menstrual cycle it was found. Describe the size of the lump – is it as small as a pea or as large as a grape or walnut?

**Does the lump feel firm but rubbery? Can you move it around? Does it ache?** A typical cancerous breast lump feels hard, gritty and painless and stays in one place.

**Is there a lump, or similar feeling of thickened tissue, in the opposite breast?** If the other breast has a similar feeling, chances are these are normal, benign breast changes.

**Is the lumpy area still there, in the same size, after your period?** If the area you found shrinks in size, or feels softer, it's probably just a normal breast change due to hormonal influences. "The ideal time to do a breast self-examination is 2 weeks after your period – always at the same time of each month," says Dr. Yankauskas. "Many doctors' surgeries have synthetic breast models where you can actually feel the size and texture of a breast lump," she adds.

## Self-Care Can Help

If you have breast lumps, and your doctor has assured you that they are nothing serious, here's what you can do to ease discomfort.

**Keep weight in check.** Women store oestrogen in body fat, so when you lose excess weight, there is less body fat where the oestrogen can be stored. This decrease of oestrogen in the body means that less of it is available to contribute to breast discomfort. "Weight loss often reduces the overall size and weight of the breast, which will also ease the discomfort," says Dr. Yankauskas.

**Walk, don't run.** "Studies have shown that women who exercise two or three times a week have fewer breast problems and lower rates of breast cancer," notes Dr. Yankauskas. "A fast-paced walk is just as beneficial as running and is gentler on the breast tissue as well as on the bones and joints." Dr. Yankauskas also recommends swimming and advises avoiding exercise that causes the breasts to bounce and jiggle, such as running or aerobic classes.

Brisk walking and swimming also help keep weight in check.

**Buy the right bra.** When exercising, be sure to wear a sports/exercise bra that supports the breasts, with wide, moderately elastic (or nonelastic) straps. "The breasts are supported by ligaments," explains Dr. Yankauskas. "The weight of the breasts, if not supported properly, will keep pulling on the ligaments, stretching them, causing pain and discomfort. The right athletic bra will keep the breasts supported, in place, and lifted, which reduces breast discomfort." Check the cups for seams, which can be irritating. If you need an underwire bra for support, make sure that it's very well padded so that it doesn't add to the friction.

**Apply heat.** "Place a warm compress, heating pad, or heated towel against the painful breast for 10 to 15 minutes, but be sure to place another towel on the skin to protect the skin from being burned," says Dr. Yankauskas. "Some women find warmth helps ease breast tenderness."

**Or reach for something cool.** "Other women feel relief if they place a cool compress against the affected breast for about 10 to 15 minutes or to their own comfort level," says Dr. Yankauskas. "Cool can help reduce the swelling that occurs when breasts retain fluid before and during the menstrual cycle. I also recommend using a bag of frozen vegetables as a cold compress – frozen peas or sweetcorn works best because the bag can be moulded to fit the shape of the breast," says Dr. Yankauskas. "It's a cheap and reusable method, and the bags hold the cold a lot longer than the average compress. Once again, use a towel to protect the skin from the cold," she adds. Experiment with either hot or cold compresses to see which works best for you.

**Take a pain reliever.** "Women with tender, painful breasts can find relief

---

## ON THE WEB & Other Resources

The main UK cancer charity is Cancer Research UK which does research and provides every sort of cancer support and advice. There are many regional offices, or contact:
**Cancer Research UK**
PO Box 123
Lincoln's Inn Fields
London WC2A 3PX
Tel: 0207 242 0200
*www.cancerresearchuk.org*

for information about this charity's work and about cancer
*www.cancerhelp.org.uk*
for information on the cancer support the charity offers

with most of the over-the-counter anti-inflammatory pain relievers, such as paracetamol, aspirin, ibuprofen and naproxen," says Dr. Yankauskas. "These pain relievers usually work best when they are taken at the first sign of discomfort," she adds.

**Try vitamin E.** "Evidence suggests that taking extra vitamin E may be effective in relieving breast tenderness and discomfort," says Dr. Yankauskas. Start with 30 IU. "If that doesn't help, increase your dose up to 200, then 400 IU per day for at least for 2 to 4 weeks. However, don't take any more than that because vitamin E is a fat-soluble vitamin, so your body stores it. You don't want to build up a high amount of vitamin E in your body because it may interfere with blood clotting." Besides supplements, vitamin E is also found in nuts, seeds and fortified breakfast cereals.

**Consider an essential oil.** Evening primrose oil can be applied to the breasts and rubbed in like a lotion, says Connie Catellani, M.D., medical director of the Miro Center for Integrative Medicine in Evanston, Illinois. The oil contains extra omega-3 fatty acids, which may help to ease discomfort, and massaging the oil into the breasts may help improve circulation and lymphatic drainage, she adds.

# Mammogram Pain

A joke making the rounds on the Internet describes how women can prepare for their mammogram. Freeze two metal bookends overnight. Strip to the waist. Invite a stranger into the room. Press the bookends against one of the breasts, and then "smash the bookends together as hard as you can." Set an appointment with the stranger for next year to do it again.

No wonder this uncomfortable yet highly valuable test has given rise to black humour.

Maryn McKenna had her first mammogram at 35, to establish a baseline of breast health.

Her doctor didn't mention that a mammogram should be scheduled early in her menstrual cycle, not just before her period, when her breasts were swollen and sensitive.

As a result, "I screamed – really screamed" when the plates came down to compress her breasts.

"The technician tried to be kind," McKenna says. "But it was her job to get the procedure done and get clear films, so there was a limit to what she could do to reduce my discomfort."

McKenna was bruised for a week afterwards, with two "nice straight-edged bruises" on the outer edge of her breasts.

Four years later, when another doctor recommended a mammogram and an ultrasound after she discovered a lump in McKenna's left breast, McKenna was terrified at the prospect of another painful mammogram.

"I went to the mammogram cold and shaky, sick with anxiety," says McKenna. "Even though it was not as painful the second time, I winced and trembled throughout the procedure." (McKenna's lump turned out to be a benign cyst.)

## Not the Worst Test of the Lot

McKenna's experience is far from unique. There is such trepidation about mammograms, some women ease the anxiety by sharing humour about the procedure.

"This is a real problem," says Marie Lugano, founder of the American Menopause Foundation in New York City. Almost 91 per cent of women over 50 experienced some degree of pain and 15 per cent reported intense pain, according to a study of 116 women conducted by Duke University's Comprehensive Cancer Center in Durham, North Carolina (one of the few studies done on the subject).

But if those figures reflect the experience of the general population, then it is also likely that many women are saying "no thanks" to repeat visits. And that could result in enormous health implications, says Emily Conant, M.D., chief of breast imaging and associate professor of radiology at the University of Pennsylvania Medical Center in Philadelphia.

Painful or not, mammograms are still the best way to detect breast cancer early and have been credited with saving thousands of lives, says Dr. Conant. About 39,000 women are diagnosed with new cases of cancer each year in the UK – and another 13,000 women die from the disease annually.

"Many other screening tests are far more uncomfortable than a mammogram – colonoscopy, for example," notes Dr. Conant. "So from my perspective, this is a relatively minor price to pay."

In Britain most women are offered mammograms from the age of 50 and are screened every three years. If there is a strong family history of the disease they may be offered mammograms at an earlier age. Anyone worried about cancer should discuss the pros and cons of mammography and other screening tests with her doctor.

## Less Painful Examinations Are in the Works

"We don't design the machines to be painful," says Joel Gray, Ph.D., vice president of business and clinical development at Lorad Corporation of Danbury, Connecticut, one of the world's largest manufacturers of mammogram machines.

Still, a mammogram has to exert pressure to do its job. Compression – which usually takes about 30 seconds – is necessary for three major reasons: it spreads out the rounded breast tissue to a more manageable 2.5 to 5-cm (1 to 2-inch) thickness that allows doctors to see the breast more clearly. It holds the breast tightly so there's little or no movement on the x-ray that could decrease the picture's clarity. And it means technicians can use less radiation – about a 0.2- to 0.3-rad dose per picture – during the process.

Researchers are working on new techniques of mammography that would involve less pain. For example, the University of Illinois is one of several institutions developing an optical mammography technique – now being tested in commercial clinical trials – that allows near-infrared light to probe breast tissue for hidden growths. Besides being painless, it also is more effective in screening cancer in women between 40 and 50 years old, whose breast tissue is denser and more difficult to read with today's conventional equipment. Today's screening mammograms miss up to one-quarter of breast cancers in women in their forties, compared with about 10 per cent of cancers in older women, according to the National Cancer Institute.

"We are very excited about these new ways that we can look through bone and soft tissue," says Enrico Gratton, Ph.D., a biomedical physicist at the University of Illinois at Urbana–Champaign. "We are making progress."

Elsewhere around the world, companies and academic circles are looking at other techniques, such as thermal imaging or electrical impulse imaging, as possible ways to increase accuracy and improve the process.

None of them have been approved officially yet, Dr. Gray points out, but in many cases the results look encouraging.

And that means the days of painful mammograms could be coming to a close.

"We're not that far away," Dr. Gratton says. "Certainly within a decade and, hopefully, within 5 years."

## Time It Right

Until then, there are a few things you can do that will certainly help to make a mammogram more bearable.

- *Try to schedule your mammogram during the first week following your period to reduce the chance of pain. At that time your breasts are least likely to be tender. Like McKenna, women who experience premenstrual syndrome – associated with excess levels of oestrogen and too little progesterone – experience less pain if they schedule the procedure in the first 10 days of their cycle. As women get older and their oestrogen levels decline, the procedure should get easier.*
- *Cut back on caffeine for at least 4 to 6 weeks before the examination, and take 200 to 400 IU of vitamin E daily, so you may experience less pain, says Connie Catellani, M.D., medical director of the Miro Center for Integrative Medicine in Evanston, Illinois.*
- *Take an over-the-counter painkiller about an hour before the examination, Dr. Conant says.*
- *Practise some form of relaxation before and while undergoing a mammogram. Breathe deeply and think about a place you feel comfortable and safe.*
- *Talk to the technician and discuss any fears you may have before the mammogram starts. Doctors say the screening also depends on the technician's skill, regardless of your age and the size and shape of your breasts. "We have women apologizing because they don't have large breasts, thinking it's more difficult to get small breasts into position for imaging. But we do mammograms on men, so breast size really shouldn't be a factor," says Dr. Conant.*

Ask the technician if there's a warming pad to make the plates less chilly. Also, the plates should never rest on bony structures, like a collarbone or breastbone. The technician should also smooth out the skin one final time before lowering the plates to make sure nothing gets pinched.

"Technicians should be asking patients, 'Are you OK' 'Can you tolerate that?' as they go," Dr. Conant says. "This also adds to the patient's feeling of 'control' over the situation."

# Cancer Prevention and Treatment

Second only to Alzheimer's disease, cancer is probably the disease women dread most. Yet the number of healthy women who are former cancer patients is a testament to fact that cancer isn't the terminal illness it was a generation ago. Nor are the causes a total mystery. Although genes do influence cancer risk, heredity alone explains only a fraction of all cancers. According to experts:

- *About one-third of the cancer deaths that occur in the UK each year can be attributed to eating an unhealthy diet and not getting enough exercise.*
- *One-third are due to cigarette smoking.*
- *The final third are due to other factors, such as infectious diseases, including the human papillomavirus, which has been closely linked with cervical cancer.*

Cancer is not just one disease but an array of more than 100 kinds of malignancy – uncontrolled growth and spread of abnormal cells that attack different organs of the body in a variety of ways. For example, lung cancer may spread to other tissues in a slightly different way than breast cancer. If the spread is not controlled, it can be life-threatening.

Cancer is caused by a combination of external forces (chemicals, radiation and viruses) and internal factors (hormones, immune conditions and inherited mutations). Often 10 or more years pass between exposures or mutations and detection of a cancer.

Researchers suspect that 5 to 10 per cent of cancers may be inherited. But in the vast majority of cases, cancer develops through a complex series of steps that include prolonged exposure to carcinogens, cancer-causing substances such as tobacco and asbestos. These carcinogens usually affect cells in specific organs.

## The Role of Hormones

Sometimes, even overexposure to a natural substance – like sunlight – is linked to an increased risk of cancer. Such seems to be the case with hormones.

"Breast, ovarian and endometrial cancers are considered hormone-related cancers because they are associated with a prolonged exposure to the hormones oestrogen and progesterone," says Carmen Rodriguez, M.D., senior epidemiologist with the American Cancer Society. A woman's menstrual cycle is divided into two phases – the first 14 days are called the follicular phase, and the second 14 days are called the luteal phase. "Around day 14 of the menstrual cycle, the luteal phase, the ovary produces high levels of oestrogen, and about 7 days later, a high level of progesterone. Researchers suspect it is the action of these hormones in some women that sometimes causes the cells to proliferate, or multiply, which is one of the principles of cancer," says Dr. Rodriguez. Not that getting your period is in the same league as smoking cigarettes, she adds.

"It's the cumulative exposure to oestrogen – and perhaps to progesterone – as a result of repeated periods over the years that may increase a woman's risk of getting hormonal cancers," explains Dr. Rodriguez.

"These ovarian hormones affect the rate of cell division." A close-up look at various reproductive system cancers explains further.

## Breast Cancer

Studies have shown that breast tissue cell proliferation rates are low during the follicular phase of the menstrual cycle, when oestrogen and progesterone levels are low. Proliferation rates are higher during the luteal phase of the cycle, when levels of these ovarian hormones are higher. "We also know that decreased exposure to oestrogens, such as during pregnancy and breast-feeding, lowers a woman's risk of breast cancer, and, conversely, getting their period at an early age (prolonging lifetime exposure to hormones produced) increases the risk," says Dr. Rodriguez.

Obesity plays a contributing a role in breast cancer, partly due to hormones. "We know that women who are very obese in premenopausal years don't ovulate regularly, and they have a lower risk of breast cancer. As soon as these obese women go through menopause, the ovaries are not functioning, and they are not producing oestrogen any more. However, obese women have a higher amount of adipose tissue than thin women do, and adipose tissue synthesizes oestrogen. So these women are still exposed to high levels of oestrogen, and they are at a higher risk of breast cancer than thin women – even after menopause."

## Ovarian and Endometrial Cancers

Each month during ovulation, the ovary produces an egg and releases it, which researchers believe causes the surface (the epithelium) of the ovary to become damaged. As a result, the ovary tries to repair itself. "Sometimes, in the process of this repair, a mutation can occur, and will eventually produce cancer," explains Dr. Rodriguez. "About 90 per cent of ovarian cancers are epithelial cancers. The more times this damage and repair happens, the greater the possibility of ovarian cancer. That's why women who have children are at a lower risk, because women don't ovulate when they are pregnant or breastfeeding."

A woman's risk of ovarian cancer also decreases when she takes oral contraceptives because they impair ovulation. "Tubal ligation, or getting the tubes tied, also lowers a woman's risk of getting ovarian cancer because the hormone production is lower," says Dr. Rodriguez.

The situation is practically the same with endometrial cancer – risk factors include taking oestrogen replacement therapy; taking tamoxifen (Nolvadex), prescribed for breast cancer; early menstruation (before the age of 12); late menopause (after the age of 50); and never having had children.

## Colon Cancer

Although breast cancer gets all the attention, colorectal cancers are the third most common cancers in women. Risk factors include a personal or family history of colorectal cancer or polyps and of inflammatory bowel disease. Other possible risk factors include physical inactivity, following a high-fat/low-fibre diet, and a low intake of fruits and vegetables.

Recent studies have suggested that oestrogen replacement therapy and nonsteroidal anti-inflammatory drugs (such as aspirin and ibuprofen) may *reduce* risk. "There are oestrogen receptors located throughout the body," explains Dr. Rodriguez. "The hormone acts differently at different parts of the body. In the case of the colon, studies show that oestrogen may be protective against colon cancer. Researchers theorize that oestrogen decreases concentrations of bile acid in the colon. Bile acids have the capability to promote tumours in the colon."

# HRT and OCs Under Scrutiny

If natural production of hormones seems to contribute to risk for cancer at some level, what about *adding* hormones as supplements, either in the form of hormone replacement therapy (HRT) at menopause, or earlier in the form of oral contraceptives (OCs)?

Not surprisingly, there does seem to be some link, for some women, under some circumstances.

As explained earlier, in chapter 11, HRT comes in many forms, including oestrogen alone or a combination therapy of oestrogen plus progesterone. "Postmenopausal women who have not had a hysterectomy, who still have their uteruses, are at a higher risk of endometrial cancer if they take oestrogen alone, without progesterone," says Dr. Rodriguez.

As for oral contraceptives, according to a well-publicized study in the

*Journal of the American Medical Association*, women with a strong family history of breast cancer who used older OCs had an increased risk of developing breast cancer. Researchers at the Mayo Clinic followed more than 400 families of women diagnosed with breast cancer between 1944 and 1952. From 1991 to 1996, the team interviewed relatives about their history of cancer and their risk factors for breast cancer. Among women whose mothers or sisters had breast cancer, those who had ever taken OCs formulated before 1975 had a three times higher risk of developing breast cancer than those who had never taken OCs. The risk was even higher in families in which five or more blood relatives had breast or ovarian cancer.

But before you stop taking the Pill, consider that Dr. Rodriguez urges women to put the study in perspective. "That's just one study, and the number of breast cancer cases among women taking oral contraceptives was very small. So they're drawing a conclusion based on a small group of women," says Dr. Rodriguez. "The data from that study suggests that it is the early formulations of the Pill, which contained very high doses of the hormones oestrogen and progestin, that increase risk. Today's contraception pills contain much lower doses. In addition, according to a recent review of studies, researchers found a very small increased risk of breast cancer in women who used oral contraceptives for a long time." And besides, oral contraceptives lower a woman's risk of ovarian cancer, she adds.

Nevertheless, women with a family history of breast cancer who have taken older oral contraceptives should be sure to practise breast self-

## THE HORMONE CONNECTION
# BREAST CANCER SURGERY: TIMING IS THE KEY

According to a British study of 112 women, those who had breast cancer surgery on day 1 or 2 or on days 13 to 32 of their menstrual cycles had a better survival rate than those who scheduled the procedure on days 3 to 12, when hormones are priming the body for ovulation.

Researchers theorize that during surgery, some cancer cells enter the bloodstream and may be stimulated by the higher oestrogen levels that naturally occur before ovulation. If your cycle is regular, it may be possible to schedule surgery during the second half to yield the best benefits and lower the risk of recurrence. Discuss it with your doctor.

examinations each month and schedule regular mammograms and clinical breast examinations.

## What You Can Do Now

Apart from the role of hormones, there's plenty else you can – and should – do lower your risk of cancers of all kinds, starting with diet.

"Epidemiological studies show very clearly that poor eating habits are linked with an increased risk of certain cancers, not to mention heart disease," says Connie Catellani, M.D., medical director of the Miro Center for Integrative Medicine in Evanston, Illinois.

And it's never too late.

"I know of some patients who even got through chemotherapy more easily because they changed their diets," says Dr. Catellani. "They switched to a diet low in fatty foods and red meat, and high in fruits and vegetables. They also cut back on refined sugars and carbohydrates, such as sweets and cakes. They found the foods in their new eating plan easier to digest and felt they had more energy and were able to tolerate the lengthy treatment better."

To lower your risk of cancer:

**Think plants.** Choose most of the foods you eat from plant sources, starting with the greengrocery aisle. "The recommendation to eat at least five servings a day of fruits and vegetables is sound advice for all cancers," says Dr. Rodriguez.

Nine are even better. "Fruits and vegetables are loaded with antioxidants, nutrients that protect cells against free radical damage. If there aren't enough antioxidants in the diet, the body can't keep up with damage from free radicals, and damage increases with time," says Dr. Catellani.

"Any change in diet which is targeted to increase the consumption of vegetables and fruits may lower a woman's risk of certain cancers, such as colon and stomach cancers. It is also good for lowering her risk of heart disease, which is the leading killer of American women," says Dr. Catellani. Her advice: stock up on the cruciferous vegetables, such as broccoli, purple sprouting broccoli, Brussels sprouts, cabbage and cauliflower. Also choose red fruits and veggies high in the cancer-fighting chemical lycopene, such as tomatoes, red grapefruit, watermelon and guava. Reach for beta-carotene-rich produce, such as winter squash, carrots and sweet potatoes. Other cancer-fighting produce include citrus fruits, such as oranges and grapefruit; dark green leafy vegetables, such as spinach, romaine lettuce, kale, spring greens and Swiss chard; and berries, such as strawberries, raspberries, blackberries and blueberries.

**Choose whole grains.** Instead of white rice, use a variety of whole grains, such as brown rice, bulgar and cracked wheat. Buy wholegrain bagels, breads, cereals, biscuits, tortillas and pasta. Both strategies maximize fibre intake, which may fight breast cancer by lowering levels of oestrogen in the body. High-fibre diets have also been associated with lower rates of colorectal cancer in some studies.

**Use your bean.** Beans, also called pulses, are rich in nutrients, like fibre, that may protect against cancer. Buy tins of bean soup and keep them in your pantry to have on hand, and toss chickpeas into salads. To make a quick black bean salad, rinse canned black beans and toss with chopped Spanish onion, olive oil, balsamic vinegar, fresh parsley, sea salt and fresh ground pepper.

**Eat more foods in their natural state.** "In addition to eating whole grains instead of refined bread and cereal products, eat fresh fruits and vegetables, instead of tinned and processed foods made with artificial chemicals that our bodies did not evolve with and cannot break down. So they accumulate in our bodies over time, and they may cause cancer later in life," says Dr. Catellani. Also, foods in their natural state have the highest amount of antioxidants.

**Opt for lean meat.** And keep portion sizes small (about the size of a deck of playing cards). "Red meat requires a lot of antioxidative action to process, so you want to keep your intake minimal," says Dr. Catellani. "Meat has also been injected with hormones, antibiotics, or other chemicals and has a high fat content. Cattle are often fed grain sprayed with pesticides. All these components of meat can be very damaging to the body and possibly increase cancer risk. When we eat meat, we're ingesting and exposing our body to all the chemicals and pesticides that that animal has been exposed to. For example, animals store these chemicals and pesticides in their fat. The more we eat, the more we're exposing ourselves to these damaging factors." (For more on the role of meat and hormone balance, see Phase 1 of the Hormone-Balancing Programme on page 258.)

**Switch to fish.** "Replace burgers and meat with fish," advises Dr. Catellani. "Beef cattle and chickens are higher on the food chain than fish, in part because they live longer. Fish, which may live a year, haven't had as much time to absorb and store as many harmful chemicals as beef cattle, which may live for several years. With a few exceptions, most fish live in the ocean in pristine conditions." In addition, the omega-3 fatty acids in fish may help fight breast cancer. Good sources of omega-3s include salmon, mackerel, tuna, sardines and herring. The next time you go out to dinner, order grilled salmon instead of a steak.

**Think of Great-Great-Grandma.** "Before you sit down to a meal, ask yourself if Great-Great-Grandma or Grandpa ate or drank this," says Dr. Catellani. "Would they be able to recognize what's on your plate? Chances are, Great-Great-Grandma did not wash down her meal with diet cola that contains aspartame, an artificial chemical." This is just one way of thinking that may help to eliminate all the recent additions of chemicals and processed foods that may possibly increase the risk of cancer, she adds.

**Serve soya.** "Soya products are rich in phyto-oestrogens, plant chemicals that seem to protect against breast cancer because they are weak oestrogens," says Dr. Catellani. "Phyto-oestrogens block harmful oestrogenic activity by occupying the oestrogen receptor sites in the body. Our bodies make three different kinds of oestrogen – oestriol, oestradiol and oestrone. Most of the oestrogen in our body is oestriol. The smallest amount is oestradiol and oestrone. Oestradiol and oestrone stimulate the breast and uterus and encourage growth of these tissues. To counter this harmful effect, oestriol tends to block those actions, so it works like a check-and-balance system. But when we get hormonal influence from our food, such as in dairy products and red meat, and the environment, through many pesticides and PCBs, which mimic oestrogen activity, it tips the balance so there's more harmful oestrogen.

"Eating soya foods helps to bring this hormonal scenario back into balance by muting the excess oestrogen," says Dr. Catellani. "In countries where soya foods are eaten in large amounts every day, like Japan and China, there's so much less breast cancer and menopausal difficulties than in the West." Soya beans contain many other potentially anticarcinogenic compounds, such as saponins, phytates and protease inhibitors.

Good food sources of soya include soya beans, soya milk, tofu and miso. Be sure to look for a label that says "not genetically modified" or "Non-GMO", and limit your intake of soya foods to one to two servings per day, says Dr. Catellani.

**Sprinkle on flaxseed.** Flax is a source of a weak anti-oestrogen that may be useful in preventing or treating oestrogen-responsive tumours found in the breast, uterus, or ovary. Flaxseed also supplies a plant form of omega-3 fatty acids. Grind the seed in a coffee grinder or a food processor for a few seconds so it's easier to digest. Then sprinkle the seed on cereal or salad.

**Drink organic, low-fat milk.** Low-fat milk, such as skimmed, has a low amount of fat, yet is a great source of a molecule called conjugated linoleic acid (CLA), which has promising anticancer activity, says Dr. Catellani. CLA is found in high amounts in dairy fat. If possible, purchase organic dairy products.

Here's another reason to linger in the dairy case. According to one study, when people at high risk for colon cancer increased their daily intake of calcium to 1200 milligrams by adding low-fat dairy products to their diet, the cells in the lining of their colons that had acted like precursors of colon cancer started acting like healthy cells. Another study found that a diet containing an average of 825 milligrams of calcium from low-fat dairy foods significantly decreased the risk for colon cancer.

**Limit alcohol.** "Alcohol raises a woman's risk of breast cancer," says Dr. Rodriguez. "Studies show that the risk of breast cancer increases with just a few drinks a week. Once again, hormones increase the effect. Alcohol increases oestrogen levels."

**Drink green tea instead.** "In countries where women drink green tea, there is less cancer," notes Dr. Catellani. "Green tea is high in antioxidants." Green tea also contains the promising anticancer activity of a compound called epigallocatechin gallate (EGCG). Green tea can be consumed either hot or cold. Instead of iced tea, make a pitcher of iced green tea today.

**Consider coenzyme $Q_{10}$.** Coenzyme $Q_{10}$ is an antioxidant that occurs naturally in the body and helps convert food into energy. Although research is preliminary, coenzyme $Q_{10}$ may help lower a woman's risk of breast cancer and may even be used as treatment for it. In a Danish study, researchers treated a group of 32 breast cancer patients with 90 milligrams of coenzyme $Q_{10}$, other antioxidants, and fatty acids. Six of the 32 patients showed partial tumour regression. In one of the six cases, the dosage of coenzyme $Q_{10}$ was increased to 390 milligrams. One month after this increase, the tumour was no longer palpable, and in another month, there was no sign of the tumour on her mammogram. A Turkish study of 21 breast cancer patients also found that coenzyme $Q_{10}$ may protect the normal breast tissue from malignant tumours.

"Several small studies have indicated that women who take coenzyme $Q_{10}$ on a regular basis seem to have a lower incidence of breast cancer," notes Dr. Catellani. "We're not sure exactly how it works, but we suspect since it's a good antioxidant, it facilitates cell damage repair.

"I recommend 30 to 60 milligrams daily of coenzyme $Q_{10}$ for women who do not have breast cancer, and 120 milligrams daily for women who do.

Women who are taking the higher dosage of coenzyme $Q_{10}$ should do so only under the direction of a doctor," she says.

**Add selenium-rich foods.** "There's been research that showed that people who live in areas where there's a high selenium content in the soil – and therefore more in the locally grown produce – seem to have a lower incidence of cancer than people who live in areas where the trace mineral is low," notes Dr. Catellani. "Researchers suspect it has antioxidant properties." Good food sources of selenium include fish, cereal grains, mushrooms, wheat germ, garlic, cucumbers, asparagus and Brazil nuts.

**Get regular exercise.** "Many studies have shown that regular exercise reduces your risk of breast cancer, and we suspect it does this by reducing oestrogen production," says Dr. Rodriguez. For example, researchers in Norway traced the health of more than 25,000 women over a 13-year period. They found that women who exercised at least 4 hours a week had a 37 per cent lower breast cancer risk than women who did no exercise at all. They also found that compared with sedentary workers, women who were very active at work, such as those whose jobs involved lots of lifting and walking, reduced their breast cancer risk by about one-quarter. A smaller, more recent study found that women who engaged in an average of 7 or more hours of physical activity per week had an 18 per cent lower chance of developing breast cancer than women who engaged in less than 1 hour per week of physical activity.

If you think you can't begin to relate to those women because you're "out of shape", or "it's too late to start an exercise programme now", think again. "Some women feel unless they exercised early in life, it's too late to offer a protective effect," says Dr. Rodriguez. "That's not true. We're finding that exercise throughout a woman's life, even in her later years, can lower her risk of breast cancer."

"I call exercising a self-activated antioxidant," says Dr. Catellani. "It gets the blood moving and steps up the process of antioxidation. If you want to detox your body and lessen your cancer risk, walk four or five times a week for 45 minutes to an hour. Or attend a dance or yoga class. What's important is that you choose something you're interested in, that you'll stick with. Women who start an exercise programme by sweating it out at the local gym for 2 hours a day usually drop the programme fairly quickly. Intense, short bursts of exercise are nowhere near as helpful as regular, long, sustained exercise at a modest pace."

**Give up the talc.** Studies have shown a small increased risk of ovarian can-

## ON THE WEB & Other Resources

The main UK cancer charity is Cancer Research UK which does research and provides every sort of cancer support and advice. There are many regional offices, or contact:

**Cancer Research UK**
PO Box 123
Lincoln's Inn Fields
London WC2A 3PX
Tel: 0207 242 0200
*www.cancerresearchuk.org*

for information about this charity's work and about cancer
*www.cancerhelp.org.uk*
for information on the cancer support the charity offers

**The British Medical Association**
Tavistock Square
London WCIH 9JP
Tel: 0845 920 0169
*www.bma.org.uk*

cer with talc use, says Dr. Rodriguez. Talc sometimes contains asbestos, a known carcinogen. Talc applied directly to the vaginal area may migrate up into the vagina and reach the ovaries. The studies did not show an increased risk in women who used talc powder on other areas of their body. Check product labels for the ingredient asbestiform fibres or contact the manufacturers for further information.

**Cool down hot flushes.** Women who have had breast cancer are sometimes advised to avoid hormone replacement therapy to ease menopausal symptoms because the additional hormones may stimulate breast cancer cells. In one small study of 27 women, the antidepressant drug paroxetine (Seroxat) reduced the frequency of hot flushes on average by 67 per cent and the severity of hot flushes on average by 75 per cent. Paroxetine is available by prescription only, so talk to your doctor if you think this might be the right thing for you.

**Clean out your emotional closet.** "Some women who are at the middle point of their lives have many issues going on at this time, such as not being able to have children anymore," notes Dr. Catellani. "The research is preliminary, but the mind-body literature suggests that people who have unresolved issues, and hold in their anger or suppress emotions, are at risk for cancer. And when they are diagnosed with cancer, they don't fare as well as those women who are at peace with themselves. Now is the time to confront that family member and open the lines of communication or to go after those secret ambitions, such as travelling, painting, or dancing. Research is showing that acting on those dreams may be good for your health."

# Jet Lag

Any woman who travels long-distance by air knows the feeling: you arrive in one place, while your body feels like it is literally "lagging" somewhere else. You wake up when everyone around you is ready for lunch. You're ready for dinner when everybody else is going to bed. Other possible effects include fatigue, headache, irritability, poor concentration, indigestion, loss of appetite and bowel irregularities.

Aptly named jet lag, this disruption of your natural body rhythms is somewhat proportional to the number of time zones you cross – and is especially pronounced if you travel "forward" in time (from west to east). If you fly from London to Oman, where there is a 3-hour time difference, chances are your body will cling to its London sleep and meal schedule for 3 or 4 days. If you fly from London to Auckland – more than a day's time difference – you're going to feel far more out of sync for a week or more.

"The rule of thumb is that it takes 1 day to recover for every time zone you have crossed when travelling east to west (where you gain time)," says Gary Zammit, Ph.D., director of the Sleep Disorders Institute at St. Luke's–Roosevelt Hospital in New York City. "When travelling west to east (where you lose time) it takes 1½ days for every time zone crossed."

But how does your body even know you are in a different time zone?

"The new environment challenges your body rhythms," explains Dr. Zammit. "When you get back to London from Oman, your body operates as though it's midnight, but everyone else is wide awake – it's only 9 p.m.. for them."

More subtly, your pineal gland, a pinecone-shaped gland located deep within your brain, "reads" shifts in light, with bright light signalling the body to wake up and darkness signalling the body to sleep. This prompts the pineal gland to release melatonin, a hormone that helps induce sleep. Normally, as the sun goes down, the pineal gland releases an increasing amount of melatonin into your bloodstream. This continues until about 2 a.m. to 4 a.m., when the hormone release begins to taper off.

Crossing time zones confuses your melatonin release schedule. So does shift work. Shift workers who work all night and emerge in the morning light also get jet lag. Flying north to south doesn't cause jet lag since you don't cross time zones and there's no change in your day–night rhythm.

Interestingly, female flight attendants seem to be more affected by jet lag at certain phases of their menstrual cycles, or their cycles may be disturbed, suggesting that hormones other than melatonin are involved.

# Natural Ways to Beat Jet Lag

Much advice concerning jet lag involves elaborate pretravel tactics to prepare your body for disruptions associated with crossing time zones and speed the transition. These involve:

- *Staying up until the bedtime in the new time zone, then sleep in as late as you can.*
- *Taking a night flight when travelling from the west to the east – say, from London to Bangkok – sleeping on the plane, and going to bed at the desired bedtime in Bangkok.*
- *Arriving a few days ahead of time when attending an important event.*
- *Planning a stopover if you are crossing several time zones.*

Those tactics may work in an ideal world. But in reality most women are pressed for time and don't have the luxury of manipulating their pretravel schedules and responsibilities to the degree suggested. If you're travelling on business, most likely you'll be gone and back in just a few days, with no time to prepare for the return leg of your trip. And of course, the stresses of travel itself contribute to jet lag.

Here's what Dr. Zammit suggests that you can do instead.

**Set your watch ahead or back.** Before you even leave on your trip, change your watch to match the time zone you will be flying to. "This helps some people get psychologically prepared," says Dr. Zammit.

**Avoid alcohol while flying.** "It can have a sedative effect and make you sleepy at the inappropriate times," says Dr. Zammit. Also, sleeping pills (benzodiazepines, like Valium) can be helpful after your arrival, although they may leave you groggy and out of sorts the next day.

**Take a walk in the sunshine.** Studies show that exposure to full-spectrum light for 30 to 60 minutes can help your pineal gland respond more quickly to your new destination. If you are travelling from west to east, do this in the early morning to give your body light when it is used to expecting it. If you are travelling from east to west, do it in the late afternoon or early evening. This will help delay the release of melatonin for a few hours and help you adjust to your new rhythm in keeping with the place you are visiting.

**Find out if your hotel can lend you a light box.** Designed for time zone travellers, these devices shine full-spectrum light on your face, simulating a walk outdoors. Sitting in front of one for at least 30 minutes while you're working is helpful.

## What about Melatonin?

Some people are more susceptible to jet lag than others. And you may find that the older you get, the more susceptible you are to the effects of time zone travel, possibly due to a natural decline in melatonin levels that occurs with age. So if the above tactics don't work as well as you like, you could consider melatonin. Although it is not available in the UK, it is widely available on-line. Do not take it without first talking to your doctor.

A synthetic version of the hormone, which is naturally released as the sun goes down, to help you sleep, melatonin supplements seem like a logical "jet lag pill". Yet melatonin doesn't seem to be the cure-all that researchers hoped for. In one study, people travelling from New York to Oslo, Norway, who took melatonin didn't suffer significantly fewer symptoms than those who took a placebo. But melatonin can help you get to sleep, which you might be grateful for when you find yourself exhausted but lying in bed with your eyes open.

- *If you're considering melatonin, try it at home ahead of time to determine what dose is best for you and to see if you experience side effects, like vivid dreams or next-day grogginess.*
- *If you tolerate melatonin well, Dr. Zammit suggests that you take it in the early evening – about 8 p.m. in your new time zone, regardless of what direction you've travelled or how many time zones you crossed.*

To be safe, don't take more than 10 milligrams of melatonin a day, depending on your degree of sleep disturbance.

# Vision Problems

The expression "She was so angry, she couldn't see straight" may have some basis in science, especially if you fly off the handle premenstrually. But emotions don't cause fuzzy vision – hormones do.

A number of common eye problems, including dryness and poor focus, are more likely to affect women during hormonally triggered events, such as menstrual cycles, pregnancy and menopause, than at other times.

The way doctors see it, there's plenty you can do.

## Help for Hormonally Dry Eyes

"The most common problem that I see among menopause-age women in my practice is dry eyes," says Eve Higginbotham, M.D., professor and chairman of the department of ophthalmology at the University of Maryland School of Medicine in Baltimore. Dry eyes can cause blurring, scratchiness, sensitivity to light and cold, a feeling of pressure and a nagging sense that there is something in your eye.

Some doctors think that with the loss of oestrogen, your eyes lose their natural ability to keep themselves moist. "Evidently, we need a certain amount of oestrogen for the lacrimal glands in the eyes to produce adequate lubrication for the eyes because so many postmenopausal women suffer from dry eyes," says Dr. Higginbotham.

Your menstrual cycle, too, can affect your vision. If you've noticed that your contact lenses don't feel quite right just before or during your period, it's not your imagination. Your cornea – the transparent exterior part of your eye that admits light to the interior – thickens as your oestrogen level peaks, changing the shape of your eye. Water retention associated with menstruation may also make your cornea more sensitive.

*Escape from* **HORMONE HELL**

# IT HURT TO BLINK

**Q:** I'm 60 years old and have had dry eyes ever since menopause. I used to wear contact lenses but gave up – they felt like cornflakes in my eyes. I don't mind wearing glasses, but my eyes are now so dry and irritated that it hurts to blink. I've tried artificial tears, but they mess up my makeup. A friend suggested taking supplements of fish oil capsules, and at this point I'm desperate. Are they worth a try?

Kirk Wilhelmus, M.D., professor of ophthalmology at Baylor College of Medicine in Houston, replies: Though no research to date suggests that fish oil can cure dry eyes, there's logic to why it might help. Fish oils are high in the omega-3 fatty acids EPA and DHA, which may increase the viscosity of oils that your body makes – mainly in the skin and eyes. The result? Less dryness.

The best way to get omega-3s is through food, not supplements. Aim to eat at least two or three servings of fish a week (tinned tuna and all varieties of salmon except smoked are good). Though supplements provide more omega-3s than these servings, you may still notice improvement in your eyes. And you're likely to reap other health benefits, too, including a lower risk of heart disease, depression and rheumatoid arthritis.

If you just can't get your lens in on the first or second try, don't persist. If you wear your lenses despite your difficulty, by the end of the day you may have dry eyes and difficulty seeing things clearly.

During pregnancy, you may have similar difficulties with lenses due to increases in another female hormone, progesterone, that produces changes in your corneas. Your vision may also change to such an extent that you may wonder if your prescription needs to be changed. Instead, sit it out, says Dr. Higginbotham: most likely your eyesight will return to normal after your baby is born (even if nothing else does).

In the meantime, here's what you can do.

**Use artificial tears.** A few drops will help provide the natural lubricant that menopause – and other hormonal upheavals – may dry up. "I usually tell the women I treat to use them four to six times a day," says Dr. Higginbotham. "If dryness is still a problem, they can increase use up to every 2 hours, or even every hour, if necessary." Artificial tears are gentle enough to be safe for long-term use and are available in chemists or wherever health aids are sold.

**If you live where it's very dry, indoors or out, use a humidifier.** It will help keep moisture in the air of your home – and in your eyes. You may find you need more than one, in difficult areas of your home.

**Talk to your eye doctor about wearing hard contact lenses, especially during pregnancy or after menopause.** "Soft contact lenses aggravate the eyes because they are competing with your eye for moisture," says Dr. Higginbotham. "Personally, I wear gas permeable lenses because they don't require moisture."

## Defence Against Cataracts, Glaucoma and Macular Degeneration

With the onset of menopause, the risk of developing cataracts and glaucoma increases. Cataracts cause a cloudy film to cover the lens of your eye, which can make your vision blurry. Often the telltale sign of glaucoma is a feeling of pressure in your eyes. However, the most common type of glaucoma, simple or open-angle, has no symptoms, according to Dr. Higginbotham. If left untreated, glaucoma can lead to irreversible blindness. Cataracts can often be removed surgically.

Researchers don't know whether these serious vision problems are a function of age or a woman's fluctuating hormones, says Dr. Higginbotham. After all, men get them, too. But some studies suggest oestrogen may play a role in these eye diseases as well.

Perhaps the most serious vision problem that may stem from the hormonal shifts of menopause is macular degeneration. Beginning with the deterioration of the part of the eye that distinguishes detail, it is the leading cause of blindness in older people; and women are twice as likely to develop macular degeneration as men.

To save your sight, experts recommend that you:

**Wear a hat and sunglasses when in direct sunlight.** Strong ultraviolet rays can increase your risk of cataracts, macular degeneration and other vision problems.

**If you smoke, quit.** "Smoking is a risk factor for macular degeneration and cataracts," says Dr. Higginbotham. (To learn how smoking affects your hormones, and much else besides, see Phase 1 of the Hormone-Balancing Programme on page 258.)

**Eat eight servings of fruits and vegetables a day, including two dark green leafy vegetables, such as spinach and kale, and two vitamin C-rich citrus fruits.** Oxidation of proteins inside the eye lens appears to play a major role

---

## THE HORMONE CONNECTION
# MOISTER EYES WITH HRT?

Could the same treatment that helps protect your bones from osteoporosis help your eyes as well? It looks that way.

A study of nearly 80 postmenopausal women aged 50 and older has revealed that those on hormone replacement therapy (HRT) had significantly fewer complaints of dry eyes and fewer other complaints than those who were not replacing the oestrogen loss that comes with menopause.

Moreover, the longer the women were on HRT, the fewer complaints they had, says Eve Higginbotham, M.D., assistant professor and chairman of the department of ophthalmology at the University of Maryland School of Medicine in Baltimore.

Precisely why HRT seems to reduce a woman's likelihood of vision problems is not yet understood. But it appears that oestrogen helps the eye produce tears, and that in turn helps lubricate the cornea, which must remain clear to transmit light.

in cataract formation. So eating foods high in vitamin C and other nutrients that act as antioxidants can potentially reduce the damaging effects of oxidation in your eyes.

Eating spinach may also deter cataracts. In the ongoing US Nurses' Health Study, researchers found that those who ate the greatest amount of foods containing lutein and zeanthin (protective nutrients related to beta-carotene) were 22 per cent less likely to develop cataracts than women who ate the least. Spinach and kale appeared to be the most protective.

**Consider supplements.** Researchers compared how much vitamin C women aged 56 to 71 consumed and found that those who'd taken vitamin C supplements for 10 years or more reduced their risk of cataracts by 77 per cent. Extrapolating from that evidence, you need more than 359 milligrams of vitamin C a day to prevent cataracts – the amount you would get in almost six 180-millilitre (6-ounce) glasses of orange juice or 1 kilogram (2.2 pounds) of cooked broccoli.

## Diabetic? Guard Your Vision

Diabetic retinopathy, a distortion of vision caused by the slowing of the flow of blood to the retina, grows more severe during pregnancy. This is because the rise in progesterone can worsen pre-existing changes in the retina related to diabetes.

Diabetic retinopathy is a long-term complication of diabetes – particularly type 1, or juvenile-onset, diabetes – and generally would not develop if you got gestational diabetes, says Mary Lake Polan, M.D., Ph.D., professor and chairman of the department of gynaecology and obstetrics at the Stanford University School of Medicine. However, if you had gestational diabetes in a previous pregnancy, you are at a higher risk for developing it in subsequent pregnancies, says Dr. Polan, and for developing diabetes as a long-term outcome after pregnancy.

If you have diabetes and plan to become pregnant:

**Take steps to control your insulin levels.** See chapter 13 for details of what you need to do.

**See your ophthalmologist and your doctor before you even begin to try to become pregnant.** They need to be sure your diabetes is well under control. The doctor will check your haemoglobin levels, and the ophthalmologist will want to do a baseline retinal examination.

**Never miss your insulin.** Obviously this is a good idea whether you have eye problems or not.

# Recovery from Surgery

Any woman facing surgery is bound to find herself worrying: how will it turn out? How much pain will I feel? How soon will my life get back to normal?

Worry won't help, of course. In fact research now shows that worrying makes it more difficult to recover from surgery.

"The more worked up you are, the harder it is on you," says Leigh Neumayer, M.D., associate professor of surgery at the University of Utah in Salt Lake City. "As it is, stress hormones rise due to surgery. How high depends on the type of surgery. With a breast biopsy, for example, they rise a little. With a hysterectomy, they go up a lot. With heart bypass surgery, they go up even more. A woman patient who is positive and informed before surgery will have an easier recovery, in most instances."

Whenever you feel anxious, your body releases two stress hormones, cortisol and adrenaline. In turn, your heart pumps faster and circulates more oxygen and blood through your body. Stress hormones also suppress your body's immune system – the last thing you want when undergoing surgery. So a growing number of doctors now recommend that you learn what to expect from an upcoming surgery and practise relaxation techniques beforehand.

Both make you feel better physically and psychologically, says Jack Rudick, M.D., professor of surgery at Mount Sinai School of Medicine in New York City. Keeping a lid on surgery-related anxiety may cut your risk of infection, lessen pain (and how much pain medication you need), and speed your recovery time.

## Presurgery Relaxation Tactics

Take the time to prepare mentally for surgery a few weeks in advance, says Dr. Rudick. It can make a world of difference.

**Ask as many questions as possible about what to expect.** "If your doctor is unwilling to answer your questions, find another doctor," says Dr. Neumayer. Your body will respond better if your mind knows what to expect. In fact one study showed that patients scheduled for hip replacement surgery who viewed a videotape of the procedure they were about to undergo were better able to cope with presurgery jitters than those who did not. The patients who watched the video also coped better with postoperative pain.

**Let your doctor know if you are extremely nervous about the surgery.**

"If you find surgery frightening, make it clear," says Dr. Neumayer. Then, if necessary, the medical staff can help you by prescribing anti-anxiety medications.

*Don't* **take antistress herbs.** Some herbs interfere with anaesthesia or pose other problems. Vitamin E, garlic, fish oil, selenium, hawthorn berry and ginkgo, for example, decrease the ability of your blood to clot, which is essential for healing. Tell your anaesthesiologist in advance about all the herbs and supplements you take. And wait until your wound has healed before resuming those supplements.

**If you have diabetes, talk to your doctor about maintaining your insulin injections after surgery.** The high levels of sugar associated with diabetes can cause bacteria and germs to grow and make it more difficult for you to recover. Controlling your insulin levels can help keep that under control.

**Practise deep breathing twice a day.** Simply sit or lie comfortably and close your eyes, says Dr. Rudick. Imagine that you have to inflate a balloon: breathe in slowly through your nose to a count of five. Then breathe slowly out through your mouth. Continue this for 5 to 10 minutes – once in the morning and once at night – every day until surgery.

**Treat yourself to a guided imagery tape.** A technique to use thoughts to deal with pain, guided imagery helps you use all your senses to distract yourself from the pain. For example, you might imagine you're on a restful beach – hear the waves, feel the breeze and smell the salty air. David Sobel, M.D., regional director of patient education in the health education department of Kaiser Permanente Medical Care Program in Oakland, California, recommends an audiotape that offers soothing music and perhaps a narra-

## THE HORMONE CONNECTION
## EXPECTING YOUR PERIOD? INFORM THE SURGEON

If you're scheduled for surgery, tell your doctor if you expect to menstruate at the time of the operation. Some doctors believe that women may bleed more from the incision site when having surgery during their menstrual cycle and, if possible, would prefer to arrange the operation for another time.

tion that invites you to picture yourself in a safe space. Continue to practise deep breathing, and listen to the tape without interruption, once in the morning and once in the evening, for several days before your surgery and the days after.

## Stress-Reduction Strategies
## for the Operating Room

**Cold? Speak up.** If you are cold in the operating room, ask for a special blanket, says Dr. Rudick. These blankets help keep patients warm in operating rooms, which are usually kept cold, and that helps keep your immune system strong.

**Just before the anaesthesia is administered, practise a little self-hypnosis.** Relax your body, breathe deeply and visualize being somewhere safe, such as a comfortable room in your home or by the seaside, says Dr. Sobel.

# Knee Injuries

Riddle: why does a woman's ability to become pregnant make her more likely to injure her knee than a man? Answer: because oestrogen, the hormone that helps her pelvis soften to accommodate a growing foetus, also may soften her knee and other ligaments, making her more vulnerable to certain knee injuries than a man.

Chances are, you won't "blow out" your knees strolling around your local area for exercise. But sports such as soccer, basketball, volleyball, or skiing, and taking aerobics or step classes, are another story. These sports require that you move quickly, then stop and make sudden turns – putting you at risk of tearing the anterior cruciate ligaments (ACL) that hold your knee in place.

Researchers have found women are at greatest risk for ACL tears when exercising during the middle of the menstrual cycle (days 10 to 14), around ovulation, when oestrogen levels are high. In contrast, you are least likely to tear your ACL if you play during the beginning of your cycle, known as the follicular phase (days 1 to 9), when oestrogen levels are lower. Oestrogen may inhibit the production of collagen, the basic building block of the ligament, though doctors aren't sure if oestrogen can affect the ligament that quickly.

Extremely low levels of oestrogen, on the other hand, can lead to another knee injury that is more common among women than men: osteoarthritis of the knees, which can cause swelling and severe pain during even the simplest activities, such as walking and standing. The risk of osteoarthritis appears to rise during or soon after menopause, when oestrogen levels drop significantly.

# Practical Tactics

"Anytime there is a difference in the prevalence of a disease between men and women, oestrogen is blamed," says Tim McAlindon, M.P.H., M.D., associate professor of medicine at Boston University School of Medicine. Whether oestrogen is truly at fault for knee injuries is still being investigated, he says.

One way to reduce your risk of tearing your ACL is to avoid exercise such as playing soccer or basketball or doing aerobics or step for the 5 days a month of your ovulation cycle. But when it comes down to it, though, how many of us can arrange competitions or ski holidays around our menstrual cycles? And skipping exercise when we're ovulating just adds one more obstacle to regular exercise. So it's a good idea – in theory.

Taking the Pill might help. Oral contraceptives help balance fluctuations in your hormones and, by keeping your knee ligaments strong, may help prevent injuries.

And if you take oestrogen supplements at menopause, you automatically compensate for the hormones you lose at that time, reducing your risk of developing osteoarthritis or slowing its development if you already have it.

If you're not taking birth control pills or hormone replacement therapy, you can still lessen knee pain and injury.

"Traditional approaches consist of first reducing the risk factors," says Dr. McAlindon. Specifically you can strengthen and help your knees in these ways.

**If you're overweight, slim down.** "Excess weight puts more pressure on your knees. But a modest loss – even a few pounds – will slow the pressure and reduce the risk of osteoarthritis," says Dr. McAlindon. Losing weight also may keep arthritis from advancing if you already have it.

**Strengthen your thighs, hips and calves.** Lift weights two or three times a week, and pay special attention to the quadriceps muscles (the large muscles on the front of your thighs). "Most people don't exercise these muscles, but they stabilize the joints and are thought to help protect the knee," says Dr. McAlindon. One good exercise for the quadriceps that won't make matters worse, especially if you are overweight, is swimming.

**Help yourself to some "therapeutic touch".** This specific kind of gentle laying on of hands, usually performed by a massage therapist or other alternative practitioner, has been found to bring the body's energy system back into balance and help reduce knee pain caused by osteoarthritis.

**Try glucosamine and chondroitin.** Available wherever nutritional supplements are sold, these two supplements seem to work in concert to slow cartilage breakdown or even repair damage in joints, thereby helping reduce inflammation, swelling and pain. Woodson Merrell, M.D., executive director of the Center for Health and Healing at Beth Israel Medical Center in New York City, suggests taking 500 milligrams of glucosamine three times a day for osteoarthritis flare-ups until the pain subsides. For chondroitin, the recommended dose is 1200 milligrams daily.

However, don't count on supplements to prevent or heal ligament tears. Once you tear your ACL, physiotherapy, surgery, or both may be necessary.

# Gum Disease

I n *Pretty Woman*, actress Julia Roberts goes into Richard Gere's hotel bathroom for what seems like a suspiciously long time. Gere, a serious businessman, wonders if Roberts, a not-so-serious hustler, is using drugs. Nervously, he opens the door. Roberts turns around and reveals: she's been flossing her teeth.

Smart woman.

Gum disease affects three out of four people over the age of 35, according to the American Dental Association. Women, moreover, are at even higher risk.

"Women are really susceptible to gum disease in part due to hormonal changes during various stages in their lives," says Barbara J. Steinberg, D.D.S., professor of surgery and medicine at Hahnemann School of Medicine in Philadelphia.

Technically, the risk of gum disease begins with plaque, a sticky film of bacteria that constantly forms on your teeth. If left on or between your teeth, plaque turns into tartar: a hard residue of food, saliva and salts. If this tartar remains, it in turn creates a space or pocket between your teeth and gums. If the condition is left unchecked, your gums and the bones that support your teeth wear away. Without treatment, you may lose some teeth.

"During puberty, menstruation and pregnancy, and while taking oral contraceptives, high levels of progesterone make your gums more sensitive to bacterial plaque," explains Dr. Steinberg. "They may swell, turn red and bleed easily – all symptoms of gum disease. Sixty to 75 per cent of all pregnant women will experience some degree of gum inflammation during their pregnancy." This is partly because progesterone occurs in saliva. That in turn can cause bacteria to grow and your gums to swell.

"Gum disease appears to put a woman at risk for having a preterm, low-weight baby" – that is, a baby born weighing less than 5.8 pounds and born before the 37th week of pregnancy, says Dr. Steinberg. "So even if you're just contemplating pregnancy, you should consult not only your physician but your dentist as well.

"Menopause is another issue," she adds. Along with causing an odd and annoying tendency for milk to taste salty, a decline in the hormone oestrogen may increase your risk of tooth loss or make gum disease more severe. If you have diabetes, you're also at increased risk for gum disease. Moreover, if you have diabetes and gum disease, bacteria that build up on your gums make absorbing oral insulin difficult.

## Basics for Everyone

Regardless of the cause, there's much you can – and should – do to help prevent and even reverse periodontal (gum) disease at its earliest stages (known as gingivitis). Here is some advice from the experts.

**Floss *before* you brush every day.** This will help bring bacteria to the surface; then you can just brush it away.

**Hold your toothbrush at a 45-degree angle, instead of parallel to your teeth.** This will help bristles clean along the gum line.

**Brush twice a day in this order.** Cover the chewing surfaces first, then the inner side of your teeth, and finally the outer side. This will make the brush its softest by the time you use it on the outer areas, where your gums are most in danger of separating from your teeth.

**Finish by brushing your tongue.** It carries hundreds of thousands of bacteria. Moreover, unless you clean your tongue, it will attract new bacteria after you brush your teeth.

**Use an antiplaque rinse either before or after you brush and floss.** This helps remove any remaining food or plaque that was dislodged during brushing.

**If you are in or past perimenopause, use a soft or medium toothbrush, not a hard one.** Because the tissues of the mouth thin at this stage of your life, a soft brush will be softer on your gums and reduce the risk that you might damage them by too-vigorous brushing.

**If you smoke, quit.** It's a definite risk factor for gum disease.

### Fend Off Hormonally Related Gum Problems

Women weighing the pros and cons of hormone replacement therapy can add to their list another potential benefit: protecting their teeth and gums. One study suggests that women who take oestrogen supplements within 5 years of the menopause may slow the progression of gum disease.

"Oestrogen seems to reduce the level of inflammation in the gums," says Richard Reinhardt, D.D.S., Ph.D., the study's lead researcher and professor of surgical specialities at the College of Dentistry at the University of Nebraska Medical Center in Lincoln. "It also tends to better preserve the bone and soft tissue that support the teeth. For women at risk for osteoporosis – which makes them more vulnerable to progressive periodontal gum and bone loss – this may be yet one more reason to be on oestrogen."

Finally, if you have diabetes, be especially diligent about keeping your glucose levels under control and, if it's prescribed, taking your insulin. "People who are not taking their insulin regularly or who have a hard time keeping their glucose levels under control have a higher incidence of gum disease," says Dr. Reinhardt. Apparently, having more infections in the mouth cause diabetics to resist the insulin. "The better you control your diabetes and clean your teeth, the less periodontal trouble you're likely to have." (For more details on controlling the hormone fluctuations that are responsible for diabetes, see chapter 13.)

# Snoring

Women who never snored before menopause are often surprised to hear complaints that they've started to snore for the first time at midlife. Or they wake up feeling tired and wonder why, never suspecting that guttural night-time episodes may be at fault.

The most common underlying problem: obstructive sleep apnoea. Simply put, airflow to or from your nose or mouth is blocked for 10 seconds to a minute.

"Up until menopause, progesterone helps stimulate normal breathing," says Joan L. F. Shaver, R.N., Ph.D., sleep researcher and dean at the College of Nursing at the University of Illinois at Chicago. It also appears to protect a woman from sleep apnoea prior to menopause. But with menopause comes a decline in the output of ovarian hormones, including progesterone – and, for many women, a rise in sleep problems. In fact, women are more likely to snore after menopause than at any other time in life. About 10 to 12 per cent of women between the ages of 40 and 59 snore, according to Dr. Shaver. By the age of 65 and beyond, that increases to 19 or 20 per cent.

Precisely how the hormonal shifts around menopause may lead to snoring and other sleep-disordered breathing problems is a question scientists are now exploring. Hormone replacement therapy doesn't seem to help. One thing, however, already appears clear: there's more at stake than quieter nights. Left untreated, sleep apnoea can be life-threatening.

"Over time, sleep breathing disorders can contribute to high blood pressure and heart problems" – possibly increasing the risk of strokes and heart attacks, says Dr. Shaver. This is because as we breathe, we acquire oxygen, which circulates throughout the blood. But when we repeatedly stop breathing, there is a drop in oxygen levels, which can strain the heart.

You may snore and not even know it. "Sleep partners don't always notice," says Dr. Shaver. "They may be snoring, too."

More reliable clues: women who have apnoea often have a morning headache, feel very tired in the daytime and find it difficult to function, says Dr. Shaver.

## One Nuisance You Don't Want to Ignore

If you have sleep apnoea, it's important to treat the underlying problem – not just snoring, its most noticeable symptom. So if you suspect you have sleep apnoea, tell your doctor or health care practitioner. She may refer you

### ON THE WEB & Other Resources

Sleep research was founded in Britain, and there are research centres of excellence in Edinburgh, Loughborough and in Sussex Universities. If you would like to know more about the research, contact:
**The British Sleep Society**
PO Box 247
Huntingdon PE28 3UZ
E-mail: *MartinKING@papworth-tr.anglox.nhs.uk*
*www.british-sleep-society.org.uk*

For a charity that helps people with sleep disorders, contact:
**The British Sleep Foundation**
10 Cabot Square
Canary Wharf
London EH14 4QB
Tel: 0207 345 3317
E-mail: *bsf@ukogilwpr.com*
*www.britishsleepfoundation.org.uk*

to a pulmonologist or other physician who specializes in treating sleep disorders. This is best done at an accredited sleep centre. If the problem is severe, you may be fitted with a mask attached to a ventilator that blows air through your nose and mouth and keeps the airway open while you sleep. For those who have a small throat, larynx and pharynx, surgery may be recommended.

For some, simpler tactics are helpful. Among them:

**If you're overweight, slim down.** "Women who are overweight are much more prone to have apnoeas," says Dr. Shaver. Excess weight can create bulkier airway tissues, making the airway smaller and making it more difficult for you to breathe. Shedding just 10 per cent of your body weight can help. For example, if you weigh about 90 kilograms (14 stone), set a goal to lose 9 kilograms (20 pounds).

**Cut out alcohol, cigarettes and sleeping pills.** All three can increase the likelihood that your throat muscles and tongue will relax during sleep to such an extent that they will block part of your airway.

**Avoid sleeping on your back.** "When you sleep, your tissues become lax and, due to gravity, can block your airway," says Dr. Shaver. Sleeping on your side prevents that. Propping a pillow behind your back can help.

**Enlist the help of your dentist.** "There are some dental devices that, when worn at night, will help keep your jaw forward and keep the airway open," says Dr. Shaver.

## PART FOUR

# Hormone Helpers

# Using Herbs and Supplements Safely

## Herbs and Their Compounds

While herbal remedies are generally safe for self-care and cause few, if any, side effects, herbalists are quick to caution that botanical medicines should be used cautiously – and knowledgeably.

First and foremost, if you are under a doctor's care for any hormonal imbalance or other health condition or are taking any medication, do not use any herb or alter your treatment regime without consulting your doctor. If you are pregnant, do not self-treat with any natural remedy without the consent of your doctor or midwife. The same applies to nursing mothers and women trying to conceive.

Some herbs may cause adverse reactions in people who are allergy-prone, have a major health condition, or are using prescription drugs, including hormones like insulin, thyroid, or oestrogen. Like any medicine, herbs can also have harmful effects if they're taken for too long or in too large amounts or if they're used improperly.

The safety guidelines presented in the following chart are based on the American Herbal Products Association's *Botanical Safety Handbook* – a recognized source of herb safety information – and on the advice of experienced herbal healers. The chart is intended to help you make informed decisions when incorporating herbs into your hormone-balancing programme. It covers only the herb or herbal compounds discussed in this book for which potential side effects, interactions, or both have been identified.

The guidelines themselves apply only to adults and usually refer to internal use. Be aware that some herbs may cause a skin reaction when applied topically. If you're trying a herb topically for the first time, your best bet is to do a patch test. Apply a small amount to your skin and monitor the area for 24 hours. If you notice any redness or a rash, discontinue use. (Note: g = grams; mg = milligrams.)

| HERB | SAFE USE GUIDELINES AND POSSIBLE SIDE EFFECTS |
|------|-----------------------------------------------|
| Black cohosh | Do not use for more than 6 months. |
| Black haw | Do not take without medical supervision if you have a history of kidney stones as it contains oxalates, which can cause kidney stones. |
| Buchu | Do not use if you have kidney disease. |
| Butterburr | Limit use to preparations that are pyrrolizidine alkaloid (PA) free. |
| Castor oil | Do not use castor oil internally if you have intestinal obstruction or abdominal pain. Do not use for more than 8 to 10 days. |
| Chasteberry (vitex) | May counteract the effectiveness of birth control pills. |
| Dandelion | If you have gallbladder disease, do not use dandelion root preparations without medical approval. |
| Dang gui (dong quai) | If you suffer from a condition that may involve heavy menstrual bleeding, such as endometriosis, do not use without the guidance of a qualified practitioner. |
| Ephedra (ma huang) | Use only under the guidance of a qualified practitioner. |
| Feverfew | If chewed, fresh leaves can cause mouth sores in some people. |
| Ginger | May increase bile secretion, so if you have gallstones, do not use therapeutic amounts of the dried root or powder without guidance from a health care practitioner. |
| Ginkgo | Do not use with antidepressant MAO-inhibitor drugs such as phenelzine sulphate (Nardil) or tranylcypromine (Parnate), aspirin or other nonsteroidal anti-inflammatory medications, or blood-thinning medications such as warfarin. Can cause dermatitis, diarrhoea and vomiting in doses higher than 240 mg of concentrated extract. |
| Hawthorn | If you have a cardiovascular condition, do not take hawthorn regularly for more than a few weeks without medical supervision. You may require lower doses of other medications, such as high blood pressure drugs. If you have low blood pressure caused by heart valve problems, do not use without medical supervision. |

| HERB | SAFE USE GUIDELINES AND POSSIBLE SIDE EFFECTS |
|---|---|
| Horse chestnut | May interfere with the action of other drugs, especially blood thinners such as warfarin. May irritate the gastrointestinal tract. |
| Horsetail | Do not use tincture if you have heart or kidney problems. May cause a thiamin deficiency. Do not take more than 2 g per day of powdered extract or take for prolonged periods. |
| Kelp | If you have high blood pressure or heart problems, use only once a day or less. Do not use if you have hyperthyroidism. Take with adequate liquid. Long-term use is not recommended. |
| Licorice | Do not use if you have diabetes, high blood pressure, liver or kidney disorders, or low potassium levels. Do not use daily for more than 4 to 6 weeks because overuse can lead to water retention, high blood pressure caused by potassium loss, or impaired heart and kidney function. |
| Marshmallow | May slow the absorption of medications taken at the same time. |
| Nettle | If you have allergies, your symptoms may worsen, so take only one dose a day for the first few days. |
| Parsley | Do not use if you have kidney disease because it increases urine flow when used in therapeutic amounts. Safe as a garnish or ingredient in food. |
| Rehmannia | Do not use if you have diarrhoea, lack of appetite, or indigestion. |
| St. John's wort | Do not use with antidepressants or other prescription medicine without medical approval. May cause photosensitivity. Avoid overexposure to direct sunlight. |
| Saw palmetto | Consult your doctor for proper diagnosis and monitoring before using to treat acne. |
| Turmeric | Do not use as a home remedy if you have high stomach acid or ulcers, gallstones, or bile duct obstruction. |
| Uva-ursi | Do not use for more than 2 weeks without the supervision of a qualified practitioner. Do not use if you have kidney disease because it contains tannins, which can cause further kidney damage. Tannins can also irritate the stomach. |
| Valerian | Do not use with sleep-enhancing or mood-regulating medications because it may intensify their effects. May cause heart palpitations and nervousness in sensitive individuals. If such stimulant action occurs, discontinue use. |
| Yarrow | Rarely, handling flowers can cause skin rash. |

## Vitamin and Mineral Supplements

Although side effects and interactions while using vitamin and mineral supplements are rare, they do occur. This guide is designed to help you use certain supplements discussed in this book safely and effectively.

Be sure to talk to your doctor before using any supplement if you have a chronic illness requiring medical supervision or medication. In fact, if you have any type of health problem, your doctor or pharmacist needs to know about any supplements you're taking before treating you with a prescription or over-the-counter medicine. If you are pregnant, nursing, or trying to conceive, use supplements only under the supervision of your doctor.

The vitamin and mineral doses listed below are the UK dietary reference values. Also given below are the safe upper limits for adults, above which harmful side effects can occur. These amounts are the total from both food and supplements. Some people may experience problems at significantly lower doses. Do not take more than the safe upper limit of any vitamin or mineral without first consulting your physician. Note that requirements for children and pregnant or lactating women may differ. (Note: mg = milligrams; mcg = micrograms; IU = international units.)

## New Supplements

Reports of adverse effects from new supplements are rare, especially when compared to prescription drugs, and supplement manufacturers are required by law to provide information on labels about reasonably safe recommended dosages for healthy individuals. Be aware that the potency and dosing strategy can very significantly among products.

You should note, however, that little scientific research exists to assess the safety or long-term effects of many new supplements, and some supplements can complicate existing conditions or cause allergic reactions in some people. For these reasons, you should always check with your doctor before taking any supplements.

We recommend that you take supplements with food for best absorption and to avoid stomach irritation, unless otherwise directed. Never take them as a substitute for a healthy diet since they do not provide all the nutritional benefits of whole foods.

And, if you are pregnant, nursing, or attempting to conceive, do not supplement without the supervision of a doctor. (Note: g = grams; mg = milligrams.)

| NUTRIENT | DIETARY REFERENCE VALUES (DRVs) FOR ADULTS | UK SAFE UPPER LIMIT *(US LEVEL GIVEN WHERE UK FIGURE DOES NOT EXIST) |
|---|---|---|
| Calcium | 700 mg | 2000 mg |
| Chromium | 25 mcg | 1000 mcg |
| Copper | 1.2 mg | 10 mg |
| Folic acid | 200 mcg (women who are or intend to become pregnant should consume an additional 400 mcg/day as a supplement | 1000 mcg |
| Iodine | 140 mcg | 1000 mcg |
| Iron | Women 11–50 years old 14.8 mg Women over 50 and men 8.7 mg | 45 mg* |
| Magnesium | Men 300 mg Women 270 mg | 350 mg* from supplements only |
| Manganese | 1.4 mg | 11 mg* |
| Niacin | Men 17 mg Women 13 mg | 35 mg* |
| Pantothenic acid | 3–7 mg | 1000 mg* |
| Riboflavin | Men 1.3 mg Women 1.1 mg | 200 mg* |
| Selenium | Men 75 mcg Women 60 mcg | 450 mcg |
| Thiamin | Men 1 mg Women 0.8 mg | 50 mg |
| Vitamin A | Men 700 mcg Women 600 mcg | 3000 mcg* |
| Vitamin B$_6$ | Men 1.4 mg Women 1.2 mg | 10 mg |
| Vitamin B$_{12}$ | 1.5 mcg | 3000 mcg* |

## CAUTIONS AND OTHER INFORMATION

Taking more than 2000 mg a day can cause serious side effects such as kidney damage. For best absorption, avoid taking more than 500 mg at one time. If you are over 50, look for a formula that contains vitamin D as well as calcium since you may need more vitamin D than is supplied by a multivitamin alone. Some natural sources of calcium, such as bonemeal and dolomite, may be contaminated with lead and other dangerous or undesirable metals.

High intakes may result in liver and kidney damage.

For best absorption, use supplements containing copper sulphate or cupric sulphate rather than copper oxide or cupric oxide.

Excess folic acid from supplements can cause progressive nerve damage in individuals – usually older people – with vitamin $B_{12}$ deficiency. When selecting a B-complex supplement, check the label for the amount of each ingredient to help you determine its safe use.

Persistently high intakes can cause hyperthyroidism and may be linked to thyroid cancer.

Avoid taking more than 18 mg a day unless a blood test indicates that you are anaemic.

Check with your doctor before beginning supplementation in any amount if you have heart or kidney problems. Doses exceeding 350 mg a day can cause diarrhoea in some people.

A healthy, balanced diet provides enough of this nutrient to meet your body's needs.

Taking more than the safe upper limit of 35 mg a day can cause flushing and itching. Because serious side effects including kidney and liver damage can occur from doses above 500 mg, high doses of niacin should be taken only under your doctor's supervision. When selecting a B-complex supplement, check the label for the amount of each ingredient to help you determine its safe use.

A healthy, balanced diet provides enough of this nutrient to meet your body's needs.

None

Excess selenium is toxic. Taking more than 400 mcg a day can cause dizziness, nausea, hair or nail loss, or a garlic odour on the breath or skin.

Persistent high intakes are associated with nerve and skin damage.

Taking more than 3000 mcg a day can cause headache, double vision, drowsiness or fatigue, nausea, or vomiting and hair loss. Excess vitamin A is stored and can cause bone and liver damage. High intakes of vitamin A are associated with an increased incidence of birth defects. Pregnant women are advised to avoid high intakes.

Taking more than 50 mg a day can cause reversible nerve damage. When selecting a B-complex supplement, check the label for the amount of each ingredient to help you determine its safe use. The UK Department of Health recommends that the maximum daily intake of $B_6$ should be 10 mg/day

None

| NUTRIENT | DIETARY REFERENCE VALUES (DRVs) FOR ADULTS | UK SAFE UPPER LIMIT *(US LEVEL GIVEN WHERE UK FIGURE DOES NOT EXIST) |
|---|---|---|
| Vitamin C | 40 mg | 1000 mg |
| Vitamin D | 10 mcg for people over age 65 | 50 mcg |
| Vitamin E | Men 4 mg Women 3 mg | None given |
| Vitamin K | 1 mcg per kg body weight | None given but high intakes are not advised |
| Zinc | Men 9.5 mg Women 7 mg | 40 mg* |

## CAUTIONS AND OTHER INFORMATION

Taking more than 1000 mg a day can cause diarrhoea and kidney stones in some people. To help maintain levels of vitamin C throughout the day, take half of the recommended dose in the morning and half at night. It is not advisable to take high doses for prolonged periods.

Taking more than 50 mcg a day can cause headache, fatigue, nausea, diarrhoea, or loss of appetite. Adults with no exposure to sunlight may need a supplement. Excess vitamin D is toxic.

Because it acts like a blood thinner, consult your doctor before taking vitamin E if you are already taking aspirin or a blood-thinning medication, such as warfarin. The safety of high levels and effects of excess vitamin E are not yet known.

Because vitamin K helps to clot blood, consult your doctor before beginning supplementation in any amount if you are already taking aspirin or a blood-thinning medication, such as warfarin. Persistent large doses are harmful and are not advised.

Taking more than 40 mg a day can cause nausea, dizziness, or vomiting. Long term intakes of high doses can lead to copper depletion.

| SUPPLEMENT | SAFE USE GUIDELINES AND POSSIBLE SIDE EFFECTS |
| --- | --- |
| Acetyl-cysteine | If you have diabetes, check with your doctor before supplementing as it may inactivate insulin. May deplete zinc and copper levels. Take with a multivitamin/mineral supplement that supplies the RDA of these minerals if supplementing for more than a few weeks. High doses may cause kidney stones in people who have cystinuria. |
| Bioflavonoids | Doses above label recommendations may cause blood thinning and increased bleeding time. |
| Bromelain | May cause nausea, vomiting, diarrhoea, skin rash and heavy menstrual bleeding. Can also increase the risk of bleeding in people taking aspirin or blood thinners. Do not take if you are allergic to pineapple. |
| Coenzyme $Q_{10}$ | Discuss supplementation with your doctor if you are taking the blood thinner warfarin. On rare occasions, it may reduce the warfarin's effectiveness. Supplementation should be observed by a knowledgeable naturopathic or medical doctor if taken for more than 20 days at levels 120 mg/day or higher. Side effects are rare but tend to be heartburn, nausea, or stomach ache, which can be prevented by consuming the supplement with a meal. |
| Cysteine | See Acetyl-cysteine. |
| DHEA | Only take under the supervision of a knowledgeable naturopathic or medical professional. May cause liver damage, acne, irritability, irregular heart rhythms, accelerated growth of existing tumours, altered hormone profiles, increased cancer risk (prostate in men and breast in women), hair loss in men and women, and growth of facial hair and deepening of the voice in women. Men and women under 35 should avoid it because it suppresses the body's natural production of DHEA. |
| Fish oil | Do not take if any of the following apply: bleeding disorder, uncontrolled high blood pressure, anticoagulants (blood thinners) or regular aspirin use, allergy to any kind of fish. People with diabetes should not take fish oil because of its high fat content. Increases bleeding time, possibly resulting in nosebleeds and easy bruising, and may cause upset stomach. Take fish oil, not fish-liver oil, because fish-liver oil is high in vitamins A and D – toxic in high amounts. |
| Flaxseed | If you are on medication, see your medical doctor before supplementing as it may negatively affect absorption. Do not supplement if you have a bowel obstruction. |
| Glucosamine | May cause upset stomach, heartburn, or diarrhoea. |
| L-tyrosine | Do not take if you are taking monoamine oxidase inhibitors (MAOI) as it can cause sweats and elevated blood pressure. |

| SUPPLEMENT | SAFE USE GUIDELINES AND POSSIBLE SIDE EFFECTS |
|---|---|
| Melatonin | Causes drowsiness; take only at bedtime and never before driving. May cause headaches, nausea, morning dizziness, daytime sleepiness, depression, giddiness, difficulty concentrating and upset stomach. May cause interactions with prescription medications. Has adverse affects on people with any of the following: a cardiovascular condition; high blood pressure; any autoimmune disease, such as rheumatoid arthritis or lupus; diabetes; epilepsy; migraine; or a personal or family history of a hormone-dependent cancer such as breast, testicular, prostate, or endometrial cancer. May cause infertility, reduced sex drive in males, hypothermia, retinal damage and interference with hormone replacement therapy. Long-term effects of melatonin supplements are unknown. (Melatonin is not available in the UK although it can be easily obtained over the Internet.) |
| Methionine | Experimental. Long-term effects unknown. Don't take without a doctor's guidance. High doses may increase the risk of heart disease in some people by elevating homocysteine levels. It's best to take in conjunction with folic acid, vitamin $B_6$, and vitamin $B_{12}$ to help control homocysteine effect. |
| Omega-3 | In some people, doses as low as 2 g may reduce blood-clotting ability, resulting in bleeding or, in extreme instances, leading to haemorrhages. |
| Phenylalanine | Experimental. Long-term effects unknown. Don't take without a doctor's guidance. *Note*: Phenylalanine supplements can raise high blood pressure to dangerous levels, especially in people taking MAO inhibitors as antidepressants. Do not take phenylalanine if you have phenylketonuria. Large amounts decrease antioxidant levels, thereby encouraging disease. |
| Pregnenolone | Experimental. Few, if any, studies have been conducted on humans. Only take under the supervision of a knowledgeable medical doctor. In doses higher than 5 to 10 mg, women may grow facial hair and men's breasts may enlarge. |
| Progesterone cream | External use only. Use intended for women 16 years of age and older. Consult your medical doctor if you experience irritation, any changes in breast symptoms, or menstrual irregularities with continuous use. |
| Quercetin (bioflavonoid) | Doses above 100 mg may dilate blood vessels and cause blood thinning in some people. Should be avoided by individuals at risk for low blood pressure or problems with blood clotting. |

# Essential Oils

Essential oils are inhaled or applied topically to the skin. With few exceptions, they're never taken internally.

Of the most common essential oils, lavender, tea tree, lemon, jasmine, and rose can be used undiluted. The rest should be diluted in a carrier base – which can be an oil (such as almond), a cream, or a gel – before being applied to the skin.

Many essential oils may cause irritation or allergic reactions in people with sensitive skin. Before applying any new oil to the skin, always do a patch test. Put a few drops on the back of your wrist. Wait for an hour or more. If any irritation or redness occurs, wash the area with cold water. In the future, use half of the amount of oil or avoid the oil altogether.

Do not use essential oils at home for serious medical problems. During pregnancy, do not use essential oils unless they're approved by your doctor. Store essential oils in dark bottles, away from light and heat and out of the reach of children and pets.

| ESSENTIAL OIL | SAFE USE GUIDELINES AND POSSIBLE SIDE EFFECTS |
| --- | --- |
| Ginger | Do not use undiluted. Do not use more than 3 drops in the bath. Avoid direct sunlight because this oil can cause skin sensitivity. |
| Lavender (true) | Can be used undiluted, but keep it away from your eyes. |
| Lemon | Do not use more than 3 drops in the bath. Avoid direct sunlight and check use-by date because this oil can cause skin sensitivity. |
| Peppermint | Do not use more than 3 drops in the bath. Do not use with other oils. Do not use undiluted. Do not use at the same time as homeopathic remedies. Do not get it near your eyes. Do not use it on the faces of infants and small children. If you have gallbladder or liver disease, do not use without medical supervision. Can be used undiluted for dental pain. |
| Sage (clary) | Do not use with alcohol because it can cause lethargy and exaggerate drunkenness. |
| Sandalwood | Can be used undiluted as a perfume, but keep it away from your eyes. |
| Ylang-ylang | Can be used undiluted as a perfume, but keep it away from your eyes. Use in moderation since its strong smell can cause nausea or headaches. |

# Women to Women:
# A Resource Guide

As recently as 10 years ago, anyone who wanted to research a health condition had to drive to a medical library and pore over shelves of medical journals. If you wanted to contact a health care association, you had only two choices – the phone or a letter.

Today, all that's changed.

Web technology has given nearly everyone access to professional and scientific resources, enabling them to do individual research, says Jackie Wootton, M.Ed., president of the Alternative Medicine Foundation in Bethesda, Maryland, and WebWatch columnist for the *Journal of Women's Health and Gender-Based Medicine*. She offers the following tips when searching Web sites for the most current health information.

1. *You can access the latest medical research literature on the MEDLINE database from the US National Library of Medicine through the PubMed Web site at: www.ncbi.nlm.nih.gov/entrez.*
2. *Government and medical sites usually offer separate resources for professionals and consumers. It is a good idea to look at both.*
3. *Web sites may be registered as .gov (government), .org (mainly nonprofit organizations), .net (networking services), .com (commercial), and so forth. Most of the unbiased information and research resources are located at .gov or .org sites.*
4. *Always look for background information on the organization behind a Web site, usually in an "About Us" section. Ask yourself: who is responsible for providing this information? Is the information compiled by several well-qualified people? Is there a reputable*

*advisory board? Who is funding the organization or the Web site?*

5. *Well-organized sites will have clearly categorized information resources listed in a sidebar. The site index, usually at either the top or bottom of the home page, may be more informative and should include an "About Us" section and contact information and give a site map.*

6. *When searching a Web site that ends with .com, indicating that it's a commercial Web site, be aware that the information resources may not be impartial. There may be underlying commercial interests. The same applies to many medical information sites, which may be sponsored by large companies.*

7. *When selecting search terms, the strategy is to narrow down your search. Putting in one keyword, such as "hormones", will bring up thousands of hits. What you are asking the search engine to do is select all Web sites that have any mention of hormones. Narrow your search by adding "autoimmune" (or whatever your area of interest).*

8. *An asterisk is useful as part of your search strategy. "Endocrin*" will find hits for endocrine disorders, endocrinology, endocrine system, and so forth.*

9. *In addition to information/research Web sites and commercial sites, there are advice sites and chat groups. Many experts will say that these are less reliable. However, they can be very useful, provided you understand that this is opinion rather than fact. After all, we all like to take several opinions and ask among friends and relatives. The Web allows us to use the global village instead, Wooten adds.*

# DIRECTORY OF USEFUL ADDRESSES

Some of these addresses have been mentioned in earlier chapters where they are particularly relevant; this chapter is a general resource for every aspect of health. For recommendations related to a specific condition, see the relevant chapter. Addresses listed here are in alphabetical order for ease of reference.

GENERAL MEDICAL

**Arthritis Care**
Offers self-help support and leaflets on various aspects of this condition
18 Stephenson Way
London NW1 2HD
020 7380 6500 (helpline)
0808 800 4050 (freephone)
*www.arthritiscare.org.uk*

**The Arthritis Research Campaign**
For free booklets on all aspects of arthritis
PO Box 177
Chesterfield
Derbyshire S41 7TQ
*www.arc.org.uk*

**BACUP**
A vast amount of information, and practical support and advice for cancer patients and their families
3 Bath Place
Rivington Street
London EC2A 3JR
020 7696 9003
*www.cancerbacup.org.uk*

**BBC**
Lots of health information very professionally presented and independent of any vested interest
*www.bbc.co.uk/health*

**British Cardiac Society**
9 Fitzroy Square
London W1P 5AH
020 7383 3887
*www.cardiac.org.uk*

**British Heart Foundation**
14 Fitzhardinge Street
London W1H 4DH
*www.bfh.org.uk*

**The British Lung Foundation**
78 Hatton Garden
London EC1B 1PX
0207 831 5831
*www.lunguk.org*

**British Medical Association**
There are BMA Family Doctor booklets on a huge range of subjects. There is also a helpful Web site run by the Association's magazine, the BMJ
Tavistock Square,
London WC1H 9JP
0845 920 0169
*www.bma.org.uk*
*www.bmj.com*

**The British Menopause Society**
The Menopause Amarant Trust
22 Barkham Terrace
Lambeth Road
London SE1 7PW
01293 413 000
*www.the-bms.org*

**The British Society for Allergy and Clinical Immunology**
66 Weston Park
Thames Ditton
Surrey KT7 0HL
020 8398 9240
*www.bsaci.soton.ac.uk*

**BUPA**
BUPA has factsheets on a wide variety of subjects on its Web site
*www.bupa.co.uk/factsheets*

**Cancer Research UK**
The main UK cancer charity formed from the merger of Cancer Research Campaign and the Imperial Cancer Research Fund. It does research and provides every sort of cancer support and advice
PO Box 123
Lincoln's Inn Fields
London WC2A 3PX
020 7242 0200
*www.cancerresearchuk.org* (for information about this charity's work and about cancer)
*www.cancerhelp.org.uk* (for information about cancer support)

**Department of Health**
Richmond House
79 Whitehall
London SW1A 2NL
020 7210 4850
*www.doh.gov.uk*

**Diabetes UK**
10 Queen Anne Street
London W1M 0BD
*www.diabetes.org.uk*

**Digestive Disorders Foundation**
3 St Andrews Place
London NW1 4LB
020 7486 0341
*www.digestivedisorders.org.uk*

**Family Heart Association**
7 North Road
Maidenhead SL6 1PL
01628 522177
*www.familyheart.org*

**Health Education Board, Scotland**
A range of fact sheets available
*www.hebs.com*

**Health Promotion England**
50 Eastbourne Terrace
London W2 3QR
*www.hpe.org.uk*

**The International Headache Society**
Linked to the World Headache Association
Oakwood
9 Willowmead Drive
Prestbury
Cheshire SK10 4BU
01625 828663
*www.@w-h-a.org*

**National Eczema Society**
163 Eversholt Street
London NW1 1BU
020 7388 4097
*www.eczema.org*

**Patients Association**
PO Box 935
Harrow
Middlesex HA1 3YJ
020 8423 9111
*www.patients-association.com*

**The Stroke Association**
Stroke House
Whitecross Street
London EC1Y 8JJ
020 7566 0300
020 7566 0330 (advisory services)
*www.stroke.org.uk*

**Women's Health Concern**
PO Box 2126
Marlow
Buckinghamshire SL7 2RY
01628 483612 (advice line)

**Women's Health Concern Ltd**
For information about the menopause
and problems associated with it
PO Box 1629
London SW15 2ZL
020 8780 3007
020 8780 3945 (fax)

**World Cancer Research Fund**
105 Park Street
London W1Y 3FB
020 7343 4200
*www.wcrf.org*

FERTILITY AND REPRODUCTIVE
MEDICINE
**The British Infertility Counselling
Association (BICA)**
69 Division Street
Sheffield S1 4GE
01342 843880
E-mail: *info@bica.net*

**The Bristol Centre for Reproductive
Medicine**
A private medical organization dealing
with fertility problems
4 Priory Road
Clifton
Bristol BS8 1TY
0117 902 1100
*www.repromed.co.uk*

**CHILD
(The National Infertility Support
Network)**
Charter House
St. Leonard's Road,
Bexhill-on-Sea
East Sussex TN40 1JA
01424 732361
E-mail: *office@child.org.uk*
*www.child.org.uk*

**The Human Fertilisation and
Embryology Authority (HEFA)**
Paxton House
30 Artillery Lane
London E1 7LS
*www.hfea.gov.uk*

**The National Fertility Association
(ISSUE)**
*www.issue.co.uk*

MENTAL HEALTH
**The Association for Postnatal Illness**
145 Dawes Road
Fulham
London SW6 7EB
020 7386 0868
*www.apni.org.uk*

**MIND
(National Association for Mental
Health)**
This Web site has all the information
needed to access resources for
people needing help with depression,
anxiety and panic disorders, as well as
more serious psychiatric problems,
such as schizophrenia and manic
depression
15–19 Broadway
London E15 4BQ
0845 766 0163
*www.mind.org.uk*

**Relate**
The organization that helps couples in trouble
Herbert Gray College
Little Church Street
Rugby
Warwickshire CV21 3AP
01788 573242
*www.relate.org.uk*

**SANE**
A charity dealing with all mental illnesses
1st Floor
Cityside House
40 Adler Street
London E1 1EE
0845 767 8000

**The Samaritans**
0845 790 9090
E-mail:*jo@samaritans.org*
*www.samaritans.org.uk*

DIET AND NUTRITION
**British Dietetic Association**
5th Floor
Charles House
148–149 Great Charles Street
Birmingham B3 3HT
0121 200 8080
*www.bda.uk.com*
**British Nutrition Foundation**
High Holborn House
52 High Holborn
London WC1V 6RQ
020 7404 6504
*www.nutrition.org.uk*

**European Herbal Practitioners Association**
*www.euroherb.com*

**Food Standards Agency**
For up-to-date information on all food-related issues in the UK
Aviation House
125 Kingsway
London WC2B 6NH
020 7276 8000
*www.foodstandards.gov.uk*

**Nutrition Society**
*www.nutsoc.org.uk*

**Vegan Society**
7 Battle Road
St-Leonards-on-Sea
East Sussex TN37 7AA
*www.vegansociety.com*

**Vegetarian Society**
Parkdale
Denham Road
Altrincham
Cheshire WA14 4QG
0161 928 0793
*www.vegsoc.org*

ONLINE SUPPLIERS
*www.biovea.co.uk*
*www.capederm.com*
*www.burstingwithhealth.co.uk*
*www.health.perception.co.uk*
*www.healthplus.co.uk*
*www.positivehealthshop.co.uk*
*www.positivenation.co.uk*

# Index

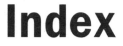

Underlined page references indicate boxed text and tables.
**Bold** references indicate photographs.

## A

# OTHER RODALE BOOKS
# AVAILABLE FROM PAN MACMILLAN

| | | | |
|---|---|---|---|
| 1-4050-0666-8 | Banish Your Belly, Butt & Thighs Forever! | *The Editors of* Prevention *Health Books for Women* | £10.99 |
| 1-4050-0665-X | Get A Real Food Life | *Janine Whiteson* | £12.99 |
| 1-4050-0667-6 | The Green Pharmacy | *Dr James A. Duke* | £14.99 |
| 1-4050-0673-0 | The Home Workout Bible | *Lou Schuler* | £15.99 |
| 1-4050-0671-4 | Laying Down the Law | *Dr Ruth Peters* | £8.99 |
| 1-4050-0672-2 | Pilates for Every Body | *Denise Austin* | £12.99 |
| 1-4050-0675-7 | The Secret Life of the Dyslexic Child | *Dr Robert Frank* | £10.99 |
| 1-4050-0669-2 | The Testosterone Advantage Plan™ | *Lou Schuler* | £12.99 |
| 1-4050-0668-4 | Whole Body Meditations | *Lorin Roche* | £10.99 |
| 1-4050-0670-6 | Win the Fat War | *Anne Alexander* | £5.99 |

All Pan Macmillan titles can be ordered from our website, *www.panmacmillan.com,* or from your local bookshop and are also available by post from:

Bookpost, PO Box 29, Douglas, Isle of Man IM99 1BQ
Credit cards accepted. For details:
Telephone: 01624 836000
Fax: 01624 670923
E-mail: bookshop@enterprise.net
*www.bookpost.co.uk*

Free postage and packing in the United Kingdom

Prices shown above were correct at time of going to press.
Pan Macmillan reserve the right to show new retail prices on covers which may differ from those previously advertised in the text or elsewhere.

RODALE

MACMILLAN